BERMAN, SNYDER

STUDY GUIDE FOR Kozier & Erb's Fundamentals of Nursing

Concepts, Process, and Practice

TENTH EDITION

PEARSON

Boston Columbus Indianapolis New York San Francisco Hoboken Amsterdam Cape Town Dubai London Madrid Milan Munich Paris Montreal Toronto Delhi Mexico City Sao Paulo Sydney Hong Kong Seoul Singapore Taipei Tokyo

Notice: Care has been taken to confirm the accuracy of information presented in this book. The authors, editors, and the publisher, however, cannot accept any responsibility for errors or omissions or for consequences from application of the information in this book and make no warranty, express or implied, with respect to its contents. The authors and publisher have exerted every effort to ensure that drug selections and dosages set forth in this text are in accord with current recommendations and practice at time of publication. However, in view of ongoing research, changes in government regulations, and the constant flow of information relating to drug therapy and drug reactions, the reader is urged to check the package inserts of all drugs for any change in indications of dosage and for added warnings and precautions. This is particularly important when the recommended agent is a new and/or infrequently employed drug.

Publisher: Julie Levin Alexander
Executive Editor: Kelly Trakalo
Project Manager: Michael Giacobbe
Program Manger: Melissa Bashe
Production Editor: Shyam Ramasubramony, S4Carlisle Publishing
Director of Marketing: David Gesell
Marketing Manager: Phoenix Harvey
Marketing Specialist: Michael Sirinides
Composition: S4Carlisle Publishing Services
Printer/Binder: Edwards Brothers Malloy

10 9 8 7 6 5 4 3 2 1

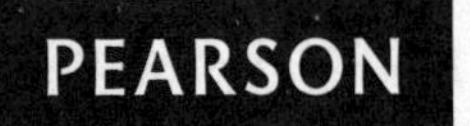
www.pearsonhighered.com

ISBN 10: 0-13-400115-X
ISBN 13: 978-0-13-400115-9

PREFACE

Students entering the field of nursing have a tremendous amount to learn in a very short time. This concise study guide has been developed to help you learn and apply key concepts and procedures, and master critical thinking skills based on ***Kozier & Erb's Fundamentals of Nursing,* Tenth Edition.**

On the nursing.pearsonhighered.com website you will find a variety of activities such as Case Studies and Application Activities that help you apply concepts to clinical scenarios.

In addition, each chapter of this study guide includes a variety of questions and activities to help you comprehend difficult concepts and reinforce basic knowledge gained from textbook reading assignments. The following is a list of features included in this edition that will enhance your learning experience:

- **Key Term Review** help you review the important terms in each chapter.
- **Key Topic Review** exercises contain matching, fill-in-the-blank, and true/false questions on key terms and key topics from each chapter.
- **Focused Study Tips** help you recall the important nursing concepts from each chapter.
- **Case Studies** provide clinical settings for critical thinking and the opportunity to apply learned processes and procedures.
- **Review Questions** are NCLEX®-style questions to help you prepare for the NCLEX®.
- **Answers** with complete rationales are included in the answer key to provide immediate reinforcement and to permit you to check the accuracy of your work.

It is our hope that this study guide will serve as a valuable learning tool and will contribute to your success in the nursing profession.

CONTENTS

CHAPTER 1

HISTORICAL AND CONTEMPORARY NURSING PRACTICE

KEY TERM REVIEW

Match each term with its appropriate definition.

1. ______ Caregiver
2. ______ Case manager
3. ______ Client
4. ______ Client advocate
5. ______ Communicator
6. ______ Consumer
7. ______ Continuing education (CE)
8. ______ Counseling
9. ______ Demography
10. ______ Florence Nightingale
11. ______ Governance
12. ______ Harriet Tubman
13. ______ Health
14. ______ In-service education
15. ______ Leader
16. ______ Manager
17. ______ Profession
18. ______ Patient Self-Determination Act (PSDA)
19. ______ Professionalism
20. ______ Socialization
21. ______ Standards of Practice
22. ______ Standards of Professional Performance
23. ______ Teacher
24. ______ Telehealth
25. ______ Telenursing

a. Degree of wellness or well-being that the client experiences

b. Role the nurse assumes to help clients learn about their health and the health care procedures they need to perform to restore or maintain their health.

c. Process of helping a client to recognize and cope with stressful psychological or social problems; to promote personal growth

d. Process by which people learn to become members of groups and societies

e. Influences others to work together to accomplish a specific goal

f. An occupation that requires extensive education

g. Recipient of nursing care

h. A role that traditionally included those activities that assist the client physically

i. Nursing role of pleading the cause of a client

j. Nurse who works with the multidisciplinary health care team to measure the effectiveness of the case management plan and to monitor outcomes.

k. A role that requires knowledge about organizational structure, leadership, advocacy, delegation, supervision, and evaluation

l. An individual who is skilled at communication and conveying concepts

m. An individual, a group of people, or a community that uses a service or commodity

n. Refers to formalized experiences designed to enhance the knowledge or skills of practicing professionals

o. The study of population, including statistics about distribution by age and place of residence, mortality (death), and morbidity (incidence of disease)

p. Also known as the "Lady with the Lamp"; work during Crimean War established hospital and procedure reform

q. The establishment and maintenance of social, political, and economic arrangements by which practitioners control their practice, their self-discipline, their working conditions, and their professional affairs

r. Requires that every competent adult be informed in writing on admission to a health care institution about his or her rights to accept or refuse medical care and to use advance directives

s. Describe behaviors expected in the professional nursing role

t. A specific type of CE program offered by an employer that is designed to upgrade the knowledge or skills of employees, as well as to validate continuing competence in selected procedures and areas of practice

u. Refers to professional character, spirit, or methods; a set of attributes, a way of life that implies responsibility and commitment

v. Provided care and safety to slaves fleeing to the North during the Civil War on the Underground Railroad

w. Use of medical information exchanged from one site to another via electronic communications to improve the patient's health status

x. The use of telecommunications and information technology to provide nursing practice at a distance

y. Describe the responsibilities for which nurses are accountable

KEY TOPIC REVIEW

1. The four functions identified within the scope of nursing practice are:

a. Promote Wellness

b. Prevent Illness

c. Restore Health

d. Care for Dying

2. The role of religious orders in the development of nursing includes:

(a) instilling the values of hard work.

b. influencing the image of nursing.

c. identifying an increased need for nurses.

(d) imprinting the profession as involving hard work.

e. improving the status of nursing.

3. The contemporary nursing leader who defined nursing is:

a. Clara Barton.

(b) Florence Nightingale.

c. Linda Richards.

d. Virginia Henderson.

4. A nurse registered to practice in one state is relocating to another neighboring state. What should this nurse do to ensure the ability to work as a nurse in the new state?

   a. Nothing. The nurse is registered as a nurse.

   b. Contact the state's department of nursing.

   c. Enroll in a school of nursing in the new state.

   d. File the paperwork to take the new state's nursing licensing examination.

5. From the following list, select the definition that best defines these terms:

a. Caregiver	F	Helps the client modify behaviors.
b. Communicator	A	This can be provided by the nurse or delegated to someone else.
c. Teacher	H	Supervises and evaluates performance.
d. Client advocate	J	Uses the outcomes of scientific study to improve the delivery of care.
e. Counselor	D	Acts to protect the client.
f. Change agent	G	Influences others to work together to reach a common goal.
g. Leader	B	Done verbally or written.
h. Manager	I	Care is oriented to the client and controls costs.
i. Case manager	E	Helps promote personal growth.
j. Research consumer	C	Assesses readiness to learn.

6. The terms used to identify the recipients of nursing are:

   a. Consumer

   b. Patient

   c. Client

7. Of the following nursing roles, select the ones that provide more autonomy within the practice of nursing.

   a. Nurse anesthetist

   b. Staff nurse on an orthopedic unit

   c. Operating room nurse

   d. Clinical nurse specialist

   e. Nurse in a physician's office

8. The process a nurse undergoes in an effort to be viewed as an integral member of the discipline of nursing is termed Professionalization

9. A nurse is interested in participating with the American Nurses Association. Participating with this organization is an example of:

   a. autonomy.

   b. governance.

   c. extended education.

   d. service.

10. The purpose of nursing students working together on projects is to:
    a. begin the process of socialization into the profession.
    b. get more work done faster.
    c. help each other through difficult courses.
    d. make new friends.
11. The payments for hospital services implemented by Medicare are termed ____________ (DRGs).
12. A nurse who provides care to a client over the telephone will need to:
    a. obtain licensure in the client's state of residence.
    b. take a course in telenursing.
    c. find out if the client's state is one of mutual recognition for licensure.
    d. do nothing.
13. The Patient Self-Determination Act requires that every client be provided with ____________ and ____________.
14. ____________ programs are the responsibility of all nurses to maintain constant professional updating and growth.

FOCUSED STUDY TIPS

1. Why is it important to review the history of nursing as one of the first steps in the education of a new nurse? What value does understanding the history of nursing provide to the contemporary nursing student?
2. What are the characteristics of a profession? How does nursing address each of these characteristics?
3. What are Benner's five stages of nursing practice? In which stage is a nurse considered proficient? Why?
4. How have economics, consumer demands, and the family structure impacted the profession of nursing?
5. A nurse who has been in the profession for over 25 years does not know how to operate a computer. What suggestions do you have to help this nurse? Why should this nurse be concerned with the inability to utilize current technology?
6. Identify the reasons for the current nursing shortage. How will this affect the future education of new nurses entering the profession?
7. The nurses in a hospital are contacting a labor union. Why do you think the nurses are contacting this union? What benefits will be gained by working with a union? What disadvantages are associated with nurses working with a union?
8. What do Sigma Theta Tau and the Association of Colleges of Nursing (ACN) represent in nursing? What are the differences between the two organizations and what are the similarities? Which organization offers continuing units for nurses? Compare these organizations with others such as the American Nursing Association (ANA) and the American Academy of Colleges in Nursing (AACN).
9. Why is it important for nurses to practice under a license? Why is a standardized licensing exam appropriate for all nurses?

CASE STUDY

A client with adult-onset asthma is attempting to quit his two-pack-per-day tobacco habit. The nurse, who has been practicing for 4 years, is assisting the client with supportive measures to improve his health status. The nurse is discussing the plan of care with the physician.

1. What role is the nurse acting in by representing the client's needs and wishes and assisting the client in behavior modification plans? Change Agent Role
2. The nurse is in the process of assisting the client to recognize and cope with both the asthma condition and the tobacco cessation program. The nurse is acting as a change agent, and what other role is the nurse representing? Client Advocate
3. According to Benner's stages of nursing expertise, in what stage is the nurse functioning? Proficient

REVIEW QUESTIONS

1. A female is considering a career as a nurse because of the aspects of caring and nurturing. This individual is using which factor of nursing to base her decision?
   1. Women's roles
   2. Religion
   3. War
   4. Economics
2. A registered nurse is considering additional education so that she can provide nonemergent acute care in an ambulatory clinic. This nurse is considering which expanded career role?
   1. Nurse anesthetist
   2. Clinical nurse specialist
   3. Nurse practitioner
   4. Nurse administrator
3. A nurse is able to provide care to several complex clients and focuses on those items that are the most important. Within which stage of Benner's stages of nursing expertise is this nurse functioning?
   1. Stage II
   2. Stage III
   3. Stage IV
   4. Stage V
4. The organization recently added a new wing to the hospital. What factor is likely to be influencing this organization related to the nursing shortage they are experiencing?
   1. Aging workforce
   2. Aging population
   3. Increased demand for nurses
   4. Workplace issues

5. Which of the following actions performed by an organization would best improve the image of nursing?
   1. Offering scholarships to high school students to attend nursing school
   2. Television commercials showing nurses and doctors providing care together
   3. A print advertisement with the statement "Nursing—The hardest job you'll ever love"
   4. An ANA-sponsored radio commercial explaining the role of nurses in society today
6. The nurse, who is working in a well-baby clinic, administers routine immunizations and recognizes this as practicing within what area of nursing practice?
   1. Promoting health and wellness
   2. Preventing illness
   3. Restoring health
   4. Providing care to the dying
7. While attending a continuing education seminar, several nurses from different states are discussing their individual state requirements for nursing licensure. Which of the following is the one common thread between all of the states' departments of nursing?
   1. Protect the public.
   2. Further nursing education.
   3. Obtain continuing education contact hours.
   4. Gain specialization.
8. A new nursing student is disappointed because classes so far are focused on topics such as communication and planning, and she wanted to be a nurse to "provide care." This nursing student is describing which role of the nurse?
   1. Teacher
   2. Client advocate
   3. Caregiver
   4. Counselor
9. The student nurse is learning how to fit into the nursing profession by learning the rules defining relationships, the behavior expected of a nurse, and to see the world in a manner similar to other nurses. This is known as:
   1. case management.
   2. professionalization.
   3. socialization.
   4. governance.
10. The nurse moves to a new area of the country and learns the new area has many people of South African descent, a higher incidence of hypertension, and people whose average age is 37. This information would be considered:
    1. news.
    2. health statistics.
    3. a targeted area of study.
    4. demography.

CHAPTER 2

EVIDENCE-BASED PRACTICE AND RESEARCH IN NURSING

KEY TERM REVIEW

Match each term with its appropriate definition.

1. I Comparative analysis
2. M Content analysis
3. A Dependent variable
4. N Descriptive statistics
5. L Evidence-based practice
6. F Hypothesis
7. G Independent variable
8. O Inferential statistics
9. P Logical positivism
10. Q Measures of central tendency
11. R Measures of variability
12. K Methodology
13. W Naturalism
14. S Pilot study
15. B Protocol
16. T Qualitative research
17. U Quantitative research
18. H Reliability
19. V Sample
20. D Scientific validation
21. E Statistically significant
22. J Target population
23. C Validity

a. A behavior, characteristic, or outcome that the researcher wishes to explain or predict

b. Detailed instructions

c. Completeness and conceptual accuracy of measures

d. Thorough critique of a study for its conceptual and methodological integrity

e. Results that are not likely to have occurred only by chance

f. A predictive statement about the relationship between two or more variables

g. The presumed cause of or influence on the behavior wished to be explained

h. Refers to the consistency of measures

i. Involves assessing study findings for their implementation potential

j. Group of individuals in which information is desired

k. The logistics or mechanics of a study

l. Using research findings and other sources of evidence to guide decisions about client care

m. Data analysis that involves searching for themes and patterns

n. Procedures that organize and summarize large volumes of data, including measures of central tendency and measures of variability

o. Involves testing hypotheses about relationships between variables or differences between groups

p. Philosophical perspective of quantitative research that maintains the "truth" is absolute and can be discovered by careful measurement

q. Statistical procedure that provides a single numerical value that denotes the "average" value for a variable

r. Statistical procedure that describes how values for a variable are dispersed or spread out

s. A "dress rehearsal" before an actual study begins

t. The systematic collection and thematic analysis of narrative data

u. The systematic collection, statistical analysis, and interpretation of numerical data

v. Source of information for a study; may be humans, events, behaviors, documents, or biological specimens

w. Maintains that reality is relative or contextual and constructed by individuals who are experiencing a phenomenon

KEY TOPIC REVIEW

1. ____________ is clinical decision making based on the simultaneous use of the best evidence, clinical expertise, and patients' values.
2. The four rights of human subjects that nurses must safeguard are:

   a.

   b.

   c.

   d.
3. The term ____________ means that any information a client relates will not be made public or available to others without the patient's consent.
4. What is the definition of research?
5. According to the "Standards of Clinical Nursing" published by the ANA (1998), is included as one of the standards of professional performance.

6. Select and mark either (1) for quantitative research or (2) for qualitative research for the following items with regard to research:

   a. ____________ Associated with naturalistic inquiry that explores subjective and complex experiences of human beings

   b. ____________ Data collection and analysis occur concurrently

   c. ____________ A systematic, logical sequence based on a specific plan designed to collect information in controlled conditions; analyzed using statistical procedures

   d. ____________ Theory or framework is developed after the data are analyzed to identify patterns and/or themes

   e. ____________ Viewed as "hard science"

7. Change in practice requires: (Select all that apply.)

   a. assessing the need for change.
   b. locating and analyzing the best evidence.
   c. providing nurses with information essential to nursing practice.
   d. integrating and maintaining the change.
   e. implementing and evaluating the practice change.

8. Correctly identify the order of the steps in conducting quantitative research.

   a. Review the related literature.
   b. Communicate conclusions and implications.
   c. Define the study's purpose or rationale.
   d. Conduct a pilot study.
   e. Analyze the data.
   f. Formulate hypotheses and define variables.
   g. Collect the data.
   h. Select the population, sample, and setting.
   i. State a research question or problem.
   j. Select a research design to test the hypothesis.

9. From the following list, select the definition that best defines the elements of an ideal study.

a. Research problem	______ Protection of human rights, standards of beneficence, respect for human dignity, approved by Institutional Review Board
b. Review of literature	______ Is appropriate, clearly informs, enhances study
c. Study framework	______ Significant, addresses an issue that is important to nursing, addresses a researchable problem, is feasible to address in a study setting
d. Data collection	______ Relevant, thorough, current, authoritative
e. Ethical considerations	______ Appropriate for variables and sample, yields appropriate level of measure, reliable and valid, safe and humane

10. Describe the two major approaches nurse researchers use to investigate client's responses to health alterations and nursing interventions.

    a.

    b.

11. The bachelor of science in nursing (BSN) is the usual level of preparation for the research nurse who:

    a. conducts independent research.

    b. focuses on the evaluation and use of research.

    c. evaluates research findings.

    d. understands and applies research findings from nursing and other disciplines in clinical practice.

12. According to the "Standards of Clinical Nursing" published by the ANA (1998), research is included as one of the standards of professional performance.

    a. True

    b. False

13. Qualitative research uses measurement in its methods.

    a. True

    b. False

14. ______ pertains to the availability of time as well as the material and human resources needed to investigate a research problem or question.

15. A ______ ______ is conducted prior to the actual study to assess the adequacy of the data collection plan and to identify any potential flaws in the study.

FOCUSED STUDY TIPS

1. What are data collection strategies that nurse researchers use?
2. Describe three research questions for which a quantitative approach to research is useful.
3. List three examples of documented nursing research in nursing magazines.
4. Which right of research study participants do you think is overlooked most often? Explain.
5. List four ways for a nurse to provide for patient confidentiality.
6. While many believe that evidence-based practice is best practice for nursing, others would argue that it has its flaws. What are two disadvantages to evidence-based practice?

CASE STUDY

The nurse, who is working on a medical unit with a large number of older adults diagnosed with diabetes, reads a research article that indicates a direct correlation between instability of blood glucose levels and age with the oldest individuals most likely to demonstrate the largest drop in blood glucose levels if they must fast for diagnostic testing.

1. Is this adequate evidence for the nurse to promote changing the practice of having clients fast in preparation for diagnostic testing?
2. What should the nurse do next?
3. The research article includes a graph with age of clients across the bottom and percentage decrease in blood sugar levels along the side axis. What type of study is this?

REVIEW QUESTIONS

1. Which of the following is a violation of a client's right to self-determination?
   1. Hidden inducements
   2. Sharing a client's information with a pharmaceutical company
   3. Providing basic care to the client
   4. Giving the client information about what participating in a study will involve
2. Upon successful completion of the NCLEX-RN®, the registered nurse is asked to participate in a research study on the coping and adjustment skills of a newly graduated registered nurse. The plan is to use an oral, recorded interview with a grounded theory. What type of research study is being conducted?
   1. Pilot study
   2. Quantitative study
   3. Qualitative study
   4. Ethnographic study
3. Which of the following activities are examples of how a professional nurse may participate in research? (Select all that apply.)
   1. Critiquing research for application to practice
   2. Identifying clinical problems suitable for nursing research
   3. Encouraging patient participation in a study without informed consent
   4. Using research findings in the development of policies, procedures, and practice guidelines for patient care
4. A nursing student documents the client's full name and date of birth on the required paperwork for a clinical course and turns it in to the instructor. Which of the following client rights is being violated?
   1. Right not to be harmed
   2. Right to full disclosure
   3. Right of self-determination
   4. Right of privacy and confidentiality
5. Which of the following identifies the "C" in PICO?
   1. Comprehension
   2. Comparison
   3. Challenging
   4. Confidentiality
6. Formulating a research problem is often facilitated by the researcher performing:
   1. a feasibility study.
   2. a literature review.
   3. a methodology evaluation.
   4. a pilot study.

7. Data analysis involves the application of which of the following procedures? (Select all that apply.)
   1. Descriptive statistics
   2. Inferential statistics
   3. Measures of central tendency
   4. Measures of variability
8. Continuing education is the responsibility of the nurse to keep abreast of ______ and ______ changes and also changes within the nursing profession.
   1. Scientific and technologic
   2. Medical and technologic
   3. Scientific and human responses
   4. Cardiac and neurologic
9. As a nurse researcher, what is involved in a research project? (Select all that apply.)
   1. Identifying a research question or problem
   2. Writing a thesis paper
   3. Collecting data using various means such as computer searches and/or questionnaires
   4. Analyzing the data and writing up the results
   5. Publishing or presenting the research findings to expand the body of nursing knowledge
10. One of the major responsibilities the nurse has when conducting nursing research is:
    1. encouraging the participation of clients in nursing research.
    2. being aware of and advocating on behalf of clients' rights.
    3. exposing clients to the possibility of injury from the research.
    4. pressuring clients into participating in the study.
11. What is the term used to describe a behavior, characteristic, or outcome that the researcher wishes to explain or predict?
    1. Dependent variable
    2. Independent variable
    3. Hypothesis
    4. Sample

CHAPTER 3

NURSING THEORIES AND CONCEPTUAL FRAMEWORKS

KEY TERM REVIEW

Match each term with its appropriate definition.

1. _______ Client
2. _______ Conceptual framework
3. _______ Critical theories
4. _______ Environment
5. _______ Grand theories
6. _______ Health
7. _______ Metaparadigm
8. _______ Midlevel theories
9. _______ Nursing
10. _______ Paradigm
11. _______ Philosophy
12. _______ Practice discipline
13. _______ Theory

a. Degree of wellness or well-being that the client experiences
b. Attributes, characteristics, and actions that provide care on behalf of, or in conjunction with the client
c. Focus on the exploration of concepts
d. A belief system
e. Those that articulate a broad range of significant relationships among the concepts of a discipline
f. Recipient of nursing care
g. A system of ideas that is proposed to explain a given phenomenon
h. Those that help elucidate how social structures affect a wide variety of human experiences
i. A group of related ideas, statements, or concepts
j. The internal and external surroundings that affect the client
k. Major concepts that can be superimposed on almost any work of nursing
l. A pattern of shared understandings and assumptions about reality and the world
m. Term used for fields of study in which the central focus is performance of a professional role.

KEY TOPIC REVIEW

1. Define theory. List two characteristics of a theory.
2. What is the main function of theory (and research) in a practice discipline?
3. During the latter half of the 20th century, disciplines seeking to establish themselves in universities had to demonstrate something that Nightingale had not envisioned for nursing—a unique body of theoretical knowledge.

   a. True　　　　b. False
4. Disciplines without a strong theory and research base were referred to as "______," a negative comparison with the "______" natural sciences.
5. What is the term encompassing the "building blocks" of theories? ______
6. A ______ ______ is a group of related ideas, statements, or concepts. It may also be called a ______ theory or ______ ______.
7. The term ______ refers to a pattern of shared understandings and assumptions about reality and the world. It includes a person's notions of reality that are largely unconscious or taken for granted.
8. What four major concepts are related to the metaparadigm for nursing?
9. According to Figure 3–1 in your text, what are some of the prevalent foundational theories in nursing?
10. Match each theorist with the appropriate term.

a. Philosophies	______	Orem
b. Conceptual models	______	Nightingale
c. Midlevel theories	______	Peplau
	______	Parse
	______	Henderson
	______	Roy
	______	Neuman
	______	Rogers
	______	Leininger
	______	Watson
	______	King

11. Who is considered to be the first nurse theorist?
12. An early effort to define nursing phenomena, ______ serves as the basis for later theoretical formulations.
13. Debates about the role of theory in nursing practice provide evidence that nursing is maturing as both an academic discipline and a clinical profession.

    a. True　　　　b. False

14. Define the following terms:
    a. Client (person)
    b. Environment
    c. Health
    d. Nursing
15. Why is nursing considered to be a practice discipline?

FOCUSED STUDY TIPS

1. Describe the two paradigms of nursing theories.
2. List the major points of the following nursing theories:
    a. Nightingale's environmental theory
    b. Peplau's interpersonal relations model
    c. Henderson's definition of nursing
    d. Roger's science of unitary human beings
    e. Orem's general theory of nursing
    f. King's goal attainment theory
    g. Neuman's systems model
    h. Roy's adaptation model
    i. Leininger's cultural care diversity and universality theory
    j. Watson's human caring theory
    k. Parse's human becoming theory
3. Read the Evidence-Based Practice feature titled "How Well Does a Levine-Based Theory Apply to the Care of Preterm Infants?" that is in this chapter in the text. Identify the implications for nursing practice.
4. Although the various nursing models have been widely used for centuries to care for clients, some may critique the use of nursing theories. Describe one critique against nursing theories that McCrae identified.

CASE STUDY

The chief executive officer (CEO) has requested that the director of nursing (DON) revise the current philosophy of nursing that is being used for both a long-term care facility and an assisted living facility. The DON wants to develop the philosophy based on a nursing theory that adequately reflects both the healthy and ill clients housed in the facilities. The facilities' mission statements embrace the ideal of clients improving and sustaining independent functions, and encourage individualized goals for all clients to meet their individual needs. The DON wants to emphasize the nurses' responsibilities during the process of nurse–client interactions as well as the outcomes of nursing care.

1. Choose the best nursing theory on which to base the revised philosophy of nursing for this particular facility.
2. Explain your rationale for using the theory that you have chosen.

REVIEW QUESTIONS

1. A supposition or system of ideas that is proposed to explain a given phenomenon or something significant is called a:
   1. concept.
   2. theory.
   3. paradigm.
   4. conceptual model.
2. Some examples of concepts, which are defined as labels given to ideas, objects, or events, are:
   1. intelligence, motivation, and obesity.
   2. comfort, fatigue, pain, depression, and/or environment.
   3. self-care, adaptation, caring, behavioral system, and/or nurse–client transactions.
   4. humanistic endeavors, unitary man, and/or learned helplessness.
3. Which theorist addresses hospice nursing issues during end-of-life care?
   1. Imogene King
   2. Callista Roy
   3. Dorothea Orem
   4. Jean Watson
4. An example of a middle-range nursing theory is:
   1. Peplau's psychodynamic nursing model.
   2. Jean Watson's model of human caring.
   3. Roy's adaptation model.
   4. Imogene King's theory of goal attainment.
5. This theorist based her theory of nursing on the principle that nursing assists clients with 14 essential functions that move them toward independence.
   1. Myra Estrin Levine
   2. Dorothea Orem
   3. Madeline Leininger
   4. Virginia Henderson
6. One of the goals of Betty Neuman's health care systems model is:
   1. maintenance of system equilibrium.
   2. assisting the client to achieve the highest level of self-care.
   3. promoting internal and external stimuli that influence the client's well-being.
   4. to heal the client and make the bed available for sicker clients.

7. Nightingale, Henderson, and Watson developed philosophies of nursing. Why are their works considered philosophies when discussed in nursing?
   1. Because they were the first three nursing theorists.
   2. Because it was an early effort to define nursing phenomena that serves as the basis for later theoretical formulations.
   3. Because they had grand theories of nursing and not middle-level theories.
   4. Because it was a late effort to define nursing.
8. Disciplines without a strong theory and research base were historically referred to as:
   1. hard.
   2. concrete.
   3. soft.
   4. medium.
9. A conceptual framework is considered to be:
   1. a group of related ideas, statements, or concepts.
   2. a pattern of shared understandings and assumptions about reality and the world.
   3. the way to elucidate how social structures affect a wide variety of human experiences, from art to social practices.
   4. a belief system, often an early effort to define nursing phenomena that serves as the basis for later theoretical formulations.
10. In the late 20th century, much of the theoretical work in nursing focused on articulating relationships among four major concepts. (Select the major concepts.)
    1. Person
    2. Environment
    3. Nursing
    4. Professionalism
    5. Health
11. Match the early nurse theorist who developed the nursing action stated below.

1. A nurse performing noncontact therapeutic touch.	a. Florence Nightingale
2. A nurse measuring the client's intake and output	b. Hildegard Peplau
3. A nurse demonstrating therapeutic communication with a client who has been diagnosed with depression	c. Martha Rogers
4. A nurse who plans care with the client to establish mutual goals and outcomes	d. Imogene King

CHAPTER 4

LEGAL ASPECTS OF NURSING

KEY TERM REVIEW

Match each term with its appropriate definition.

1. _______ Assault
2. _______ Autopsy
3. _______ Battery
4. _______ Breach of duty
5. _______ Burden of proof
6. _______ Causation
7. _______ Civil law
8. _______ Common law
9. _______ Complaint
10. _______ Contract
11. _______ Defamation
12. _______ Euthanasia
13. _______ False imprisonment
14. _______ Informed consent
15. _______ Injury
16. _______ Interstate compact
17. _______ Liability
18. _______ Libel
19. _______ Living will
20. _______ Mandated reporters
21. _______ Plaintiff
22. _______ *Respondeat superior*
23. _______ Right
24. _______ Tort law
25. _______ Unprofessional conduct

a. Laws evolving from court decisions
b. Harm that occurred as a direct result of failure to follow standards of care
c. Examination of the body after death
d. Agreement between competent persons, on sufficient consideration to do or not do a legal act
e. Communication that is false, and results in injury to the reputation of a person
f. Defines and enforces duties and rights among private individuals that are not based on contractual agreements
g. Defamation by means of print, writing, or pictures
h. The requirement that, by law, requires nurses to report abuse, neglect, or exploitation
i. Document filed by a person claiming that legal rights have been infringed upon
j. A standard of care that is not observed
k. The willful touching of a person that may or may not cause harm
l. An attempt or threat to touch a person unjustifiably
m. Deals with relationships among individuals
n. The duty of proving an assertion of wrongdoing
o. The unjustifiable detention of a person without legal warrant to confine the person
p. Type of harm

q. A privilege or fundamental power to which an individual is entitled unless revoked by law or given up voluntarily

r. State of being legally responsible for one's obligations and actions, and to make financial restitution for wrongful acts

s. Provides specific instructions about what medical treatment the client chooses to omit or refuse in the event that the client is unable to make those decisions

t. Includes incompetence or gross negligence, conviction for practicing without a license, falsification of client records, illegally obtaining, using, or possessing controlled substances

u. Person who claims that his or her rights have been infringed on by one or more persons

v. Legal relationship by which the employer assumes responsibility for the conduct of the employee

w. Agreement by a client to accept a course of treatment after being provided complete information

x. The mechanism used to create mutual recognition among states

y. The act of painlessly putting to death people suffering from an incurable or chronically painful disease

KEY TOPIC REVIEW

1. Why is it important for nurses to know the basics of legal concepts?
2. What is accountability, and what are two reasons it is needed in nursing?

   a.

   b.

3. Name two functions of laws in nursing.

   a.

   b.

4. The Constitution of the United States is the supreme law of the state.

   a. True b. False

5. Regulation of nursing is a function of state law.

   a. True b. False

6. List two types of laws and give the definition of each type.

   a.

   b.

7. Choose the correct definition of criminal action, the correct example of criminal action, and the potential results if a person is found guilty in a criminal trial. (Select all that apply.)

   a. Deals with the relationships among individuals in society.

   b. Deals with disputes between an individual and the society as a whole.

   c. If found guilty, the defendant may have to pay a sum of money.

   d. If found guilty, the defendant may lose money, be jailed, be executed, and/or lose any professional licenses.

   e. One example of this type of legal infraction is a nurse who deliberately delivers a lethal dose of medication to a client.

   f. One example of this type of legal action is a malpractice suit.

8. The action of a lawsuit is called ______________.

9. Organize the five steps in the civil judicial process according to the procedural rules.
   a. A document, called a complaint, is filed by an individual referred to as the plaintiff, who claims that his or her legal rights have been infringed on by one or more other individuals or entities referred to as defendants.
   b. In the trial of the case, all the relevant facts are presented to a jury or only to a judge.
   c. The judge renders a decision, or the jury renders a verdict. If the outcome is not acceptable to one of the parties, an appeal can be made for another trial.
   d. Both parties engage in pretrial activities, referred to as discovery, in an effort to obtain all the facts of the situation.
   e. A written response, called an answer, is made by the defendants.
10. What is the legal purpose for defining the scope of nursing, licensing requirements, and standards of care? (Select all that apply.)
    a. For the protection of the nurse
    b. For the protection of the client
    c. For the protection of the public
    d. To maintain client confidentiality
    e. For the protection of the physician
11. Each state has an obligation to define its scope of nursing practice and licensing requirements.
    a. True b. False
12. The name of the newly developed regulatory model is the ________ ________ model. It allows for multistate licensure for nurses. Nurses can practice in states bordering their own state if both states have an ________ compact.
13. ________ is the voluntary practice of validating that an individual nurse has met minimum standards of nursing competence in specialty areas such as maternal–child health, pediatrics, metal health, gerontology, and school nursing.
14. Define standards of care and list the two classifications.
    a.
    b.
15. List four examples of external standards of care:
    a.
    b.
    c.
    d.
16. A written contract cannot be changed legally by an oral agreement.
    a. True b. False
17. Describe the difference between an expressed contract and an implied contract. Give an example of each type.
18. Explain the difference between a right and a responsibility and give an example of each.
19. A ________ is an organized work stoppage by a group of employees to express a grievance, enforce a demand for changes in conditions of employment, or solve a dispute with management. Usually, it is a result of failed collective bargaining between the parties.

20. What are the two types of informed consent?

    a.

    b.

21. It is the nurse's responsibility to have the informed consent form signed prior to an invasive procedure.

    a. True b. False

22. What three things does the nurse's signature confirm with the signed consent form?

    a.

    b.

    c.

23. If a client refuses to sign the consent form, what actions does the nurse need to take?

24. What are two reasons for nurses to be knowledgeable regarding the Nurse Practice Act in their state of practice?

25. Nurses are included as mandated reporters of violence, abuse, and/or neglect.

    a. True

    b. False

26. How is the nurse involved in the Americans with Disabilities Act? Explain your answer.

27. State laws regulate the distribution and use of controlled substances such as narcotics, depressants, stimulants, and hallucinogens.

    a. True b. False

28. _________ is cited as one of the main reasons for chemical dependence in health care workers.

29. Define the terms and list any nursing responsibilities about the following legal issues surrounding death:

    a. Advance directives

    b. Autopsies

    c. Certification of death

    d. Do-not-resuscitate orders (DNRs)

    e. Euthanasia

    f. Inquests

    g. Organ donation

30. _________ law is usually involved with nursing liability.

31. Choose the types of invasion from which the client must be protected. (Select all that apply.)

    a. Reporting the number of births that occurred in the hospital for statistical analysis

    b. Reporting of infections and communicable diseases

    c. Taking photographs or having nursing students observe the client's care without the client's consent

    d. Revealing the name of a client who was treated for domestic violence

    e. Reporting violent incidents to the local authorities

32. What is the Health Insurance Portability and Accountability Act (HIPAA) of 1996, and why is it important? What are the four specific areas of HIPAA? Refer to the HIPAA website found on the Companion Website.

33. What are four categories that nurses must question to protect themselves legally when carrying out health care provider's orders?

FOCUSED STUDY TIPS

1. Define and give an example of the following laws. Which is the highest level of law?

   a. Civil law

   b. Common law

   c. Contract law

   d. Law

   e. Private law

   f. Public law

   g. Statutory law

   h. Tort law

2. Refer to Figure 4–1 in the text. Describe how laws are created from constitutions, statutes, administrative agencies, and decisions of courts.

3. Why is it important to know the state legislators who represent your state? Name the state legislators for your state. How do you contact your legislators, and why is it necessary to contact them regarding nursing issues?

4. State your position on having malpractice insurance as a registered nurse. Is it your responsibility or the responsibility of your employer? Under what circumstances could you use the malpractice insurance? Refer to the Application Activity: Nurse Practice Act on the Companion Website.

5. What are the procedures that occur when a nursing license is revoked in the state in which you will practice?

6. Go to the NCSBN website and list the states that have passed the NLC legislation. Refer to Box 4–1 in the text for additional information.

7. What are the statutes in your state for "consent"? What is considered the legal age of consent?

8. Discuss the areas of potential liability in nursing and define the following terms: malpractice, intentional torts, crime, felony, manslaughter, misdemeanors, duty, and torts.

9. Determine the difference between defamation and slander. Give an example of each that might occur in the health care setting. Who could bring a defamation/slander lawsuit?

10. What are some legal protections in nursing practice to protect the nurse from litigation? Is the Good Samaritan Act designed for nurses? What are the responsibilities of nurses who choose to render emergency care? Does your state require nurses to assist in emergencies?

11. Discuss and defend your position on professional liability insurance. Is it a requirement for all nurses? List the advantages of maintaining professional liability insurance.

12. Why is nurse documentation so important? What is the purpose of nurse documentation? How can it be used in a court of law? Does the nurse need to document if an incident report is filled out in the client's chart? Refer to the text, Chapter 4, Figure 4–5, for additional information.

13. What measures can nursing students implement in order to fulfill responsibilities to clients and to minimize the chances for liability? Refer to Boxes 4–5 and 4–6 in Chapter 4 of the text.

14. The nurse is caring for a client who has been declared legally brain dead. The client did not specify if he wishes to be an organ donor. What is the nurse's best action?

15. Discuss the difference between a crime and a tort.

CASE STUDY

A client was scheduled for the surgical removal of the left ovary. During the surgery, the surgeon noticed that the appendix of the client was inflamed. He decides to remove it to prevent further problems. The client's consent for surgery only listed removal of the left ovary.

1. Did the surgeon adhere to the signed consent form that the client signed before the surgery?

2. Under the circumstances, what type of tort is the surgeon liable for?

3. What was the operating nurse's role in this incident?

REVIEW QUESTIONS

1. Which nurse would be considered to be the "best expert witness" for the defense in a case regarding an obstetric patient who died after delivery complications?
   1. A nurse who holds a bachelor's degree in nursing and has been practicing for 2 years
   2. A nurse who holds a master's degree in nursing and has a certification in emergency nursing
   3. A nurse who holds a doctorate of nursing science in pediatric care
   4. A nurse who holds a master's degree in nursing and a state certification in maternal–infant nursing
2. Which clients could make decisions regarding health care? (Select all that apply.)
   1. A woman who arrives in the emergency department with an altered mental state and the aroma of ethyl alcohol
   2. The parents of a 14-year-old girl involved in a car collision
   3. A middle-aged man who has the mental capacity of an 8-year-old
   4. A 10-year-old boy who has arrived with friends and has a shallow laceration needing three sutures
   5. A competent older adult who requires surgery on a prolapsed bladder
3. A client was discharged after having a 1-day surgery on her gallbladder. The nurse discharging the client failed to give the client oral or written discharge instructions. This failure to carry out the provision of discharge instructions could result in charges of:
   1. malpractice.
   2. negligence.
   3. assault.
   4. battery.

4. Which statement indicates that the client understands informed consent of a surgical procedure?
    1. The nurse discovers the signed informed consent form on the bedside table before the surgeon discusses the procedure with the client.
    2. The client's oldest son stated that he explained the procedure to the client and the client told him that he wanted the surgery.
    3. The client states that the surgeon explained the procedure to him, allowed him to ask questions, and explained the risks of not permitting the surgery.
    4. The client been declared legally incompetent; however, the client states understanding of the surgical procedure.
5. While reviewing the transfer papers of a client, the nurse notes that the client has both a living will and a durable power of attorney. A living will differs from a durable power of attorney in that a living will:
    1. describes how the client wants his wishes carried out in the event of a terminal illness.
    2. designates who should make medical decisions if the client is incapable of making independent decisions.
    3. determines which relative gets the house.
    4. allows a health care provider to make decisions if the client is unable to make decisions.
6. A nurse threatens to give a loud, disruptive client an injection that will "knock the client out." The nurse follows through on the threat and gives the injection without the client's consent. What has the nurse committed?
    1. Threat, assault
    2. Battery, invasion of privacy
    3. Assault, invasion of privacy
    4. Assault, battery
7. A nurse documents in the client's chart that the health care provider is incompetent because the health care provider did not respond promptly to the nurse's call regarding the client. This is an example of __________ and __________.
    1. defamation
    2. slander
    3. libel
    4. battery
    5. unprofessional conduct
8. Conviction for practicing nursing without a license, incompetence or gross negligence, falsification of client records, and illegally obtaining, using, or possessing controlled substances is called:
    1. libel.
    2. slander.
    3. unprofessional conduct.
    4. assault.

9. Most statutes include conscience clauses that are designed to protect hospitals and nurses in matters dealing with abortion services. These clauses allow the nurse to be protected from:

   1. prejudicial statements.
   2. discrimination or retaliation.
   3. defamation or unjust prejudice.
   4. legal liability.

10. Identify the element that is NOT one of the functions of the law in the nursing environment.

    1. Accountability helps to maintain a minimum standard of nursing practice.
    2. Law differentiates nurses' responsibilities from those of other health care professionals.
    3. Law specifies which nursing actions are legal in caring for clients.
    4. Law specifies which hospital policies are legal in caring for clients.

CHAPTER 5

VALUES, ETHICS, AND ADVOCACY

KEY TERM REVIEW

Match each term with its appropriate definition.

1. D Accountability
2. G Active euthanasia
3. F Advocate
4. M Assisted suicide
5. A Attitudes
6. S Autonomy
7. O Beliefs
8. N Beneficence
9. P Bioethics
10. J Code of ethics
11. K Fidelity
12. B Justice
13. Q Moral development
14. T Moral distress
15. R Moral rules
16. E Nonmaleficence
17. H Nursing ethics
18. I Passive euthanasia
19. L Personal values
20. C Veracity

a. Mental positions or feelings
b. Fairness
c. Telling the truth
d. Answerable to self and others for one's own actions
e. Do no harm
f. One who expresses and defends the cause of another
g. Actions that bring about the client's death directly
h. Rules governing the behavior of nurses related to the morality of human behavior.
i. Withdrawing or withholding life-sustaining therapy
j. A formal statement of a group's ideals and values
k. To be faithful to agreements and promises
l. An individual's enduring beliefs or attitudes about the worth of a person, object, idea, or action
m. Process of client taking his or her own life with help from another individual
n. The concept of "doing good" for the benefit of others
o. Interpretations or conclusions that people accept as true
p. Ethics as applied to human life or health
q. Process of learning to tell the difference between right and wrong and of learning what should and should not be done
r. Specific prescriptions for action based on an individual's principles or beliefs.
s. The right to make one's own decisions
t. Conflict that arises when what the nurse believes needs to be done cannot be carried out due to an obstacle such as client wishes, personal beliefs, or facility regulations.

KEY TOPIC REVIEW

1. Define values and describe why values are important in nursing. Worth of a person, Influence decisions
2. Describe the difference between values and beliefs. Beliefs = opions, values = Direction
3. Attitudes are mental positions or feelings toward a person, object, or idea.
4. List five values identified by the American Association of Colleges of Nursing (AACN, 2008). Refer to Box 5–1 in the text.
   a. Altruism
   b. Autonomy
   c. Human. Dignity
   d. Integrity
   e. Social Justice
5. When should the nurse use values clarification as a nursing intervention? When it conflicts with Health
6. Which type of ethics is used when nurses make decisions about the acts of abortion or euthanasia? Nursing Ethics
7. What is the term that is similar to *ethics* and often used interchangeably? Morality
8. Moral development is the process of learning to tell the difference between right and wrong. It begins in young adulthood and continues through life.
   (a.) True b. False
9. Match the following three moral framework theories with the correct descriptive terms.
   a. Consequence-based (teleological) theories
   b. Principles-based (deontological) theories
   c. Relations-based (caring) theories

   ______ These theories involve logical and formal processes.

   ______ These theories look to outcomes or consequences of an action.

   ______ These theories promote the common good or the welfare of the group.

   ______ These theories stress individual rights.

   ______ One form of these types of theory is called utilitarianism.

   ______ These theories focus on issues of fairness.

   ______ These theories stress courage, generosity, commitment, and the need to nurture and maintain relationships.

   ______ These theories involve logical, formal processes and emphasize individual rights, duties, and obligations.

10. Within recent years, what statements regarding ethics have been made broader in scope or added to the *Code of Ethics for Nurses*? Refer to Box 5–3 in the text. Compassion
11. What is the goal of ethical reasoning within the context of nursing? Mutual peaceful agreement
12. What are three functions of the advocacy role that nurses assume? Inform, Support, Mediate
13. Beneficence means "doing good."

14. Justice is often referred to as fairness.

15. Veracity refers to telling the truth.

16. Accountability means "answerable to oneself and others for one's own actions," while Responsibility refers to "the specific accountability or liability associated with the performance of duties of a particular role."

FOCUSED STUDY TIPS

1. What are your values regarding life, death, health, and illness?
2. Practice assisting someone (a friend, parent, significant other, etc.) in clarifying their values and identifying behaviors that may need further clarification by using the seven values clarification steps listed in Box 5–2 of the text.
3. What are some factors that have led to increased ethical concerns? Why do ethical concerns even exist?
4. List 6 of the 12 rights of the Bill of Rights for clients receiving health care. As a nurse, what are your responsibilities in promoting the Bill of Rights?
5. What common ethical issues do health care professionals currently face? How do some hospitals resolve ethical issues?
6. Define harm. Give one example of unintentional harm and one example of intentional harm.
7. When caring for a client with acquired immunodeficiency syndrome (AIDS), what is the moral obligation of the nurse according to the ANA position statement?
8. Define veracity. What is the moral obligation of the nurse to use veracity, even when it is known that using veracity will cause harm?
9. Compare and contrast accountability and responsibility as applied to the nursing profession.

CASE STUDIES

1. You are the nurse caring for a 45-year-old client who is in the end stages of acquired immunodeficiency syndrome (AIDS). She is married and has two children, ages 14 and 17. The client is unable to perform the care needed for her children and spouse, and she had to take a leave of absence from employment 8 months ago due to her advanced AIDS. Her family is experiencing emotional turmoil and financial stress due to her prognosis and inability to fully function in her roles as a contributor to income, mother, and wife. The client requests your assistance in deciding what end-of-life decisions she should make. Her family and friends want her to do everything in her power to survive; however, she tells you that she is "so tired."

   a. What considerations should you take into account in assisting the client to make these decisions?
   Client/Family outlook
   b. In what way could you assist the client in reaching decisions about further health care?
   Make their own Choice
   c. Would an ethics committee be involved in this matter?
   Yes
   d. What principles of autonomy are applied to this situation?
   Final Sayso

2. A well-known government official is in the hospital for cosmetic surgery. A story and photograph of the client and his medical information appear in the local paper. The client feels that his privacy has been invaded.

   a. What are his rights as a client? Privacy
   b. Could he take legal actions? Yes

REVIEW QUESTIONS

1. When distinguishing between morality and legal correctness, what indicators would the nurse recognize as reflecting the morality of a situation? (Select all that apply.)
   1. Feelings such as shame, guilt, or hope
   2. Tendency to respond to the situation with words such as *should*, *right*, *ought to*, or *good*
   3. Legislative regulations requiring or preventing a specific action
   4. Infringement on an individual's human rights
   5. Fear of imprisonment
2. What is the best example of altruism exhibited by a nurse?
   1. Turning the bed-bound client every 4 hours
   2. Withholding scheduled pain medication to a client who has a level 6 pain scale rating
   3. Insisting that a client use the bedpan instead of assisting the client to the restroom because it is easier for the nurse
   4. Allowing a Catholic client to keep his rosary beads within reach as a comfort measure
3. What client behavior might indicate unclear self-values?
   1. A client with coronary heart disease who follows the recommended diet plan to reduce cholesterol and fat
   2. A mother with a child diagnosed with asthma stops smoking tobacco
   3. A client who has multiple admissions to the chemical dependency program
   4. A client with diabetes who monitors finger-stick blood sugars and other health concerns relating to the diabetic condition
4. What statement is true regarding ethical committees and the role these committees play in dealing with health care conflicts?
   1. Ethical committees ensure that relevant facts of a case are presented
   2. Ethical committees are not designed to reduce the institution's legal risk
   3. Ethical committees decide when laws have been violated.
   4. Nurses usually do not serve as team members on ethical committees.
5. What moral framework is the nurse operating under if she refuses to participate in a surgery for a 93-year-old client who has stated on numerous occasions that he does not want further surgery? His family and surgeon are insisting on the client having the surgery. The nurse's rationale is that the nurse–client relationship commits her to protecting him and meeting his needs.
   1. Relationships-based theory
   2. Consequences-based theory
   3. Deontological-based theory
   4. Principles-based theory
6. Which clinical scenario is an example of nonmaleficence and unintentional harm?
   1. Not locking a wheelchair and transferring a client into the wheelchair
   2. Catching a client who is falling and bruising the client's arm
   3. A client's allergic reaction to a prescribed medication
   4. Administering oxygen at 6 L/min to a client when the order is for 2 L/min

7. Identify behaviors that would be classified as an invasion of privacy for a client. (Select all that apply.)
   1. A nurse who removes articles from a bedside table in order to “clear out some of that junk”
   2. A middle-aged, mentally alert client who requests a nursing assistant to “get rid of a bedpan, used ketchup container, and other unused items”
   3. A nursing student who documents the client’s name and address on paperwork to hand in to the clinical faculty member
   4. A cousin who wants to review the chart for lab results and the health care provider’s orders
8. What is the correct action by the nurse if a health care provider asks the nurse to perform a task in which the nurse does not have adequate knowledge or experience performing?
   1. Inform the health care provider about the lack of education and experience, and then perform the task.
   2. Do not inform the health care provider and carry out the task.
   3. Inform the health care provider regarding the lack of education and/or experience necessary to safely perform the task. Refuse to do the task.
   4. Inform the health care provider, and then both parties can attempt to figure it out.
9. What is the best example of documentation by the nurse in the client’s record?
   1. All facts and information regarding a person’s condition, treatment, care, progress, any refusal or consent of treatment, and response to illness and treatment are noted.
   2. All facts and information regarding a person’s condition, treatment, care, progress, and response to illness and treatment are noted.
   3. All facts and information regarding a person’s condition, treatment, care, progress, any refusal or consent of treatment, physician’s competence, and response to illness and treatment are noted.
   4. All facts and information regarding a patient that the nurse feels are appropriate are noted.
10. Organ donation prohibits the: (Select all that apply.)
    1. donation of organs in clients diagnosed with brain death.
    2. sale of body organs.
    3. marketing of body organs.
    4. donation of cartilage and bones.

CHAPTER 6

HEALTH CARE DELIVERY SYSTEMS

KEY TERM REVIEW

Match each term with its appropriate definition.

1. _______ Case management
2. _______ Coinsurance
3. _______ Critical pathways
4. _______ Diagnosis-related groups (DRGs)
5. _______ Differentiated practice
6. _______ Health care system
7. _______ Health maintenance organization (HMO)
8. _______ Independent practice associations (IPAs)
9. _______ Integrated delivery system (IDS)
10. _______ Licensed vocational (practical) nurse (LVN/LPN)
11. _______ Managed care
12. _______ Medicaid
13. _______ Medicare
14 _______ Patient focused care
15. _______ Preferred provider arrangements
16 _______ Preferred provider organization
17. _______ Supplemental Security Income

a. Similar to HMOs, care is provided in offices, where the client pays a fixed amount
b. Provides direct client care under the direction of a registered nurse, physician or other licensed practitioner
c. A delivery model that brings services and providers to the clients
d. Incorporates acute care services, home health care, extended and skilled care facilities, and outpatient services
e. A health care system whose goals are to provide cost-effective, quality care
f. National and state health insurance program for older adults
g. Federal public assistance program that provides health care coverage to people who require financial assistance
h. The percentage share of a government-approved charge that is paid by the client
i. A classification system that establishes pretreatment diagnosis billing categories
j. Health care plan that contracts with a group of providers or agency that provides services at a discounted rate
k. Involves multidisciplinary teams that assume collaborative responsibility for planning, assessing needs, and coordinating, implementing, and evaluating care for groups of clients.
l. An interdisciplinary plan or tool that specifies assessments, interventions, treatments, and outcomes for health-related conditions across a time line
m. A group health care agency that provides health maintenance and treatment services to voluntary enrollees

n. Government-funded benefits available to people with disabilities

o. The totality of services offered by all health disciplines

p. System in which the best use of nursing personnel is based on the personnel's educational preparation and skill sets

q. Health care plan that contracts with individual health care providers

KEY TOPIC REVIEW

1. What are the three types of health care services?

   a.

   b.

   c.

2. What is the purpose of primary prevention health care systems?

   a. Health promotion and illness prevention

   b. Rehabilitation, health restoration, and palliative care

   c. Diagnosis and treatment

   d. To promote the World Health Organization

3. What is the purpose of secondary prevention?

   a. Health promotion and illness prevention

   b. Rehabilitation, health restoration, and palliative care

   c. Diagnosis and treatment

   d. To promote the World Health Organization

4. What is the purpose of tertiary prevention?

   a. Health promotion and illness prevention

   b. Rehabilitation, health restoration, and palliative care

   c. Diagnosis and treatment

   d. To promote the World Health Organization

5. What are the primary goals of *Healthy People 2020*?

   a.

   b.

   c.

   d.

6. Which is an example of a secondary prevention health care service?

   a. Health care providers' offices

   b. Weight control programs

   c. Blood pressure clinics

   d. Rehabilitation hospitals

7. ________ is the official agency at the federal level for public health.

8. What is the function of an occupational health clinic? Give some examples of the types of roles that a nurse might perform in that environment.

9. Name four factors affecting health care delivery in today's health care environment.

   a.

   b.

   c.

   d.

10. According to the U.S. Census, the expected number of individuals over age 85 will be the ________ growing population segment in the United States and will number over ________ million by 2020 and ________ million by 2030.

11. What impact does the Health Insurance Portability and Accountability Act (HIPAA) of 1996 have on the health care system?

12. What are critical pathways, and how are critical pathways used in case management and managed care?

13. What are two advantages of ambulatory care centers?

    a.

    b.

FOCUSED STUDY TIPS

1. Discuss the World Health Organization (WHO) project and *Healthy People 2020.*
2. What role does the federal government have in providing care to veterans and merchant mariners?
3. Define the roles of the following providers of health care:
   a. Registered nurse
   b. Licensed vocational nurse or licensed practical nurse
   c. Advanced practice nurse
   d. Complementary care provider
   e. Case manager
   f. Dentist
   g. Dietitian
   h. Occupational therapist
   i. Paramedical technologist
   j. Pharmacist
   k. Physical therapist
   l. Physician
   m. Physician assistant
   n. Podiatrist
   o. Respiratory therapist
   p. Social worker
   q. Spiritual support personnel
   r. Unlicensed assistive personnel

4. Discuss in depth the uneven distribution of health services in the United States. What are two facets of this problem?

5. Discuss the relationship between technological advances and the rising costs of health care in the United States.

CASE STUDIES

1. The nurse is collecting a health and physical assessment from an 80-year-old client who is blind and was recently admitted to the acute care facility.
   a. What type of health care coverage is the client almost guaranteed of carrying?
   b. If the client's income is below the poverty level, what type of coverage could also be included in the health care coverage plan?
2. The client is getting ready for discharge. The health care provider has written an order for physical therapy after discharge. In addition, the health care provider requests that a dietitian follow up with additional education regarding the client's newly diagnosed type 2 diabetes.
   a. What roles do the physical therapist and dietitian fulfill?
   b. Where could the client receive the services, and what type of coverage could possibly pay for these services?
3. Refer to the Evidence-Based Practice feature in the text (Box-21) to answer the following questions regarding the types of nurses and delivery models in hospitals and how those factors influence patient outcomes.
   a. What is the true regarding clients with chronic conditions or disabilities and access to care?
   b. What are the nursing implications when caring for clients with chronic conditions or disabilities?

REVIEW QUESTIONS

1. Which two frameworks for care are used for the delivery of nursing care that supports continuity of care and cost-effectiveness? (Select all that apply.)
   1. Managed care
   2. Nonfunctional method
   3. Secondary nursing
   4. Team nursing
2. Medicare is divided into two divisions, Part A and Part B, and one supplemental plan. Part A is the:
   1. voluntary prescription drug plan that began in January 2006.
   2. voluntary plan that provides partial coverage of outpatient and health care provider services to those who are eligible.
   3. plan section providing insurance toward hospitalization, home care, and hospice care.
   4. plan section providing very limited financial coverage to low-income persons.
3. Medicare is divided into two divisions, Part A and Part B, and one supplemental plan. Part B is the:
   1. voluntary prescription drug plan that began in January 2006.
   2. voluntary plan that provides partial coverage of outpatient and health care provider services to those who are eligible.
   3. plan section providing insurance toward hospitalization, home care, and hospice care.
   4. plan section providing very limited financial coverage to low-income persons.

4. Medicare is divided into two divisions, Part A and Part B, and one supplemental plan. Part D is the:
   1. voluntary prescription drug plan that began in January 2006.
   2. voluntary plan that provides partial coverage of outpatient and physician services to people eligible.
   3. plan section providing insurance toward hospitalization, home care, and hospice care.
   4. plan section providing very limited financial coverage to low-income persons.
5. Medicaid is described as:
   1. a voluntary prescription drug plan that began in January 2006.
   2. a voluntary plan that provides partial coverage of outpatient and health care provider services to those who are eligible.
   3. a plan providing insurance toward hospitalization, home care, and hospice care.
   4. a plan providing very limited financial coverage to low-income persons.
6. Which individuals are eligible for Supplemental Security Income (SSI)? (Select all that apply.)
   1. Individuals who are blind
   2. Individuals not eligible for Social Security
   3. Children from low-income families that are covered under Medicaid
   4. Anyone over age 65
   5. Anyone with a diagnosed disability
7. What is the name of the classification system that prospective payment systems utilize?
   1. Medicare
   2. Medicaid
   3. State Children's Health Insurance Program (SCHIP)
   4. Diagnosis-related groups (DRGs)
8. Third-party reimbursement refers to the insurance company that pays the client's (first party) bill to the provider (second party). This component is part of the:
   1. private health insurance plan.
   2. diagnosis-related group (DRG).
   3. group health insurance plan.
   4. preferred provider organization.
9. Prepaid group plans for insurance include:
   1. Medicare and Medicaid.
   2. Blue Cross and Blue Shield.
   3. HMOs, PPOs, PPAs, IPAs, and PHOs.
   4. Social Security and Supplemental Security Income.
10. What is an example of illness prevention?
    1. Immunizing children against chickenpox
    2. Caring for a dying client
    3. Assisting a stroke victim to the highest rehabilitation level possible
    4. Secondary prevention

CHAPTER 7

COMMUNITY NURSING AND CARE CONTINUITY

KEY TERM REVIEW

Match each term with its appropriate definition.

1. _______ Collaboration
2. _______ Community
3. _______ Community-based health care
4. _______ Community-based nursing
5. _______ Community health nursing
6. _______ Community nursing centers
7. _______ Continuity of care
8. _______ Discharge planning
9. _______ Integrated health care system
10. _______ Population
11. _______ Primary care
12. _______ Primary health care

a. Provides health-related services in places where people spend their time
b. Provides primary care to specific populations and is staffed by nurse practitioners and community health nurses
c. Composed of people who share some common characteristic but who do not necessarily interact with each other
d. Provision of integrated, accessible health care services by clinicians who are accountable for addressing a majority of personal health care services
e. A philosophy of nursing that guides nursing care provided for individuals and families wherever the individuals are, including where they live, work, play, or go to school
f. Emphasizes the promotion and preservation of the health of groups
g. A collegial working relationship with another health care provider in the provision of patient care
h. Health care based on practical, scientifically sound and socially acceptable methods and technology made accessible to individuals and families
i. A collection of people who share some attribute of their lives
j. Process of preparing a client to leave one level of care for another
k. Coordination of health care services by health care providers for clients moving from one health care setting to another.
l. Makes all levels of care available in an integrated form—primary care, secondary care, and tertiary care

KEY TOPIC REVIEW

1. What are four of the factors motivating change in the health care system?
   a. Escalating health care costs
   b. Decreasing technology
   c. Changing patterns of demographics
   d. Shorter hospital stays
   e. Decreased patient acuity
   f. Limited access to health care
2. List four characteristics of primary care.
   a.
   b.
   c.
   d.
3. List four characteristics of primary health care.
   a.
   b.
   c.
   d.
4. A ________ is a collection of people who share some attribute of their lives and interact with each other in some way. It is also defined as a social system in which the members interact formally or informally and form networks that operate for the benefit of all people in the community.
5. A ________ is composed of people who share some common characteristics but do not necessarily interact with each other.
6. List four types of community-based frameworks and give the definition of each.
   a. Type:
      Definition:
   b. Type:
      Definition:
   c. Type:
      Definition:
   d. Type:
      Definition:
7. Easy access is needed for an effective community-based health care system.
   a. True b. False

8. Choose the community-based settings for nursing practice. (Select all that apply.)
   a. Community nursing centers
   b. Long-term care facilities
   c. Parish nursing
   d. Telehealth
   e. Hospitals
9. Community-based nursing focuses on care of individuals in geographically local settings, whereas community health nursing emphasizes the promotion and preservation of the health of groups.
   a. True b. False
10. Both primary health care and primary care strive for universal access to and affordability of health care.
   a. True b. False

FOCUSED STUDY TIPS

1. What do the Pew Health Professions Commission competencies for future practitioners include? What are the competencies (listed in the text) that the health care practitioner would require?
2. Primary health care involves five principles. List and explain the five principles in detail.
3. Identify the essential aspects of home health nursing. What makes this community-based role especially challenging?
4. How does the community health care setting differ from traditional settings?
5. Define community-based health care (CBHC). Where is the care directed, and what is involved in CBHC?
6. How are consumers effecting major changes in health care delivery systems?

CASE STUDY

A nurse has been working as the case manager in a pediatric unit and decides that she wants to be involved in community nursing.

1. What are some types of community nursing that could be considered?
2. What skills would be needed for community nursing that might not be used in the pediatric unit?

REVIEW QUESTIONS

1. The key elements necessary for collaboration among health care providers include:
   1. Mutual respect, trust, and negotiation.
   2. Communication skills, mutual respect, and shared decision making.
   3. Negotiation, conflict management, and mutual respect.
   4. Conflict management, trust, and decision making.

2. As a nurse collaborator, which actions will the nurse perform? (Select all that apply.)
    1. Sharing personal expertise with other nurses and eliciting the expertise of others to ensure quality client care
    2. Seeking opportunities to collaborate with and within professional organizations
    3. Offering expert opinions on legislative initiatives related to health care
    4. Collaborating with other health care providers and consumers on health care legislation to best serve the needs of the public
3. When does discharge planning begin for a client?
    1. Prior to discharge
    2. On admission
    3. Two days after admission
    4. Two hours before discharge
4. Which client would be identified before discharge as needing a referral to a community-based health care facility?
    1. An older adult client who has no caregivers to provide the necessary oversight of care
    2. A child who has had an uncomplicated removal of the tonsils
    3. A mother who delivered a 7-pound baby vaginally the previous day
    4. A client who has a well-healed surgical wound to the abdomen
5. What is the major focus of integrated health care systems?
    1. Primary health care in the event of an emergency
    2. Health promotion and disease prevention
    3. Chronic disease management
    4. Long-term care of disabilities
6. Choose the correct responses that identify the function of a community (Select all that apply.)
    1. Individual support
    2. Social control
    3. Socialization
    4. Production of goods
7. Choose the correct responses that identify the parish nurse's roles. (Select all that apply.)
    1. Personal health counselor
    2. Health educator
    3. Referral source
    4. Integrator of faith and health
8. Which population represents the individuals most likely to be cared for by an advanced practice nurse? (Select all that apply.)
    1. Incarcerated adults
    2. Healthy school-age children
    3. Homeless individuals
    4. Healthy adults

CHAPTER 8

HOME CARE

KEY TERM REVIEW

Match each term with its appropriate definition.

1. _______ Caregiver role strain
2. _______ Durable medical equipment (DME) company
3. _______ Home care
4. _______ Home health care nursing
5. _______ Hospice nursing
6. _______ Registry

a. Health services provided in the home setting

b. Nursing services and products provided to clients in the home

c. Support and care of the terminally ill person and his or her family

d. Provides health care equipment to the client at home

e. State of altered health and well-being due to the physical, emotional, social, and financial burdens of caring for another.

f. Contracts with individual care providers to care for the client in the home

KEY TOPIC REVIEW

1. Identify factors that have contributed to the increase and growth in home health care.
2. What does home care involve in today's health care system?
3. _________ nursing is support and care of the terminally ill person and his or her family, and is considered a subspecialty of home health nursing.
4. What are three advantages of home health nursing?

   a.

   b.

   c.

5. What are three disadvantages of home health nursing?

   a.

   b.

   c.

6. List four duties that a home health nurse might perform in the home setting.

   a.

   b.

   c.

   d.

7. Any individual involved with the care of a client may identify the need for home health.

   a. True b. False

8. Match the following types of home health agencies with the appropriate description.

a. Official or public agencies	_________	Institutions that rely on private pay sources or "third-party" reimbursement
b. Voluntary or private not-for-profit agencies	_________	United Way
c. Private, proprietary agencies	_________	Hospital home health agencies
d. Institution-based agencies	_________	State health department

9. List four topics regarding infection control that the home health nurse will educate the patient on in the home.

   a.

   b.

   c.

   d.

FOCUSED STUDY TIPS

1. What is the Visiting Nurse Associations of America's definition of a home health nurse?
2. Describe the unique aspects of home health nursing. What is involved in the practice of home health nursing? List additional providers in home health and describe their duties or roles.
3. What does the home health referral process entail? What is necessary from the physician in order to begin home health care? What are the nurse's responsibilities?
4. How is home health reimbursed? What criteria or guidelines for reimbursement are required by Medicare or Medicaid?
5. Why is documentation especially critical in home health?
6. Explain the concept of infection control in the home setting. What is the nurse's major role? How can the nurse minimize risk of infection?
7. How can infection prevention present a challenge to the home health nurse?

CASE STUDY

The home health nurse is caring for Maria Campos, a 72-year-old who has recently been diagnosed with type 2 diabetes. Mrs. Campos has a history of hypertension and hyperlipidemia and has not adhered to her prescribed medication regimen in the past. She speaks very little English. Answer the following questions based on the clinical scenario presented.

1. What interventions will the home health nurse likely perform when caring for Mrs. Campos?
2. What unique cultural considerations will the nurse take when caring for Mrs. Campos?
3. What age-related considerations will the nurse plan?

REVIEW QUESTIONS

1. What type of company provides health care equipment for home health clients?
   1. Hospice
   2. Private home health agency
   3. Durable medical equipment (DME)
   4. Durable equipment
2. The home health nurse is functioning as an educator during a home health visit. Which action or intervention best exemplifies this role?
   1. Changing an indwelling Foley catheter
   2. Discussing living wills and durable power of attorney and obtaining a social work consultation
   3. Instructing a client on a diabetic diet
   4. Documentation of care provided by the agency
3. The home health nurse is functioning as an advocate during an initial assessment. Which action or intervention best exemplifies this role?
   1. Changing an indwelling Foley catheter
   2. Discussing living wills and durable power of attorney and obtaining a social work consult
   3. Instructing a client on a diabetic diet
   4. Documentation of care provided by the agency
4. The home health nurse is functioning as a caregiver during a home health visit. Which action or intervention best exemplifies this role?
   1. Changing an indwelling Foley catheter
   2. Discussing living wills and durable power of attorney and obtaining a social work consult
   3. Instructing a client on a diabetic diet
   4. Documentation of care provided by the agency
5. What is considered to be the core concept of home health care?
   1. Advocating
   2. Caregiving
   3. Case managing
   4. Educating

6. Identify the clinical manifestations of caregiver role strain. (Select all that apply.)
   1. Decreased energy
   2. Anxiety
   3. Difficulty concentrating
   4. Difficulty performing routine tasks
7. An example of a home health service provided by nurses is:
   1. Housekeeping duties for the client.
   2. Providing a hospital bed for the client.
   3. Performing daily wound care for the client.
   4. Writing the living will for the client.
8. Hospice nursing provides:
   1. Intravenous therapy for nutrition such as total parental nutrition (TPN).
   2. Tracheotomy care for a client with COPD.
   3. Care to the terminally ill client.
   4. Education about acute conditions such as diabetes.
9. When is the most appropriate time for the client and family members to be involved in obtaining home health services?
   1. On the initial home health assessment visit by the registered nurse.
   2. On admission to the hospital.
   3. Prior to discharge from the hospital.
   4. When the client is terminally ill.

CHAPTER 9

ELECTRONIC HEALTH RECORDS AND INFORMATION TECHNOLOGY

KEY TERM REVIEW

Match each term with its appropriate definition.

1. _______ Clinical decision support systems
2. _______ Computer-based patient records
3. _______ Data warehousing
4. _______ Distance learning
5. _______ Electronic health records (EHRs)
6. _______ Health informatics
7. _______ Hospital information system (HIS)
8. _______ Management information system (MIS)
9. _______ Nurse informaticist
10. _______ Nursing informatics
11. _______ Telemedicine

a. The science of using computer information systems in the practice of nursing
b. Expert who combines computer, information, and nursing science to develop policies and procedures that promote effective and secure use of computerized records by nurses and other health care professionals
c. Uses technology to transmit electronic data about clients to persons at distant locations
d. Electronic forms that incorporate evidence from literature into particular client situations that guide care planning
e. Organizes data from various areas in the hospital such as admissions, medical records, clinical laboratory, pharmacy, order entry, and finance
f. Permit electronic client data entry and retrieval by caregivers, administrators, accreditors, and other persons who require the data
g. The management of health care information, using computers
h. Facilitates the structure and application of data to manage an organization or department
i. Educational opportunities delivered under situations in which the teacher and learner are not in the same place at the same time
j. Accumulation of large amounts of data that are stored over time
k. Permit electronic client data entry and retrieval by caregivers, administrators, accreditors, and other persons who require the data

KEY TOPIC REVIEW

1. List three areas on which the Technology Informatics Guiding Education Reform (TIGER) Initiative focuses.

   a.

   b.

   c.

2. Client concerns regarding _________ and _________ of health records have arisen as electronic databases and communications have proliferated.

3. What are the two most common types of information systems used by nurses?

   a.

   b.

4. What areas of a hospital may use HIS to organize data?

   a.

   b.

   c.

   d.

   e.

   f.

5. List six examples of the use of bedside data entry.

   a.

   b.

   c.

   d.

   e.

   f.

6. The term _________ refers to a computer being connected to other computers in a _________.

7. Indicate one type of computer software used in nursing and list one application used with that software.

8. The _________ established legal requirements for the protection, security, and appropriate sharing of patient personal health information (referred to as protected health information or PHI).

9. Name four ways in which computers have enhanced nursing education.

   a.

   b.

   c.

   d.

10. List the four functions of nursing informatics.

    a.

    b.

    c.

    d.

FOCUSED STUDY TIPS

1. Discuss the criteria for evaluating Internet health information. How has the widespread availability of information impacted health care today?

2. What is the difference between distance education courses and web-enhanced or hybrid courses?

3. What are the advantages of taking the National Council Licensure Examination (NCLEX®) on a computer? When did the test change from pen-and-paper administration to computer administration?

4. Telemedicine (or telehealth) uses technology to transmit electronic data about clients to persons at distant locations. What are some of the advantages of telemedicine? What are the disadvantages?

5. One of the main concerns with health care and information technology is privacy issues. As a nurse, how can you impact changes on the state and federal level regarding privacy? Refer to the ANA position statement on privacy. What is the nurse's role in the privacy issue?

6. How has the implementation of HIPAA presented a challenge to nurses?

CASE STUDY

A 45-year-old client is scheduled to have a hysterectomy later this week. She is at the hospital to get her preoperative nursing assessment, several laboratory exams, and chest x-ray. The nurse and laboratory technologist are using a computerized data entry system that is managed on a handheld device.

1. If the client's results are entered into computer-based patient records (CPRs), who would be able to legally access her medical information?

2. The chest x-ray is abnormal and the primary care provider wishes to consult a respiratory specialist. If he sends the x-ray film electronically to the consulting primary care provider, that is an example of what type of medicine?

3. What are the advantages of this type of consultation?

4. Does the client have to sign any consent forms with regard to her electronic medical records?

REVIEW QUESTIONS

1. What is an advantage of having "paper" medical records for clients?

    1. Paper medical records have had legal standards in place that have been tested effective.

    2. Paper medical records are often standardized and thorough.

    3. Paper medical records take up less space when being stored.

    4. Paper medical records ensure client health information is protected.

2. The World Wide Web (WWW) refers to:
   1. Documents accessed electronically.
   2. Complex links among web pages or websites.
   3. Universal resource locators.
   4. A network designed to facilitate the organization and application of data.
3. Universal resource locators (URLs) are also called:
   1. Television stations.
   2. Addresses.
   3. Links among web pages or websites.
   4. Rural addresses.
4. Which of the following computerized systems would assist a physician in Russia to consult with a physician in the United States?
   1. Distance learning
   2. Computer-based client records
   3. Telemedicine
   4. Local-area network
5. What does the designation ".org" in a URL denote?
   1. Commercial sites
   2. Organizations
   3. Educational institutions
   4. Government sites
6. A group of nursing students located at different sites for a nursing class are participating in classes through two-way audio and video transmissions. In addition, the students use chat and instant messaging. This is an example of which type of distance learning model?
   1. Asynchronous distance learning
   2. Synchronous distance learning
   3. Simultaneous distance learning
   4. Self-study distance learning
7. What is one way in which a nurse administrator might use a computer?
   1. Following client's health status during the hospital stay
   2. Managing a budget
   3. Obtaining the latest information on cardiac diseases
   4. Participating in a research study
8. How is computer-assisted instruction (CAI) used in nursing?
   1. It makes it easier to adjust to the use of software programs.
   2. It allows nurses to share health care information with clients.
   3. It is used to test nursing students for the NCLEX.
   4. It is used as a bookkeeping system.

9. What role does the Health Insurance Portability and Accountability Act (HIPAA) play in client confidentiality?
   1. It provides a database for insurance agencies to utilize.
   2. It provides for data standardization.
   3. It provides for data classifications.
   4. It provides for privacy and confidentiality for clients in health care.
10. Electronic medical records (EMRs) or computer-based records (CPRs) permit electronic client data retrieval by caregivers, administrators, creditors, and other persons who require the data. What agency or act sets legal requirements for the protection, security, and appropriate sharing of client personal health information?
    1. Hospitals
    2. Patient bill of rights
    3. State governments
    4. HIPAA

CHAPTER 10

CRITICAL THINKING AND CLINICAL REASONING

KEY TERM REVIEW

Match each term with its appropriate definition.

1. _______ Clinical judgment
2. _______ Clinical reasoning
3. _______ Cognitive processes
4. _______ Concept map
5. _______ Creativity
6. _______ Critical analysis
7. _______ Critical thinking
8. _______ Deductive reasoning
9. _______ Inductive reasoning
10. _______ Intuition
11. _______ Metacognitive processes
12. _______ Nursing process
13. _______ Problem solving
14. _______ Socratic questioning
15. _______ Trial and error

a. A process for clarifying the nature of a problem, suggesting possible solutions, and evaluating the solutions for the best possible choice to implement

b. Generalizations are formed from a set of facts or observations

c. Process of working from general premises to reach a specific conclusion

d. Understanding of things without conscious use of reasoning

e. A technique one can use to look below the surface to differentiate what one knows from what one merely believes

f. A number of approaches are tried until a solution is found

g. An intentional higher level reasoning that is delineated by several factors as a guide for rational judgment and action

h. Thinking that results in the development of new ideas and products

i. Application of a set of questions to a particular situation to determine essential information and discard unneeded information

j. A decision-making process to ascertain the right nursing action to be implemented at the appropriate time in the client's care

k. Graphic representation of linear and nonlinear relationships for representing critical thinking

l. A systematic client-centered method for structuring nursing care

m. The analysis of a clinical situation as it unfolds or develops

n. The thinking processes based on the knowledge of aspects of client care

o. Include reflective thinking and awareness of the skills learned by the nurse in caring for the client.

KEY TOPIC REVIEW

1. Critical thinking consists of high-level cognitive processes that include ____________ ____________ and ____________ ____________.
2. Define the following problem-solving methods:
   a. Trial and error
   b. Intuition
   c. Nursing process
   d. Scientific method
   e. Modified scientific method
3. ____________ ____________ is a purposeful mental activity that guides beliefs and actions.
4. Define inductive and deductive reasoning in critical thinking.
5. ____________ ____________ is a technique one can use to look beneath the surface, recognize and examine assumptions, search for inconsistencies, examine multiple points of view, and differentiate what one knows from what one merely believes.
6. List five characteristics that most critical thinkers have.
   a.
   b.
   c.
   d.
   e.
7. ____________, at every step of critical thinking and nursing care, helps examine the ways in which the nurse gathers and analyzes data, makes decisions, and determines the effectiveness of interventions.
8. Identify the sequential steps to the decision-making process.
   a.
   b.
   c.
   d.
   e.
   f.
   g.
   h.
9. What is the definition of decision making? Give one example of decision-making.
10. Critical thinkers are willing to admit what they do not know; they are willing to seek new information and to rethink their conclusions in light of new knowledge.
    a. True b. False

11. Identify and define the four types of concept maps.

    a.

    b.

    c.

    d.

FOCUSED STUDY TIPS

1. What are the four stages of critical thinking?
2. Describe Maslow's hierarchy of basic human needs. Why is this concept important to nursing?
3. List the characteristics of critical thinking. What are the skills needed by one who uses critical thinking?
4. List and describe the three methods used with critical thinking when problem solving during the nursing process.
5. Why must the nursing process occur in the chronological order of assessment, diagnosing, planning, implementing, and evaluating?

CASE STUDY

The student nurse should begin using critical thinking in daily life by using it in the clinical environment and during everyday situations. To clarify the critical thinking process for the nursing student, a nonnursing case study will be used for this case study.

A close friend states that she is habitually overdrawing her bank checking account. She has asked you for advice with this problem. Using the Socratic questions listed in Box 10–3 of the text, analyze this problem.

a. Questions about the decision or problem:

b. Questions about assumptions:

c. Questions about point of view:

d. Questions about evidence and reasons:

e. Questions about implications and consequences:

REVIEW QUESTIONS

1. What is the least effective decision-making process?
    1. Analyzing the data
    2. Formulating conclusions
    3. Establishing assumptions
    4. Synthesizing information
2. What does the trial-and-error method of problem solving lack?
    1. Effectiveness
    2. Organization
    3. Thoughtfulness
    4. Exactness

3. The research process of problem solving is:
   1. Most effective when used by experienced nurses. .
   2. Least effective when used by experienced nurses.
   3. Illogical at times.
   4. Lacking in formality.
4. Why is the nursing process method used in nursing? (Select all that apply.)
   1. It allows the nurse to work independently without collaboration.
   2. It involves the interaction between the client and nurse as they work together.
   3. It is used to identify potential or actual health care needs, set goals, devise a plan to meet the client's needs, and evaluate the plan's effectiveness.
   4. It is designed to work well in all environments.
5. What does critical thinking allow nurses to do during emergency situations?
   1. Establish teamwork with other disciplines.
   2. Maintain a calm demeanor.
   3. Meet the physician's needs.
   4. Recognize important cues.
6. If a child cannot grasp the mechanics behind using an incentive spirometer, the nurse could give the client balloons and/or a jar of bubbles to blow. What does this best demonstrate? (Select all that apply.)
   1. Modified scientific method
   2. Scientific method
   3. Creativity
   4. Critical thinking
7. While working in the critical care unit, a nurse is caring for a client after cardiac bypass surgery. The nurse feels that "something is wrong" even though the client has no outward signs or symptoms. What is this an example of?
   1. Intuition
   2. Trial and error
   3. Research process
   4. Scientific method
8. In the emergency department, the nurse observes that a client is actively bleeding from an abdominal gunshot wound. The nurse assumes that the client is at an increased risk for hypovolemic shock after observing frank red blood spurting from the wound. What is this an example of?
   1. Creativity
   2. Deductive reasoning
   3. Inductive reasoning
   4. Critical analysis

9. While attending a nursing educator's conference, a nursing instructor obtains information about the use of concept maps and clinical pathways. The nursing instructor returns to work at the university and discusses the new techniques with the other instructors. What is this an example of?
    1. Creating an environment that supports critical thinking
    2. Seeking information regarding new educational promotions
    3. Intellectual humility
    4. Judgment
10. What is the definition of the nursing process?
    1. A skill essential to safe, competent, skillful nursing practice
    2. A type of thinking that results in the development of new ideas and products
    3. A critical thinking process for choosing the best actions to meet a desired goal
    4. A systematic, rational method of planning and providing individualized nursing care
11. How are nursing cognitive skills learned?
    1. Through reading and applying health-related literature
    2. Through the use of critical thought
    3. Through the application of content the nurse has previously learned
    4. Through the application of clinical scenarios the nurse has experienced

CHAPTER 11

ASSESSING

KEY TERM REVIEW

Match each term with its appropriate definition.

1. _______ Assessing
2. _______ Cephalocaudal
3. _______ Clinical signs
4. _______ Clinical symptoms
5. _______ Closed questions
6. _______ Cues
7. _______ Data
8. _______ Database
9. _______ Directive interview
10. _______ Inferences
11. _______ Interview
12. _______ Leading question
13. _______ Neutral question
14. _______ Nondirective interview
15. _______ Objective data
16. _______ Rapport
17. _______ Review of systems
18. _______ Screening examination
19. _______ Subjective data
20. _______ Validation

a. Usually closed, and directs the client's answer
b. Highly structured, elicits specific information
c. Planned communication
d. An understanding between two or more people
e. Systematic and continuous collection, organization, validation, and documentation of data
f. Generally require only a yes or no answer
g. Double checking data, ensuring that objective and related subjective data agree
h. Information relayed by the client that cannot be seen or measured by the nurse but must be accepted as the client's perception
i. A client can answer without direction or pressure; is open ended
j. Subjective data
k. Objective data
l. Head to toe
m. Subjective or objective data that can be observed by the nurse
n. A physical examination briefly conducted of all systems that does not include an in-depth exam of any one system
o. All information about a client
p. Also known as information
q. A brief review of essential functioning of various body parts
r. Rapport-building interview
s. Nurse's interpretation or conclusions based on cues
t. Detectable by an observer, can be measured or tested

KEY TOPIC REVIEW

1. What are the three purposes of the nursing process?

   a.

   b.

   c.

2. The nursing process is both interpersonal and collaborative between the nurse and the client.

   a. True b. False

3. Assessing is a continuous process carried out through all the phases of nursing.

   a. True b. False

4. What are the four different types of assessment?

   a.

   b.

   c.

   d.

5. According to The Joint Commission, each client must have an initial assessment within __________ hours of admission.

6. What are the four activities involved in the assessment process?

   a.

   b.

   c.

   d.

7. Determine if the following information is subjective (S) or objective (O) assessment data.

   a. __________ "I feel tired all the time."

   b. __________ Skin warm and dry to touch

   c. __________ "I am itching all over."

   d. __________ Smell of ammonia in urine

   e. __________ Purplish discoloration on left forearm

   f. __________ Temperature of 102 degrees orally

8. Distinguish between the primary (P) and secondary (indirect) (S) sources of data in the assessment process.

   a. __________ "My son has vomited for three days."

   b. __________ "I have been coughing for two weeks."

   c. __________ "My wife is forty-five years old."

   d. __________ "I have a rash."

9. When does the observation portion of data collection occur?
   a. On the initial assessment
   b. Prior to the initial assessment
   c. It is an ongoing process.
   d. Observation is not part of data collection.
10. An ___________ is a planned communication or conversation with a purpose.

FOCUSED STUDY TIPS

1. Explain the difference between the medical model of problem solving and the nursing process. What are the parallels between the two models?
2. Why would it be important to review data from client records such as occupation, religion, marital status, and so on before beginning the nurse health history?
3. Why is sharing of information important in health care? What is pertinent information that needs to be relayed between nursing shifts?
4. Compare and contrast the body systems and cephalocaudal approaches to assessment. What are the advantages and disadvantages to both approaches?
5. Compare and contrast Orem's self-care model and Roy's adaptation model.

CASE STUDY

A client is being transferred to the unit from the recovery room after having an abdominal tumor removed. The recovery room nurse gives a verbal report on the client's condition, stating that the dressing is dry and intact, vital signs stable, IV of normal saline infusing at 100 mL per hour in the left forearm, intact and patent, medications given, and that the client has no complaints of pain. During the initial assessment, the medical–surgical nurse notes that the abdominal dressing has bright red drainage. The client stated, "I am really hurting bad!" The vital signs are 140/86 mmHg, RR 24/min, T 36.8°C (98.2°F) orally, and pulse of 90 beats/min.

1. What is the objective data?
2. What is the subjective data?
3. Who is considered the primary source?
4. Who is considered the secondary source?

REVIEW QUESTIONS

1. The nurse is assessing the sputum characteristics of a client with pneumonia. What are the senses that the nurse may use in the assessment of the sputum? (Select all that apply.)
   1. Vision
   2. Smell
   3. Hearing
   4. Touch

2. What phases of the nursing process are identified by the most current *Scope and Standards of Nursing Practice* that are not recognized by the national licensure examination for registered nurses (NCLEX-RN)?
   1. Outcomes identifications and diagnosis
   2. Analysis and diagnosis
   3. Outcomes identifications and analysis
   4. Assessment and evaluation
3. During the process of data collection, the nurse must be aware of the different cultural aspects in health care. In the interview phase, what will the nurse consider may have a cultural implication? (Select all that apply.)
   1. Time of the interview
   2. Setting of the interview
   3. Physical distance between the nurse and client
   4. Seating arrangement
4. What is an example of an open-ended question that the nurse may use in the interview process?
   1. "Did you take your medication today?"
   2. "Have you ever had to undergo surgery?"
   3. "Are you a student at the local college?"
   4. "How have you been feeling lately?"
5. What is the name of the head-to-toe approach that usually begins the nurse physical examination?
   1. Review of systems
   2. Screening examination
   3. Cephalocaudal
   4. Caudal approach
6. What framework is based on 11 functional health patterns and collects data about dysfunctional and functional behavior?
   1. Orem's self-care model
   2. Gordon's functional health patterns
   3. Roy's adaptation model
   4. The wellness model
7. After completing the health history and the physical assessment, the nurse identifies discrepancies in the information. What is this process called?
   1. Assessing
   2. Diagnosing
   3. Validating
   4. Evaluating
8. A client presents to the emergency department with complaints of chest pain. The nurse takes the client's vital signs. The nurse is performing which phase of the nursing process?
   1. Assessing
   2. Diagnosing
   3. Planning
   4. Implementing

9. The nurse reassesses a client's temperature 45 minutes after administering acetaminophen. This is an example of what type of an assessment?
    1. Ongoing
    2. Intermittent
    3. Terminal
    4. Routine
10. The nurse is measuring the drainage from a Jackson–Pratt drain. What is considered objective data?
    1. The client is complaining of abdominal pain.
    2. The drainage measurement is 25 mL.
    3. The client stated, "I did not empty the drain."
    4. The client stated that he has a pain level of 5.

CHAPTER 12

DIAGNOSING

KEY TERM REVIEW

Match each term with its appropriate definition.

1. _______ Defining characteristics
2. _______ Dependent functions
3. _______ Diagnosis
4. _______ Diagnostic labels
5. _______ Etiology
6. _______ Health promotion diagnosis
7. _______ Independent functions
8. _______ Norm
9. _______ Nursing diagnosis
10. _______ PES format
11. _______ Qualifiers
12. _______ Risk factors
13. _______ Risk nursing diagnosis
14. _______ Standard
15. _______ Syndrome diagnosis
16. _______ Taxonomy

a. Relates to the client's preparedness for implementing behaviors to improve his or her health condition
b. Generally accepted measure, rule, model, or pattern
c. Basic three-part diagnostic statement
d. A cluster of signs and symptoms that indicate the presence of a particular diagnostic label
e. Describes a cluster of nursing diagnoses that have similar interventions
f. A classification system or set of categories arranged based on a single principle or set of principles
g. Added words to give additional meaning to a diagnostic statement
h. Causal relationship between a problem and its related or risk factors
i. Statement or conclusion regarding the nature of a phenomenon
j. Areas of health care that are unique to nursing
k. Variables that indicate that increased likelihood that a problem could arise
l. Clinical judgment that a problem does not exist; rather, a problem is likely to develop without nursing intervention
m. Generally accepted norm
n. Client's problem statement, plus etiology
o. Standardized NANDA names for diagnoses
p. The nurse's obligation to carry out physician-prescribed therapies and treatments

KEY TOPIC REVIEW

1. What is the first stage of the nursing process?
2. What is the second stage of the nursing process?
3. A __________ is a classification system or set of categories based on a single principle or set of principles.
4. What are the parts of the North American Nursing Diagnosis Association (NANDA) nursing diagnosis?

   a.

   b.

   c.

5. All nurses are responsible for making nursing diagnoses according to the ANA Standards of Practice.

   a. True b. False

6. The nursing diagnosis is a judgment made only after thorough, systematic data collection.

   a. True b. False

7. What are the five types of nursing diagnoses?

   a.

   b.

   c.

   d.

   e.

8. To enhance clinical usefulness, diagnostic labels must be as _________ as possible.
9. What five words are identified as qualifiers to give additional meaning to a diagnostic statement?

   a.

   b.

   c.

   d.

   e.

10. What is the definition of etiology? What is the purpose of the etiology statement?
11. Risk diagnoses do not have subjective or objective indications of the presence of the diagnosis found during the assessment phase.

    a. True b. False

12. For actual nursing diagnoses, the defining characteristics are the client's signs and symptoms in the assessment phase of the nursing process.

    a. True b. False

FOCUSED STUDY TIPS

1. A nursing diagnosis has three components. List the three components and give an example of each.
2. Why is it important to differentiate among the possible causes in the nursing diagnosis? (Refer to Table 12–2 in the text.)
3. What are the differentiating factors between a nursing diagnosis and a medical diagnosis?
4. Describe characteristics of the nursing diagnosis. What is a two-part diagnostic statement? What is a three-part diagnostic statement?
5. List two examples each of a one-part, two-part, and three-part diagnostic statement. Refer to the PES diagnosis in the text.
6. Compare and contrast dependent and independent nursing functions.

CASE STUDY

A newly admitted client will be your responsibility as the registered nurse. The client is a 47-year-old male of Native American heritage with type 2 diabetes. He states that he has not been taking his medication because it doesn't make him feel better; he also has difficulty remembering to take the medication. The following information pertains to this client:

- Fingerstick blood sugar = 213 mg/dL
- BP 150/90 mmHg; temp 37°C (98.6°F) oral; respirations 24/min; pulse 78 beats/min.
- "I use the bathroom about eight times per day."
- Ht 6 feet 4 inches; weight 284 pounds

1. What is an actual nursing diagnosis for this client?
2. What is a potential nursing diagnosis for this client?
3. Identify one subjective and one objective assessment to substantiate the nursing diagnosis.
4. What is the outcome goal for the client?
5. What are two independent functions the nurse might perform when caring for this client?

REVIEW QUESTIONS

1. What is the purpose of data collection and analysis?
   1. To carry out the plan of care.
   2. To collect and then analyze data.
   3. To identify actual or potential health concerns.
   4. To identify a client's response to care.

2. Which statement is a nursing diagnosis?
    1. Fever of unknown origin
    2. Pancreatitis
    3. Potential for sleep-pattern disturbances
    4. Congestive heart failure
3. What is the purpose of a nursing diagnosis?
    1. To define a taxonomy of nursing language.
    2. To promote a taxonomy of nursing language.
    3. To identify a client's problem and its etiology.
    4. To establish a set of principles.
4. Choose the appropriate activities that the nurse may perform during the diagnosing component of the nursing process. (Select all that apply.)
    1. Compare data against current nursing standards.
    2. Obtain a nursing health history.
    3. Cluster or group the data to generate a tentative hypothesis.
    4. Review the client records and nursing literature.
    5. Identify gaps and inconsistencies in the data.
5. What is a nursing function during the diagnosing phase of the nursing process?
    1. Clarify all inconsistencies in the data before making inferences.
    2. Identify Gordon's functional health patterns and compare with the client.
    3. Review the literature and review professional journals and textbooks.
    4. Document the health assessment in a specific form.
6. *Readiness for Enhanced Parenting* is an example of which type of diagnosis?
    1. Wellness diagnosis
    2. Health-seeking diagnosis
    3. Two-part diagnosis
    4. Three-part diagnosis
7. Which of the following nursing diagnostic statements is correct?
    1. *Fluid Replacement* related to fever
    2. *Impaired Skin Integrity* related to immobility
    3. *Impaired Skin Integrity* related to ulceration of sacral area
    4. *Pain* related to severe headache
8. How does the nurse begin a diagnostic label for a collaborative problem?
    1. *Readiness for Enhanced Spiritual Well-Being*
    2. *Alteration of Respiratory Status*
    3. *Potential Complication for Pneumonia: Atelectasis*
    4. *Impaired Respiratory System*

9. The PES format for writing a nursing diagnosis is used for which of the following?
    1. Actual nursing diagnoses
    2. Potential nursing diagnoses
    3. Risk for nursing diagnoses
    4. Wellness diagnoses
10. Choose the correct example of a qualifier for a nursing diagnosis.
    1. *Syndrome*
    2. *Potential*
    3. *Deficient*
    4. *Risk for*
11. Identify and select the advantages of using a taxonomy of nursing diagnoses. (Select all that apply.)
    1. A taxonomy of nursing diagnoses would promote a classification system or set of categories for a single or set of principles for professional nurses.
    2. A taxonomy of nursing diagnoses can be used by physicians to define diagnostic nursing terminology.
    3. A taxonomy of nursing diagnoses enhances the professional practice of the nurse in generating and completing a nursing care plan.
    4. A taxonomy of nursing diagnoses consists of nursing diagnoses for a single principle or set of principles that were developed by other nursing professionals.
12. Identify the components of a nursing diagnosis. (Select all that apply.)
    1. Related factors
    2. Risk factors
    3. Problem
    4. Definition
    5. Defining characteristics
    6. Medical conditions

CHAPTER 13

PLANNING

KEY TERM REVIEW

Match each term with its appropriate definition.

1. _______ Collaborative care plans
2. _______ Collaborative interventions
3. _______ Concept map
4. _______ Critical pathways
5. _______ Dependent interventions
6. _______ Discharge planning
7. _______ Formal nursing care plan
8. _______ Goals/desired outcomes
9. _______ Independent interventions
10. _______ Indicator
11. _______ Individualized care plan
12. _______ Informal nursing care plan
13. _______ Multidisciplinary care plan
14. _______ Nursing interventions
15. _______ Nursing Interventions Classification (NIC)
16. _______ Nursing Outcomes Classification (NOC)
17. _______ Policies
18. _______ Priority setting
19. _______ Procedures
20. _______ Protocols
21. _______ Rationale
22. _______ Standardized care plan
23. _______ Standing order

a. Activities that nurses are licensed to initiate on the basis of their knowledge and skills

b. Developed to govern the handling of frequently occurring situations

c. Actions that a nurse performs to enhance client outcomes

d. Process of establishing a preferential sequence for addressing nursing diagnoses and interventions

e. Actions the nurse carries out in conjunction with other health team members

f. Collaborative care plan that sequences care that must be given

g. Process of anticipating and planning for release from a facility

h. A taxonomy of nursing outcome statements

i. Specific patient state that is most sensitive to nursing interventions and measurable

j. Similar to protocols; specify what is to be done

k. Gives the nurse authority to carry out specific actions under certain circumstances

l. Strategy for action that exists in the nurse's mind

m. Tailored to meet unique needs of a specific client

n. Outlines care required for clients to include nursing interventions as well as medical treatments to be performed by other members of the health care team

o. A critical pathway that sequences care required for client with common conditions

p. Activities carried out under the orders or supervision of a licensed physician or other health care provider

q. Actions commonly required for a particular group of clients

r. Written or computerized guide that organizes information

s. Describe what the nurse hopes to achieve by implementing the nursing interventions

t. Formal plan that specifies the nursing care for groups of clients with common needs

u. Evidence-based principle given as the reason for selecting a particular nursing intervention

v. Visual tool in which ideas or data are enclosed in circles or boxes connected by lines or arrows to indicate relationships

w. A taxonomy of nursing interventions

KEY TOPIC REVIEW

1. __________ __________ are the actions that a nurse performs to achieve client goals.
2. When does planning begin?
3. Who is responsible for developing the initial comprehensive plan of care, and when is it initiated?
4. List the four purposes the nurse uses to guide daily planning by utilizing ongoing assessment data.
   a.
   b.
   c.
   d.
5. What four tasks do the nurse and client complete during the planning stage of the nursing process?
   a.
   b.
   c.
   d.
6. Match the four different types of nursing care plans with their correct definitions.

a. Informal nursing care plan	_________	Tailored to meet the unique needs of a specific client—needs that are not addressed by the standardized plan
b. Standardized care plan	_________	A strategy for action that exists in the nurse's mind
c. Individualized care plan	_________	A written or computerized guide that organizes information about the client's care
d. Formal nursing care plan	_________	A formal plan that specifies the nursing care for groups of clients with common needs

7. Refer to Figure 13–2 in the text. What documents may be included in a complete plan of care?
   a.
   b.
   c.
   d.
   e.
   f.
   g.

8. Refer to the standards of care for thrombophlebitis in Figure 13–3 of the text. How are standards of care different than individualized care plans? What are the advantages and disadvantages of standards of care?

9. Define concept map and rationale. Why are students asked to complete pathophysiology flow sheets, concept maps, or care plans with rationales?

10. What do the client goals or desired outcomes describe? What is the Nursing Outcomes Classification (NOC)?

FOCUSED STUDY TIPS

1. What is planning? What phase of the nursing process is planning? What is the end product of planning called? Who is involved in the planning process?

2. Discuss the three types of planning and list the significant tasks that registered nurses must do during each of the types/stages of planning.

3. Differentiate between protocols, policies, procedures, and standing orders.

4. What are the 10 guidelines for writing nursing care plans? Why is each guideline important?

5. What is meant by the activity of priority setting in the planning process? What factors need to be considered when assigning priorities?

6. What is the purpose of desired goals and/or outcomes?

7. What is the purpose of assigning priorities of care when planning client interventions?

8. Compare and contrast Nursing Interventions Classification (NIC) and Nursing Outcomes Classification (NOC).

CASE STUDIES

Outcomes should be SMART (specific, measurable, appropriate, realistic, and timely). Analyze the following nursing care plan:

A client has stage 4 pressure ulcers on the coccyx, left and right malleolus, and both heels. He is unable to turn himself in the bed. His daughter states, "This happened so suddenly; he did not have these sores until he had the stroke and quit eating." The nurse assesses the client and notes that he is an older adult, appears emaciated, and is immobile with the previously stated pressure ulcers.

a. What are the subjective and objective data?
b. What nursing diagnosis will fit this situation?
c. What are the realistic short-term and long-term goals for this client?
d. What are four nursing orders or interventions that can be used for this client?

REVIEW QUESTIONS

1. "Client will walk to end of hallway without assistance by Friday" is an example of a:
   1. Long-term goal.
   2. Short-term goal.
   3. Nursing intervention.
   4. Rationale.

2. "Client will ambulate 20 yards without assistance in 8 weeks" is an example of a:
   1. Long-term goal.
   2. Short-term goal.
   3. Nursing intervention.
   4. Rationale.
3. The nurse instructs the preoperative client to cough and deep breathe postoperatively to avoid respiratory complications. This is what type of nursing intervention?
   1. Independent intervention
   2. Dependent intervention
   3. Collaborative intervention
   4. Variable intervention
4. The nurse instructs the client on turning, coughing, and deep breathing q2h. What is the relationship of nursing interventions to problem status?
   1. Health promotion interventions
   2. Treatment interventions
   3. Prevention interventions
   4. Observation interventions
5. The home health registered nurse needs to assign a person to insert a Foley catheter on a client. To whom can she delegate this task?
   1. The unlicensed personnel with extensive training
   2. The licensed practical/vocational nurse
   3. The physician
   4. The client's daughter
6. Planning consists of which component?
   1. Reassessing the client
   2. Analyzing data
   3. Selecting nursing interventions
   4. Determining the nurse's need for assistance
7. Consider the following nursing diagnosis: *Imbalanced Nutrition: Less Than Body Requirements* related to inability to feed self. What is an example of a short-term goal for this client?
   1. The client will eat 75% of his meals by Friday (September 20) with the use of modified eating utensils to feed self with minimal assistance.
   2. The client will learn about nutritious meal planning as exhibited by choosing one correct menu.
   3. The client will acquire competence in managing cookware designed for clients with handicaps.
   4. The client will learn preparation techniques that are quick and easy to manage.

8. The nurse admits a client in active labor to the labor and delivery unit of the hospital. When does the planning for client care start?
   1. After the physician has delivered the baby
   2. After the admission process
   3. When the client is discharged to the postpartum unit
   4. During the initial meeting
9. Which component is part of the permanent client record?
   1. Nursing protocols
   2. Client care plan
   3. Procedures for client care
   4. The nurse's notebook of daily notes to herself
10. When caring for a client with stage 4 pressure ulcers on the coccyx, the nurse turns the client every 2 hours while in bed. What part of the nursing process is being carried out?
    1. Assessment
    2. Diagnosis
    3. Implementation
    4. Evaluation
11. What are the benefits of a nursing intervention classification system? (Select all that apply.)
    1. It helps demonstrate the impact that nurses have on the health care delivery system.
    2. It assists educators to develop curricula that better articulates with clinical practice.
    3. It standardizes and defines the knowledge base for nursing curricula and practice.
    4. It facilitates the appropriate selection of a nursing intervention and communication of nursing treatments to other nurses and other providers.
12. A taxonomy of nursing outcome statements is developed to describe measurable states, behaviors, or perceptions to respond to which part of the nursing process?
    1. Nursing assessments
    2. Nursing interventions
    3. Nursing goals
    4. Nursing outcomes

CHAPTER 14

IMPLEMENTING AND EVALUATING

KEY TERM REVIEW

Match each term with its appropriate definition.

1. _______ Audit
2. _______ Cognitive skills
3. _______ Concurrent audit
4. _______ Evaluating
5. _______ Evaluation statement
6. _______ Implementing
7. _______ Interpersonal skills
8. _______ Outcome evaluation
9. _______ Process evaluation
10. _______ Quality assurance (QA) program
11. _______ Quality improvement (QI)
12. _______ Retrospective audit
13. _______ Root cause analysis
14. _______ Sentinel event
15. _______ Structure evaluation
16. _______ Technical skills

a. Process for identifying the factors that bring about deviations in practices that lead to a sentinel event

b. Evaluation of a client's record after discharge from an agency

c. Focuses on the setting in which the care was given

d. Focuses on demonstrable changes in the client's health status as a result of nursing care

e. Unexpected event that involves death or serious physical or psychological injury, or risk thereof

f. Purposeful hands-on skills

g. Include problem solving, decision making, thinking and creativity

h. All of the activities, verbal and nonverbal, individuals use when interacting directly with one another

i. A process used to sure the best possible care is delivered with the resulting optimal outcomes

j. Review of a client's health care while the client is still receiving care

k. Focuses on how care was given

l. Planned ongoing activity in which the client and health care professionals determine the client's progress toward achievement of goals and effectiveness of nursing care plan

m. Consists of two parts: a conclusion and supporting data

n. Review of records

o. Consists of doing and documenting the activities that are specific nursing actions needed to carry out the interventions

p. Ongoing, systematic process designed to evaluate and promote excellence in the health care provided to clients

KEY TOPIC REVIEW

1. The nursing process is _________ oriented, _________ _________, and _________ directed.
2. According to NIC terminology, _________ consists of doing and documenting the activities that are specific nursing actions needed to carry out the interventions.
3. _________, _________, and _________ skills are used to implement nursing strategies.
4. When does the implementing phase terminate?
5. The first three nursing phases of _________, _________, and _________ provide the basis for the nursing actions performed during the implementing step.
6. Match the type of skill with the following activities.

   a. Cognitive skills
   b. Interpersonal skills
   c. Technical skills

   ______ "May I help you to the restroom?"
   ______ Creativity
   ______ Problem solving
   ______ Nurse working effectively with members of the health care team
   ______ Taking a blood pressure
   ______ Caring for a dying patient
   ______ Need self-awareness and sensitivity to others to perform this skill
   ______ Bandaging a client's leg

7. What is included in the five processes of implementing?

   a.
   b.
   c.
   d.
   e.

8. Nursing activities are communicated verbally as well as in writing.

   a. True b. False

FOCUSED STUDY TIPS

1. What are the guidelines for implementing nursing interventions?
2. What are the five components of the evaluation process?
3. What are the two components of an evaluation statement?
4. Explain the difference between quality improvement and quality assurance.
5. Why should the nurse never document in advance?

6. "How are quality improvement and quality assurance similiar? When would these concepts be used in clinical practice?"

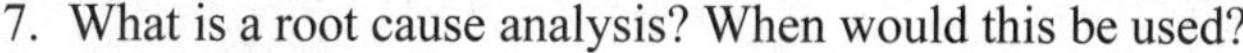

7. What is a root cause analysis? When would this be used?

CASE STUDY

Mr. Raymond Sanchez is a 57-year-old man who has been diagnosed with pancreatic cancer. He has been hospitalized due to weight loss and acute pain. No further chemotherapy or treatment is planned. Answer the following questions about Mr. Sanchez.

1. List different potential nursing diagnoses for Mr. Sanchez, give an example of subjective and objective data, and list one nursing intervention for each diagnosis.

2. List other comfort measures that the nurse may implement for Mr. Sanchez.

REVIEW QUESTIONS

1. Evaluation of the client's health care while the client is still receiving care from the agency is called a:
   1. Retrospective audit
   2. Audit
   3. Concurrent audit
   4. Peer review
2. Basic nursing interventions are based on:
   1. Scientific knowledge, nursing research, and evidence-based practice
   2. Creative thinking and intuition
   3. Physician's orders
   4. Client's wishes and nursing research
3. What is the fifth and last phase of the nursing process?
   1. Evaluating
   2. Assessment
   3. Planning
   4. Implementing
4. The nurse documents that the goal or desired outcome was met, partially met, or not met. What part of the evaluation statement is the nurse documenting?
   1. Supporting data
   2. Collecting data
   3. Finale
   4. Conclusion

5. While implementing the plan of care for the client, the nurse should: (Select all that apply)
   1. Supervise unlicensed support personnel who provide care to the client.
   2. Complete every task for the client.
   3. Supervise and direct the physician providing care.
   4. Evaluate the client's reactions to the planned interventions.
6. Which skills best describe nursing interpersonal skills?
   1. Problem solving, decision making, critical thinking, and creativity
   2. All of the activities, verbal and nonverbal, used when interacting directly with others
   3. Manipulating equipment, giving injections, and bandaging
   4. Leadership management and delegation
7. Which situation will the nurse need assistance with implementing the nursing interventions?
   1. Applying Buck's traction for the fifth time
   2. Documenting care delivered over the past hour
   3. Turning the client in bed without the client experiencing discomfort
   4. Transferring a bilateral amputee form bed to chair
8. What are two nursing phases that overlap each other in the nursing process?
   1. Assessing; diagnosing
   2. Planning; implementing
   3. Implementing; evaluation
   4. Evaluating; assessing
9. The nurse writes an evaluation statement after determining whether a nursing goal or client outcome has been met. What are the two parts in an evaluation statement?
   1. Conclusion and implementation
   2. Conclusion and supporting data
   3. Implementation and summary
   4. Implementation and data analysis
10. A quality-assurance (QA) program evaluates and promotes excellence in the health care provided to clients. Select the three components of care that are reviewed during this process:
    1. Structure evaluation
    2. Process evaluation
    3. Outcome evaluation
    4. Internal processes and external agency evaluations

CHAPTER 15

DOCUMENTING AND REPORTING

KEY TERM REVIEW

Match each term with its appropriate definition.

1. _______ Change-of-shift report
2. _______ Chart
3. _______ Charting
4. _______ Charting by exception (CBE)
5. _______ Client record
6. _______ Discussion
7. _______ Documenting
8. _______ Flow sheet
9. _______ Focus charting
10. _______ Handoff communication
11. _______ Kardex
12. _______ Narrative charting
13. _______ PIE
14. _______ Problem-oriented medical record (POMR)
15. _______ Problem-oriented record (POR)
16. _______ Progress note
17. _______ Record
18. _______ Recording
19. _______ Report
20. _______ SOAP
21. _______ Source-oriented record
22. _______ Variance

a. Chart entry made by all health professionals involved in a client's care

b. Also known as a chart

c. Concise method of organizing and recording data about a client making information quickly accessible to all health professionals

d. Client health record

e. Consists of notes that include routine care, normal findings, and client problems

f. Chart or record that can be written or computer based

g. Process in which information about patient care is communicated in a consistent manner including an opportunity to ask and respond to questions

h. A goal not met in a critical pathway

i. Problem-oriented record

j. Data are arranged according to the problems a patient has rather than the source of the information

k. Process of charting or documenting

l. Uses specific assessment criteria in a particular format

m. Acronym for subjective, objective, assessment, and plan

n. Makes client concerns and strengths the focus of care, usually using three columns

o. Informal oral consideration of a subject by two or more health care personnel to identify a problem or establish strategies to resolve a problem

p. Each person or department makes notations in a separate section of the client's chart

q. Process of charting or recording

r. Communication tool used to provide continuity of care for clients by providing critical information to oncoming nurses

s. Process of making an entry in a client record

t. Documentation system in which only abnormal or significant findings are recorded

u. Acronym for problems, interventions, and evaluation of nursing care

v. Oral, written, or computer-based communication intended to convey information to others

KEY TOPIC REVIEW

1. The client's record is protected legally as a private record of the client's care. Access to the client's record is limited to:

   a. Family members.

   b. The physician.

   c. The physician and client.

   d. Health care professionals delivering care and the client.

2. The nurse has a _________ to maintain confidentiality of all patient information.

3. Identify four purposes of client records:

   a.

   b.

   c.

   d.

4. What are the five requirements established by The Joint Commission regarding client record documentation?

   a.

   b.

   c.

   d.

   e.

5. What measures should be taken when faxing confidential health information? Is consent needed? What should be done before hitting the "Send" button?

6. Students or graduates are not bound by a strict ethical code and legal responsibility to hold all information in confidence.

   a. True b. False

7. Describe source-oriented records. What is a traditional part of a source-oriented record?

8. List two advantages and three disadvantages of source-oriented charting.

9. What is a problem-oriented medical record (POMR) or problem-oriented record (POR)? What are the four components of POMR?

10. List two advantages and two disadvantages of POMR charting.
11. What is the SOAP format that is used in charting and progress notes? What is meant by the acronyms SOAPIE and SOAPIER?
12. Explain how charting by exception (CBE) works, and explain why some nurses are uncomfortable with this method. What are the three elements of CBE?
13. List four advantages and one disadvantage of case management.

FOCUSED STUDY TIPS

1. Explain the Security Rule of the Health Insurance Portability and Accountability Act (HIPAA) of 1996.
2. Name four suggestions for ensuring confidentiality and security of computerized records.
3. What is the PIE system of charting?
4. How does focus charting work? What are its advantages?
5. Refer to Box 15–2 in the text. Review the pros and cons of computer documentation. Do you agree with this information?
6. What are the requirements for documentation in a long-term care facility?
7. What is a variance? Explain how the nurse will document a variance in the client's record.

CASE STUDIES

1. While charting, you notice that you have made an error. You did not write the correct oral temperature down. It should have been 98 degrees orally instead of 101 degrees orally.

   a. What is the correct method to fix this error?

   b. Identify an incorrect method for fixing errors in client records. Why is this method incorrect?

2. The nurse has been caring for Michael Branson, a 47-year-old male who. was admitted for the treatment of alcohol withdrawal and is experiencing delirium tremens. It has been 2 days since Mr. Branson's last intake of alcohol. The client has an infusing IV, is in a room kept dark and quiet to reduce stimuli, and has been monitored closely. The client has been having auditory and visual hallucinations throughout the day, which are reduced following sedative administration. When hallucinations are minimized, the client is alert and oriented to person, place, time, and date. During periods of hallucinations, the client becomes agitated and his blood pressure, pulse, and respiratory rate increase. When preparing the change-of-shift report for this client, what kind of specific data would you want to report to the oncoming nurse assigned to Mr. Branson's care?

REVIEW QUESTIONS

1. What is used to organize client data, allowing quick access for health care professionals to review information regarding the client?

   1. End-of-shift report
   2. SOAPIER notes
   3. Variance reports
   4. Kardex

2. In long-term care facilities, what two types of care are provided? (Select all that apply.)
   1. Easy
   2. Skilled
   3. Intermediate
   4. Unskilled
3. Which client will require more frequent documentation by the nurse?
   1. A stable client who is 2 days postvaginal delivery of a term infant
   2. A client presenting to the emergency department with signs/symptoms of a viral respiratory problem
   3. An older adult client who is postoperative day 4 of a hip replacement
   4. A client admitted to the ICU after a major myocardial infarction
4. If the nurse makes an error while charting, what is the recommended method to correct the mistake?
   1. Use "correction fluid" and obliterate the error.
   2. Draw one line through the error and write "mistaken entry" above it, then sign your name or initials beside it.
   3. Draw one line through the error and write "error" above it, then sign your initials beside it.
   4. Do nothing and hope no one notices the error.
5. The client has refused to have a Foley catheter inserted after surgery. What would need to be charted in the client's chart?
   1. The client refused the Foley catheter. The client was educated about the need for the Foley and the consequences of refusing the treatment; client verbalized understanding of the education.
   2. The client stubbornly refused the Foley catheter insertion.
   3. The client was medicated and the Foley was inserted without difficulty.
   4. The client refused the Foley catheter.
6. Identify the purposes of charting. (Select all that apply.)
   1. To fill up the nurse's spare time.
   2. To communicate care and responses to care.
   3. To create a legal document.
   4. To demonstrate what the nurse did every moment of the shift.
   5. To provide a basis for evaluation.
7. The student nurse is learning to chart effectively in the clinical setting. Which action by the student nurse increases the student's knowledge about effective charting?
   1. Chart and hope it is correct.
   2. Practice charting and hope it will improve with time.
   3. Do nothing now and learn charting after graduation.
   4. Read charts to learn from actual situations.
8. Which example of documentation is most correct when charting a client's behavior?
   1. The client was shouting, "I am so mad that I am going to hit you if you come any closer."
   2. The client seems angry and moderately aggressive.
   3. The client is angry and shouting.
   4. The client stated that he was mad and wanted to hit someone.

9. During the change-of-shift report, the nurse reports that the client is having "respiratory difficulty." What should the nurse add to this report?

   1. "But she seems okay."
   2. "Her respiratory rate is up to 28 breaths/min; oral temperature is 100 degrees; heart rate is 96 beats/minute; O2 saturation of 90%."
   3. " I put her on 3 liters of oxygen."
   4. "I called the doctor but he didn't do anything."

10. When the nurse places a check mark or a dash in an allocated space and uses an asterisk to reflect other pertinent information that has been recorded elsewhere on the chart, this is an example of what type of documentation?

    1. Multidisciplinary charting
    2. Charting by exception
    3. Focus charting
    4. Flow sheet charting

11. What measures can the nurse take to maintain confidentiality of client records? (Select all that apply.)

    1. Personal passwords are not shared with anyone else.
    2. Never leave the computer unattended after logging into the system.
    3. Do not leave paperwork with the client's information in an unsecured location.
    4. Discard all unneeded computer-generated worksheets in the trash can.

12. Identify examples that health care professionals may use in order to communicate specific information regarding the client or the client's care. (Select all that apply.)

    1. Change-of-shift report
    2. Discussing the client's care in the cafeteria
    3. Contacting the physician via telephone regarding new orders for medication to decrease an increased temperature
    4. Care plan conferences

CHAPTER 16

HEALTH PROMOTION

KEY TERM REVIEW

Match each term with its appropriate definition.

1. _______ Action stage
2. _______ Boundary
3. _______ Closed system
4. _______ Contemplation stage
5. _______ Disease prevention
6. _______ Feedback
7. _______ Health promotion
8. _______ Health protection
9. _______ Health risk assessment (HRA)
10. _______ Holism
11. _______ Homeostasis
12. _______ Input
13. _______ Maintenance stage
14. _______ Negative feed-back
15. _______ Open system
16. _______ Output
17. _______ Positive feed-back
18. _______ Precontemplation stage
19. _______ Preparation stage
20. _______ Primary prevention
21. _______ Psychological homeostasis
22. _______ Secondary prevention
23. _______ Self-regulation
24. _______ Termination stage
25. _______ Tertiary prevention

a. Stimulates change

b. Focuses on early identification of health problems and prompt intervention

c. Assessment and educational tool that indicates a client's risk for disease or injury during the next 10 years

d. Occurs when the person actively implements behavioral and cognitive strategies

e. Generalized health promotion and specific protection against disease

f. Energy, matter, and information move into and out of the system through the system boundary

g. Inhibits change

h. Person acknowledges having a problem, seriously considers changing a specific behavior, and verbalizes a plan to change

i. Person does not think about changing his or her behavior in the next 6 months

j. Its focus is to help rehabilitate individuals and restore them to an optimum level of functioning within the constraints of the disability.

k. Mechanism by which some of the output of a system is returned to the system as input

l. Information, material, or energy that enters the system

m. Emphasizes the whole person and how one area of concern relates to the entire person

n. Person strives to prevent relapse by integrating adopted behaviors into his or her lifestyle

o. Homeostatic mechanisms come into play automatically

p. Energy, matter, or information given out by the system as a result of its processes

q. Behavior motivated by a desire to actively avoid illness

r. Disease prevention

s. Behavior motivated by the desire to increase well-being

t. Describes the relative constancy of the internal processes of the body

u. The person intends to take action in the immediate future

v. Does not exchange information with its environment

w. The ultimate goal of the transtheoretical model.

x. A real or imaginary line that differentiates one system from another

y. Emotional or psychological balance

KEY TOPIC REVIEW

1. List four main characteristics of homeostatic mechanisms.

 a.

 b.

 c.

 d.

2. The nurse must consider all components of health in order to ensure holistic health care. What are the five components of health?

 a.

 b.

 c.

 d.

 e.

3. Abraham Maslow, a renowned needs theorist, ranks human needs on five levels. List the levels in ascending order and give an example of a need in each level.

   a.

   b.

   c.

   d.

   e.

4. What did Richard Kalish add to Maslow's hierarchy of needs, where did he add it, and why did he add it?

5. *Healthy People 2020: Understanding and Improving Health* (U.S. Department of Health and Human Services, 2010) presents a comprehensive strategy for promoting health and preventing illness, disability, and premature death.

   a. True b. False

6. List the two major goals of *Healthy People 2020* and what is reflected by those goals.

   a.

   b.

7. Health-promoting behavior is directed toward attaining positive health outcomes for the client.

   a. True b. False

8. How do health promotion plans need to be developed to encourage clients to participate in their care?

9. To encourage a client to quit smoking, what strategy of implementation should the nurse use?

10. Which of the following should be included in a client's lifestyle assessment that would be relevant to his or her health care? (Select all that apply.)

    1. Nutrition
    2. Physical activity
    3. Drug, alcohol, and cigarette smoking habits
    4. Marital status

FOCUSED STUDY TIPS

1. How does understanding developmental stage theories enable the nurse to provide knowledgeable care?

2. As a nurse, what is your role in health promotion? How can you enhance health promotion actions in your community?

3. Discuss the Health Promotion Model. Refer to the text, Figure 16–4.

4. When exploring the stages of change, is change always linear? Why or why not? Why is it important for nurses to understand the stages of change?

5. What is the nurse's role in health promotion? Do you believe that the nurse should be a good role model for healthy living? How would you feel if a nurse who never exercises is attempting to instruct you (a client) in the importance of exercise?

6. Compare and contrast health promotion and disease prevention. Give one example of each concept.

CASE STUDY

You are caring for Benjamin Conner, a 65-year-old who presents with acute chest pain and shortness of breath. Upon assessment, you learn that Mr. Conner is a 40-pack-year smoker and leads a sedentary lifestyle. After Mr. Conner's condition has been stabilized, you are planning education to provide to Mr. Conner.

1. What health promotion education will you provide?
2. When providing education to Mr. Conner, what type of prevention will you be demonstrating?

REVIEW QUESTIONS

1. A client reports that he believes he will "never kick the habit" of smoking because he has tried before and failed. Using the transtheoretical model (TTM), what stage of health behavior change is the client functioning in?
    1. Preparation stage
    2. Contemplation stage
    3. Termination stage
    4. Precontemplation stage
2. Identify which of the following are basic types of health promotion activities. (Select all that apply.)
    1. A billboard promoting abstinence to prevent sexually transmitted infections and unplanned pregnancies
    2. A wellness assessment program
    3. A nurse who models healthy lifestyle behaviors
    4. A school of nursing that is holding a blood pressure fair
3. The nurse refers a new below-the-knee (BKA) amputation client to a support group for amputees. This is an example of what type of prevention?
    1. Primary
    2. Secondary
    3. Tertiary
    4. Terminal
4. The nurse is providing health education about injury and poisoning prevention to a group of young mothers at a health fair. What type of prevention is the nurse conducting?
    1. Primary prevention
    2. Secondary prevention
    3. Tertiary prevention
    4. Limited prevention
5. A client had surgery for gastrointestinal problems and required a colostomy. What type of preventive care would this client need at this stage?
    1. Primary prevention
    2. Secondary prevention
    3. Tertiary prevention
    4. Limited prevention

6. A community health nurse is teaching a group of older adults about self-examination techniques for breast and testicular cancer. What type of health care prevention is the nurse teaching?
   1. Primary prevention
   2. Secondary prevention
   3. Tertiary prevention
   4. Limited prevention
7. Which client would benefit from Pender's health promotion model? (Select all that apply.)
   1. An active 21-year-old client who does not smoke or drink alcohol
   2. A 50-year-old client who exercises four times a week
   3. A 32-year-old who has yearly breast exams and other routine health screenings
   4. An overweight 29-year-old who engages in risky behaviors
8. A client has complete confidence that she has learned health behaviors that will enable her to maintain her current health status by exercising three to five times a week, monitoring her dietary intake, and by no longer engaging in risky behaviors. What stage of health behavior change is this client experiencing?
   1. Maintenance
   2. Action
   3. Preparation
   4. Termination
9. The client is attending Alcoholics Anonymous (AA) meetings for support to assist in remaining sober. It is anticipated that the client will remain in this group for several years. What stage of health behavior change is this client experiencing?
   1. Maintenance
   2. Action
   3. Preparation
   4. Termination
10. Who is responsible for developing health promotion plans?
    1. Physician
    2. Family
    3. Client
    4. Nurse

CHAPTER 17

HEALTH, WELLNESS, AND ILLNESS

KEY TERM REVIEW

Match each term with its appropriate definition.

1. ___G___ Acute illness
2. ___I___ Adherence
3. ___H___ Chronic illness
4. ___K___ Disease
5. ___A___ Etiology
6. ___J___ Exacerbation
7. ___N___ Health
8. ___R___ Health behaviors
9. ___M___ Health beliefs
10. ___P___ Health status
11. ___O___ Illness
12. ___F___ Illness behavior
13. ___E___ Lifestyle
14. ___C___ Locus of control
15. ___B___ Remission
16. ___Q___ Risk factors
17. ___D___ Well-being
18. ___L___ Wellness

a. Cause of a disease or condition

b. When symptoms dis-appear

c. A concept from social learning theory that nurses can use to determine whether clients are likely to take action regarding health

d. A subjective perception of vitality and feeling well that can be described, experienced, and measured

e. Refers to a person's general way of living

f. Ways in which individuals describe, monitor, and interpret symptoms, take actions, and use the health care system

g. Characterized by symptoms of relatively short duration

h. Characterized by symptoms that last for an extended period, usually 6 months or more

i. The extent to which an individual's behavior coincides with medical or health advice

j. When symptoms reappear

k. Alteration in body functions resulting in a reduction of capacities or a shortening of the normal life span

l. A state of well-being

m. Concepts about health that an individual believes are true

n. A state of complete physical, mental, and social well-being, and not merely the absence of disease or infirmity

o. A highly subjective state that may or may not be related to disease

p. State of health of an individual at a given time

q. Practices that have potentially negative effects on health

r. The actions people take to understand their health state, maintain an optimal state of health, prevent illness and injury, and reach their maximum physical and mental potential

KEY TOPIC REVIEW

1. What is the difference between illness and disease? Disease Alters Body Function
2. Match the theorist with the correct theory of the stages and aspects of illness.
   a. Parsons ___B___ Outlined five stages of illness
   b. Suchman ___A___ Described four aspects of the sick role
3. How is a client's usual pattern of behavior changed with illness or hospitalization? Disrupts
4. Explain the internal variables in biologic, psychological, and cognitive dimensions. Biologic, Psychologic, Cognitive
5. Explain the differences between well-being and wellness. (Well Being = Feeling Well) (Wellness = Choices to feel well)
6. What are three external influences on health? Environment, Standards of living, Family, Social
7. List the seven dimensions of wellness that Anspaugh, Hanrick, and Rosato proposed. Physical, Social, Emotional, Intellectual, Spiritual, Occupational, Environmental
8. The causation of a disease is called its etiology.
9. What are the four aspects of the sick role that Parson describes?
   a. Not Responsible for their condition
   b. excused from certain Social Roles & Tasks
   c. Get well as quickly as possible
   d. Seek competent Help
10. Define the following.
    a. Locus of control: Likely to take action for their own Health
    b. Exacerbation: Increase in severity
    c. Health behaviors: Stay Healthy Actions
    d. Health beliefs: Concepts Individuals Believe True
    e. Health status: Level of Health
    f. Acute illness: Short duration
    g. Remission: Lessening of symptoms
    h. Risk factors: Negative affects on Health

FOCUSED STUDY TIPS

1. How are health belief and behavior models useful in nursing? What are two models used for nursing?
2. How can nurses enhance health care adherence?
3. Why do nurses have to be aware of their own personal definitions of health? How can that enhance their nursing practice?
4. Explore the various theorists who have described stages and aspects of illness. How does Parson describe the sick role?

5. Illness affects the entire family. How can the nurse best explain the effects on the family to the significant others of the ill person?

6. Describe the three elements of the Leavell and Clark agent–host–environment model of health and illness. Discuss the model's concept of illness prevention and wellness promotion.

CASE STUDY

A 52-year-old female with a family history of lung cancer requests information about smoking cessation. The client admits that she smokes one pack per day and has smoked for approximately 32 years.

1. With consideration of the goals of *Healthy People 2020*, how can the nurse assist the client?

Provide her with Stop Smoking Info, Groups

REVIEW QUESTIONS

1. A client has severe arthritis, yet she still works 40 hours per week and takes care of her family. This is an example of which health model?
   1. Clinical model
   2. Adaptive model
   3. Role performance model
   4. Eudemonistic model
2. Which health model describes illness as a condition that prevents self-actualization?
   1. Clinical model
   2. Adaptive model
   3. Role performance model
   4. Eudemonistic model
3. Osteoporosis and autoimmune diseases are examples of what type of biologic dimension that influences a person's health?
   1. Genetic makeup
   2. Gender
   3. Age
   4. Developmental levels
4. During the first years of life, infants lack physiological and psychological maturity, so their defenses against diseases are lower. This is an example of what type of biologic dimension that influences a person's health?
   1. Genetic makeup
   2. Gender
   3. Age
   4. Developmental levels
5. The impact of illness on an individual may cause: (Select all that apply.)
   1. The client to become dependent on the health care provider..
   2. The client to have role changes within the family.
   3. The client to become more outgoing and friendly.
   4. The client's self-esteem to greatly increase.

6. A nursing student is instructing a female client on healthy lifestyle choices. What are the correct examples of healthy lifestyle choices? (Select all that apply.)

   1. Tobacco use of 1 pack per day
   2. Exercising 3 to 4 days per week for 1 hour
   3. Regular dental checkup
   4. Seat belt use

7. A client who was obese has lost a large amount of weight in order to feel better about himself. What health belief model could the nurse use to assist the client?

   1. Health locus of control model
   2. Rosenstock's health belief model
   3. Becker's health belief model
   4. Pender's health belief model

8. A client reports that she has been practicing yoga for the past 2 years in order to reduce stress and increase muscle flexibility. What part of wellness is this client participating in?

   1. Physical and emotional
   2. Physical and social
   3. Social and emotional
   4. Intellectual and emotional

9. The nurse is attempting to instruct a client with chronic obstructive pulmonary disease on the benefits of not smoking, yet the nurse admits that she also smokes one pack a day. What might be a factor in the client's refusal to quit smoking at this time?

   1. The client is distressed about quitting the habit of smoking.
   2. The nurse is not modeling healthy lifestyle choices.
   3. The perceived benefits of not smoking are inconclusive at this time.
   4. The client's cultural heritage demands that he smoke two packs of cigarettes per day.

10. Diabetes mellitus is an example of:

    1. Acute illness.
    2. Adherence.
    3. Chronic illness.
    4. Exacerbation.

CHAPTER 18

CULTURALLY RESPONSIVE NURSING CARE

KEY TERM REVIEW

Match each term with its appropriate definition.

1. _______ Acculturation
2. _______ Assimilation
3 _______ Biomedical health belief
4 _______ Cultural broker
5. _______ Cultural competence
5. _______ Culturally responsive care
6. _______ Culture
7. _______ Discrimination
8. _______ Diversity
9. _______ Ethnicity
10. _______ Ethnocentrism
11. _______ Folk medicine
12. _______ Generalizations
13. _______ Health disparities
14. _______ Heritage
15. _______ Holistic health belief
16. _______ Magico-religious health belief
17 _______ Nationality
18. _______ Prejudice
19. _______ Race
20. _______ Racism
21. _______ Religion
22. _______ Scientific health belief
23. _______ Subculture
24 _______ Transcultural nursing

a. Refers to the fact or state of being different

b. Preconceived notion or judgment that is not based on sufficient knowledge

c. Biomedical health beliefs

d. The thoughts, communications, actions, customs, beliefs, values, and institutions of racial, ethnic, religious, or social groups

e. Things passed down from previous generations

f. Belief in the superiority of one's own culture and lifestyle

g. Differential and negative treatment of individuals on the basis of their race, ethnicity, gender, or other group membership

h. Composed of people who have a distinct identity and yet are related to a larger cultural group

i. Holds that the forces of nature must be maintained in balance or illness results

j. One who engages both parties effectively and efficiently in accessing the nuances and hidden sociocultural assumptions embedded in each other's language

k. Social and cultural characteristics as well as ancestry

l. Beliefs and practices relating to illness and healing that derive from cultural traditions rather than from modern medicine's scientific base

m. Based on the belief that life is controlled by physical and biochemical processes that can be manipulated by humans

n. Differences in care experienced by one population compared with another population

o. Statements about common cultural patterns

p. Process by which an individual develops a new cultural identity

q. Relationship between individuals who believe that they have distinctive characteristics that make them a group

r. A system of beliefs, practices, and ethical values about divine or superhuman power worshipped as the creator and rulers of the universe

s. Centered on the client's cultural perspectives, integrating the client's values, and beliefs into the plan of care

t. The ongoing process in which the health care professional continuously strives to achieve the ability and availability to work effectively within the cultural context of the patient (individual, family, community)

u. Generally refers to the sovereign state or country where an individual has membership, which may be through birth, through inheritance (parents), or through naturalization

v. View in which health and illness are controlled by supernatural forces

w. Involuntary process occurs when people incorporate traits from another culture

x. Assumption held about racial groups that includes belief that races are inherently unequal

y. Centered on client's cultural perspectives, integrating client's values and beliefs into the plan of care

KEY TOPIC REVIEW

1. What is culture? How does it define health?
2. The term ____________ refers to things passed down from previous generations.
3. What is the purpose of the U.S. Department of Health and Human Services (USDHHS), in terms of culture?
4. What is a goal of the Centers for Disease Control and Prevention (CDC), in terms of culture?
5. What is the purpose for the National Center on Minority Health and Health Disparities (NCMHD)?
6. Describe what influence the Racial and Ethnic Approaches to Community Health Across the United States (REACH U.S.) program has on nursing care?
7. What is one of the goals of *Healthy People 2020?*
8. How does the *National Healthcare Disparities Report* influence current nursing practice?
9. Differentiate between culturally sensitive, culturally appropriate, and culturally competent care in professional nursing.
10. ____________ is credited with creating the theory of culture care diversity and universality.

FOCUSED STUDY TIPS

1. What are the core practice competencies of culturally competent nursing care?
2. What does the magico-religious health belief view entail? Give an example.
3. How do scientific or biomedical health beliefs differ from holistic health beliefs?
4. How does ethnocentrism differ from cultural beliefs?
5. Describe the LEARN model and the four C's of culture used in cultural assessments.

CASE STUDIES

1. While caring for an Asian client who became ill while visiting relatives in the United States, the nurse notices an unusual bruised circular pattern on the trunk of the client.
   a. If the nurse is culturally competent, what would be an appropriate comment?
   b. If the nurse has xenophobia, what comment might the nurse make regarding the coining or cupping that occurred?
   c. Give an example of an ethnocentric statement from the nurse.
   d. What nursing action would be considered discrimination?
2. A nurse is taking care of a traditional Hispanic client on a medical–surgical unit following a laparotomy appendectomy. Review Box 18–2 in the text for an overview of the health-related practices of different cultures.
   a. If the client does not return direct eye contact, is this indicative of a cultural difference or a result of a "shifty," evasive client?
   b. The client's family desires to spend as much time with him as possible, including staying after hours. How does the nurse handle this situation?
   c. The client does not want to take his preventive medication to prevent stress ulcers. He states that his life and recovery status are in God's hands, and that he "has no need of pharmaceutical medications." What action should the nurse take at this time?

REVIEW QUESTIONS

1. The major factor contributing to the increased emphasis on the need for proficiency in cultural nursing practice in the United States is which of the following?
   1. An increasing birth rate
   2. Increased access to health care services
   3. Demographic changes
   4. A decreasing rate of immigration
2. A client who has a French mother and an Italian father is described as having a(n) __________ identification.
   1. Bicultural
   2. Diversity
   3. Subculture
   4. Acculturation
3. A client who is homosexual is described as having:
   1. Biculturalism.
   2. Acculturation.
   3. Diversity.
   4. Subculture.
   5. Assimilation.

4. The involuntary process of _________ occurs when people adapt to or borrow traits from another culture.
   1. Biculturalism
   2. Acculturation
   3. Diversity
   4. Subculture
   5. Assimilation
5. If a citizen of Japan permanently moves to America, then _________ may occur when that individual becomes an American citizen.
   1. Biculturalism
   2. Diversity
   3. Assimilation
   4. Subculture
   5. Acculturation
6. A nurse caring for a Chinese client orders rice for every meal without consulting the client. What may the nurse be displaying?
   1. Prejudice
   2. Discrimination.
   3. Stereotyping.
   4. Racism.
7. Using the HEALTH traditions model, which would be considered an example of spiritual and mental health?
   1. Avoiding persons who can cause illnesses
   2. Special foods and drinks
   3. Acupuncture
   4. Healing rituals
8. While caring for a Latin American client who cannot speak or understand English, the nurse recognizes that she will need a(n) _________ in order to care for the client.
   1. Family member
   2. Translator
   3. Representative
   4. Interpreter
9. While caring for a diverse cultural population, the nurse must recognize that cultural beliefs and behaviors may lead to:
   1. Stereotyping.
   2. Ethnocentrism..
   3. Placement of the nurse's culture onto others.
   4. Being confused regarding the many values and beliefs of different cultures.

10. Identify which nursing interventions would be beneficial when communicating with clients who have limited knowledge of English. (Select all that apply.)

    1. Use slang words, limited medical terminology, and no abbreviations.
    2. Speak slowly, in a respectful manner, and at a normal volume.
    3. Use nonverbal communication, which uses silence, touch, eye movement, facial expressions, and body posture that is acceptable to that particular culture.
    4. Ask a member of the client's family, especially a child or spouse, to act as interpreter.
    5. Address the client, not the interpreter.

11. Campinha-Bacote's model of cultural competence is based on a framework that integrates transcultural nursing, medical anthropology, and multicultural counseling. Identify three of the five constructs of this model of cultural competence.

    1. Cultural awareness
    2. Cultural appearance
    3. Cultural desires
    4. Cultural skills
    5. Cultural experiences

CHAPTER 19

COMPLEMENTARY AND ALTERNATIVE HEALING MODALITIES

KEY TERM REVIEW

Match each term with its appropriate definition.

1. _______ Acupressure
2. _______ Acupuncture
3. _______ Allopathic medicine
4. _______ Alternative medicine
5. _______ Aromatherapy
6. _______ Ayurveda
7. _______ Biofeedback
8. _______ Biomedicine
9. _______ Chiropractic
10. _______ Complementary medicine
11. _______ Guided imagery
12. _______ Herbal medicine
13. _______ Holism
14. _______ Homeopathy
15. _______ Hypnotherapy
16. _______ Imagery
17. _______ Massage therapy
18. _______ Meditation
19. _______ Music therapy
20. _______ Naturopathic medicine
21. _______ Qigong
22. _______ Reflexology
23. _______ T'ai chi
24. _______ Traditional Chinese medicine
25. _______ Yoga

a. Application of a trance state in which an individual's concentration is focused and distraction is minimized

b. Conventional or allopathic medicine

c. A self-healing system, assisted by small doses of remedies or medicines

d. Therapies other than biomedicine used to promote health and wellness

e. Therapeutic use of essential oils of plants in which the odor or fragrance plays a key role

f. Use of music to induce relaxation or distract clients

g. Technique of applying pressure or stimulation to specific points on the body using needles

h. Chinese discipline consisting of breathing and mental exercises combined with body movement

i. System of medicine that emphasizes the interdependence of the health of the individual and the quality of societal life

j. Scientific manipulation of the soft tissues of the body

k. Form of acupressure commonly performed on the feet

l. The use of plants in treating illness

m. Method for life that includes ethical models for behavior and mental and physical exercises aimed at producing spiritual enlightenment

n. Method by which a person can learn to control certain physiological responses of the body

o. Discipline that combines physical fitness, meditation, and self-defense

p. Health profession that believes that health is a state of balance, especially of the nervous and musculoskeletal systems

q. Alternative medicine

r. System based on the premise that the body's qi circulates through pathway meridians and can be accessed and manipulated

s. General term for a practice that involves relaxing the body and easing the mind

t. The belief that people are more than physical bodies, that the combined mental, emotional, spiritual, relationship, and environmental components play a crucial role in a person's health

u. A state of focused attention that encourages changes in attitudes, behavior, and physiological reactions

v. A system of medicine and way of life that emphasizes client responsibility, client education, health maintenance, and disease prevention

w. Technique of applying pressure or stimulation to specific points on the body using finger pressure

x. A two-way communication between the conscious and unconscious mind that involves the whole body and all of its senses

y. Western medicine

KEY TOPIC REVIEW

1. ______ is the combination of mental, emotional, spiritual, relationship, and environmental factors.

2. What is the mission of the American Holistic Nurses Association (AHNA)?

3. How can the nurse create a healing environment in health care?

4. Identify three methods of self-healing for nurses.

   a.

   b.

   c.

5. Identify which of the following are manual methods of healing: (Select all that apply.)
   a. Massage
   b. Meditation
   c. Hypnotherapy
   d. Chiropractic
   e. Hand-mediated biofield therapies
   f. Aromatherapy

6. ______ is viewed as the force that integrates the body, mind, and spirit, and connects everything.

7. What is the third largest independent health profession in the Western world after conventional medicine and dentistry?

8. Match the type of prayer with its correct definition.

a. Intercessory prayer	______ No specific outcome is requested during prayer time
b. Nondirected prayer	______ An informal talk with God—like talking with a good friend
c. Ritual prayer	______ Individual who is praying asks for a specific outcome
d. Colloquial prayer	______ Asking God for things for oneself or others
e. Directed prayer	______ The use of formal prayers or rituals such as prayers from a prayer book or Jewish siddur
f. Meditation prayer	______ Contemplative prayer

9. What are the contraindications for magnetic therapy and, on principle, does this therapy work?

10. Describe chelation therapy and how it works in the body.

FOCUSED STUDY TIPS

1. Discuss the six concepts that are common to most alternative practices.

2. Describe the different mind–body therapies and the benefits of each.

3. What issues arise with animal-assisted therapies in health care? Describe the benefits of animal-assisted therapy.

4. Differentiate between conventional medicine, biomedicine, allopathic methods, and alternative or complementary medicines.

5. How are herbs used in medicine? What are some nursing guidelines for herbs used in conjunction with over-the-counter (OTC) medications?

6. Differentiate between mind–body therapies and manual healing methods.

CASE STUDIES

1. The nurse is conducting the initial assessment interview for Roberta Sinclair, a 72-year-old female.,
   a. What type of questions should the nurse ask to investigate Ms. Sinclair's use of complementary and alternative therapies?

2. Gabe Santos, a 57-year-old client, is admitted to the hospital with uncontrolled hypertension. Mr. Santos states that he takes his antihypertension medication as directed, exercises, and watches his sodium intake. Mr. Santos also reports taking an enteric-coated aspirin daily. However, Mr. Santos states he has noted more bruising than usual lately. Refer to the "Practice Guidelines" in the text to answer the following questions.
   a. Which popular herbal preparations could interfere with Mr. Santos's current medication regimen?
   c. Which additional complementary and alternative healing modalities might the nurse suggest to Mr. Santos to help treat his hypertension?

REVIEW QUESTIONS

1. Concepts that are common to most alternative practices include: (Select all that apply.)
   1. Holism.
   2. Balance.
   3. Spirituality.
   4. Prescription medications.
   5. Technology and instrumentation.
2. What is the name of the system of medicine that emphasizes client responsibility, client education, health maintenance, and disease prevention?
   1. Naturopathic medicine
   2. Nutritional medicine
   3. Homeopathic medicine
   4. Chiropractic medicine
3. What nursing action is most correct regarding the use of alternative and complementary therapies?
   1. Recommend hydrotherapy for the older adult clients.
   2. Recommend colonics for clients with Crohn's disease.
   3. Encourage the client to discuss the use of herbs, teas, vitamins, or other natural products.
   4. Encourage the client in using alternative therapies, such as acupuncture and yoga.
4. The nurse suggests to a client with osteoarthritis to participate in Pilates. What are the benefits of Pilates for this client?
   1. It will give the client an activity to perform to lessen boredom.
   2. It encourages a spiritual connection.
   3. It may improve flexibility and joint health, and relieve muscle aches.
   4. It cleanses the colon and promotes a healthy feeling.

5. Which of the following therapies stimulates the production of catecholamines, hormones, and endorphins? It can be used in establishing relationships, relieving tension and anxiety, and even facilitating learning.
    1. Music therapy
    2. Hypnotherapy
    3. Guided imagery therapies
    4. Humor and laughter therapy
6. The American Holistic Nurses Association and an organization called "Beyond Ordinary Healing" offer a nurses' certificate program in complementary and alternative medicine (CAM).. After successfully passing the certification, what is the nurse certified to perform?
    1. Music therapy
    2. Hypnotherapy
    3. Guided imagery therapies
    4. Humor and laughter therapy
7. What do meditation, biofeedback, and guided imagery have in common?
    1. The process of physical resting and rhythmic breathing
    2. The process of physical activity and music therapy
    3. The process of relaxation and sleep
    4. The process of utilizing aromatherapy
8. Which of the following genres of music are used to induce relaxation and distract clients from pain?
    1. Rap music
    2. Opera music
    3. Piano and flute melody playing quietly
    4. Country music with yodeling
9. A client is on complete bed rest and complains of back pain from lying "in the bed all the time." What is a nursing intervention that uses a nonpharmacologic method to ease the discomfort? (Select all that apply.)
    1. Administering a dose of morphine for pain
    2. Assisting the client to a bedside chair
    3. Giving the client a back massage
    4. Instructing the client that the health care provider will see him tomorrow night
    5. Using music that contains no words
    6. Instructing the client in guided imagery

CHAPTER 20

CONCEPTS OF GROWTH AND DEVELOPMENT

KEY TERM REVIEW

Match each term with its appropriate definition.

1. _______ Accommodation
2. _______ Adaptation
3. _______ Adaptive mechanisms
4. _______ Assimilation
5. _______ Attachment
6. _______ Cognitive development
7. _______ Defense mechanisms
8. _______ Development
9. _______ Developmental stages
10. _______ Developmental task
11. _______ Ego
12. _______ Fixation
13. _______ Growth
14. _______ Id
15. _______ Libido
16. _______ Maturation
17. _______ Moral
18. _______ Moral behavior
19. _______ Moral development
20. _______ Morality
21. _______ Personality
22. _______ Superego
23. _______ Temperament
24. _______ Unconscious mind

a. Arises at a certain period in the life of an individual, successful achievement of which leads to success with later tasks

b. Resides in the unconscious, and seeks immediate pleasure and gratification

c. Contains the conscience

d. The way in which individuals respond to their external and internal environments

e. The way a person perceives the requirements of living in society and responds to them

f. The pattern of change in moral behavior with age

g. The manner in which people learn to think

h. The outward expression of the inner self

i. The result of conflicts between the id's impulses and the anxiety created by the conflicts due to social and environmental restrictions

j. A process of differentiation and refining of abilities and skills

k. The part of a person's mental life of which the person is unaware

l. Refers to the requirements necessary for people to live together in society

m. Relating to right and wrong

n. Inability of the personality to proceed to the next stage because of anxiety

o. Theory that proposes that life is a series of levels of achievement

p. Process through which humans encounter and react to new situations by using the mechanisms they already possess

q. Adaptive mechanisms

r. Process of change whereby cognitive processes mature sufficiently to allow the person to solve problems that were unsolvable before

s. Ability to handle demands made by the environment

t. The realistic part of the person

u. Physical change and increase in size

v. Lasting, strong emotional bond

w. An increase in the complexity of function and skill progression

x. Underlying motivation to human development

KEY TOPIC REVIEW

1. What is meant by the term *growth*? What indicators of growth are used?
2. Define development.
3. List four factors that influence growth and development.

   a.

   b.

   c.

   d.
4. What is meant by psychosocial development?
5. Sigmund Freud introduced a number of concepts about development. What are the major concepts in his theory? Define the terms used in his theory.
6. Describe social learning theory.
7. Describe Kohlberg's theory on moral development.
8. What does the behaviorist learning theory emphasize?
9. Which two theorists describe stages of spiritual development or faith? Describe their concepts in depth.

10. Define the following terms:
    a. Accommodation
    b. Adaptation
    c. Assimilation
    d. Developmental task

FOCUSED STUDY TIPS

1. What is the definition of personality? Why is it hard to define?
2. Describe Erik Erikson's stages of development.
3. What are Freud's five stages of development?
4. Describe the moral theories of Kohlberg and Gilligan.
5. Describe Piaget's phases of cognitive development.
6. Describe the concept of temperament and its relationship to growth and development.

CASE STUDY

The nurse is caring for a 6-month-old infant at a well-child clinic. Using Piaget's phases of cognitive development, answer the following questions:

1. What primary abilities will the infant use in this phase of cognitive development?
2. Describe the significant behavior noted in this phase of cognitive development.

REVIEW QUESTIONS

1. In which direction does growth and development occur from birth if it starts from the head and moves to the trunk, the legs, and the feet?
    1. Proximodistal direction
    2. Simple to complex direction
    3. Peripheral to medial direction
    4. Cephalocaudal direction
2. The nurse prepares to give an antibiotic injection to a 3-year-old child who has an infection. When the child views the nurse with a needle, he begins to cry and say "no-no" while reaching for his mother. According to Piaget's phases of cognitive development, what stage/phase is the toddler experiencing?
    1. Primary circular phase
    2. Concrete operations phase
    3. Preconceptual phase
    4. Initiative versus guilt phase

3. While caring for a 72-year-old client, the nurse suspects that the client may be experiencing depression when the client states that he feels like he is "falling apart because of age." According to Robert Peck's theory regarding adult development, what task is the client struggling with?
   1. Ego differentiation versus work-role perception
   2. Body transcendence versus body preoccupation
   3. Ego transcendence versus ego preoccupation
   4. Integrity versus despair
4. A school nurse is teaching high school students about sexually transmitted infections and pregnancy prevention in a health education course. According to Havighurst's age periods and developmental tasks, why is this the appropriate age to introduce this discussion?
   1. Adolescents are achieving new and more mature relations with their peers and are trying to assert their independence.
   2. Adolescents are finding a congenial social group and selecting mates.
   3. Adolescents are developing a conscience, morality, and a set of values.
   4. Adolescents are establishing satisfactory affiliations with one's age group.
5. A pregnant adolescent client tells the nurse that abortion is wrong, and that it is for this reason the client decided to continue her pregnancy. What concept does the adolescent's comment reflect?
   1. Morals
   2. Spirituality
   3. Religion
   4. Psychological development
6. The nurse is exploring activities that would enhance an older adult client's retirement, per the client's request. Which theorist would explain this type of adult development?
   1. Freud
   2. Piaget
   3. Kohlberg
   4. Peck
7. According to Gould's study, which is the best example of stage 4?
   1. A 19-year-old leaving for college
   2. A 25-year-old in the military
   3. A 30-year-old graduate student
   4. A 65-year-old retired schoolteacher
8. A 26-year-old female client makes the statement that she realizes that she has been selfish in her life and she needs to "do more" for her aging parents. According to Carol Gilligan's research, what stage of moral development is the client in?
   1. Stage 1
   2. Stage 2
   3. Stage 3
   4. Stage 4

CHAPTER 21

PROMOTING HEALTH FROM CONCEPTION THROUGH ADOLESCENCE

KEY TERM REVIEW

Match each term with its appropriate definition.

1. _______ Amblyopia
2. _______ Apgar scoring system
3. _______ Apocrine glands
4. _______ Denver Developmental Screening Test (DDST-II)
5. _______ Embryonic phase
6. _______ Emmetropic
7. _______ Failure to thrive
8. _______ Fetal phase
9. _______ Hyperopic
10. _______ Identification
11. _______ Introjection
12. _______ Lanugo
13. _______ Menarche
14. _______ Myopic
15. _______ Primary sexual characteristics
16. _______ Puberty
17. _______ Repression
18. _______ Sebaceous glands
19. _______ Secondary sexual characteristics
20. _______ Separation anxiety
21. _______ Stereognosis
22. _______ Strabismus
23. _______ Teratogen
24. _______ Vernix caseosa

a. Occurs when the child perceives self as similar to another person and behaves like that person

b. Fine downy hair that covers the body of the fetus

c. Occurs in the second and third trimester of pregnancy

d. Onset of menstruation

e. Differentiate male from female but not directly related to reproduction

f. Provides a numeric indicator of the baby's physiological capacities to adapt to extrauterine life

g. Protective covering that develops over the fetal skin

h. Failure to establish normal neuropathways of vision that leads to reduced visual acuity in one eye

i. Ability to identify an unseen object by touch

j. A condition in which the infant shows substandard growth and development

k. The ability of the eye to refract light normally

l. Fear and frustration that comes with parental absences

m. Release sweat onto the skin in response to emotional stimuli only

n. Removing experiences, thoughts, and impulses from awareness

o. Standardized test used to screen development of children from birth to 6 years of age

p. First stage of adolescence

q. Anything that adversely affects normal cellular development in the embryo or fetus

r. Eight-week period during which the fertilized ovum develops into an organism with most of the features of the human

s. Secrete sebum

t. Organs necessary for reproduction

u. Cross eye

v. Assimilation of the attributes of others into oneself

w. Farsighted

x. Nearsighted

KEY TOPIC REVIEW

1. How long does prenatal development last?

2. ______ are the three periods of pregnancy that last about ______ months.

3. Identify the trimester and/or phases of fetal development and describe what is taking place with the fetus during that time.

   a.

   b.

   c.

4. What are the five maternal factors that contribute to higher risks of low-birth-weight babies?

   a.

   b.

   c.

   d.

   e.

5. Birth weight ______ by the ______ month and ______ by the ______ month.

6. For the infant, how does cognitive development occur?

7. List three milestones that toddlers develop between ages 12 months to 3 years.

   a.

   b.

   c.

8. According to Erickson, what task are preschoolers, ages 4 to 5, engaged in?

9. In the school-age period the skills learned are particularly important in relation to work later in life and the willingness to try new tasks.

   a. True

   b. False

10. Choose the major landmarks of the adolescent period. (Select all that apply.)

    a. Rapid growth in height

    b. Deciduous teeth are shed

    c. Sexual maturity

    d. Increasing dependence on the family

    e. Leading causes of death are motor vehicle crashes, homicides, suicides, and other unintentional injuries

FOCUSED STUDY TIPS

1. Why is it important for the nurse to know the normal developmental tasks for each age group?
2. Identify nursing activities to assess and promote health of the fetus and the developmental milestones, noting the average time of occurrence.
3. Identify nursing activities to assess and promote health of the toddler and the developmental milestones, noting the average time of occurrence.
4. Identify nursing activities to assess and promote health of the preschooler and the developmental milestones, noting the average time of occurrence.
5. Identify nursing activities to assess and promote health of the adolescent and the developmental milestones, noting the average time of occurrence.
6. Describe how vision changes from infancy to adulthood.

CASE STUDIES

1. The nurse is discussing infant growth and development with the parents of a newborn. The nurse discusses several reflexes that are found in the normal neonate.

   a. What reflex disappears after 8 months of age?

   b. If the Babinski reflex persists after 1 year and remains positive, what does that indicate?

2. The mother of a 15-year-old girl is talking with the pediatric nurse and says, "I don't know what is wrong with my daughter. She was always such a good kid, but now she talks back, only wants to be with her friends, and won't participate in family activities."

   a. What explanation might the nurse give this mother to explain the adolescent's behavior?

   b. What anticipatory guidance will the nurse provide this mother to prepare her for future changes she is likely to see in her daughter?

3. The nurse is performing an Apgar score on a newborn who has been born via cesarean section. The newborn's heart rate is 110 beats/min and respirations are regular. The newborn is crying and active. The newborn's skin color is pink, except for the extremities, which are blue in color.

   a. At what time(s) will the nurse perform the Apgar score?

   b. What is the newborn's current Apgar score?

REVIEW QUESTIONS

1. The nurse is instructing a group of pregnant women about ways to reduce the risks of birth defects. Which of the following statements indicates a need for further instruction and/or clarification?

   1. "It is okay for me to use the sauna at the health club but not the hot whirlpool bath."
   2. "I should continue taking the folic acid my health care provider prescribed prior to the confirmation of my pregnancy."
   3. "I need to stop smoking and try to avoid secondhand smoke."
   4. "I should stop drinking alcohol while I am pregnant."

2. A 10-year-old client has terminal cancer. What does the nurse expect to be the normal concept of death at this age?

   1. There is no concept of death at this age.
   2. Death only happens to old people.
   3. The dead can return, much like a family member returns from a trip.
   4. Death is a final and inevitable outcome of life.

3. The most common health risk occurring in today's environment for school-age children is:

   1. Falls.
   2. Obesity.
   3. Colic.
   4. Unprotected sex.

4. A woman who is approximately 5 months pregnant tells the nurse that she is beginning to feel a fluttering in her lower abdomen. She is worried that she is having a miscarriage. Based on the nurse's knowledge of prenatal development, what is the best response by the nurse?

   1. "Is your back hurting bad?"
   2. "Fetal movements may be felt around 5 months by the mother."
   3. "Fetal movements start around 3 months and mothers may feel the movement."
   4. "Fetal movement begins at 8 months and you may be feeling that movement."

5. The Denver Developmental Screening Test (DDST-II) measures the abilities of a child compared to those of an average group of children of the same age. What are the areas of development screened? (Select all that apply.)

   1. Growth and weight
   2. Personal-social development
   3. Fine motor adaptive development
   4. Language
   5. Gross motor skills
   6. Fine motor skills

6. A teenage mother questions the nurse about why her "newborn baby's head is dented and pointed." The nurse's best response is:
    1. "His head is dented and pointy looking, almost like an eraser."
    2. "This is a normal process and the head shape will return to normal in 6 months."
    3. "The head will return to a normal shape in approximately 1 week. The baby's head is often misshapen because molding occurs during vaginal deliveries."
    4. "He looks deformed. I will get a health care provider to check him immediately."
7. While conducting a newborn assessment, the nurse notes that the newborn baby has a positive Babinski reflex. How does the nurse elicit the Babinski reflex?
    1. By holding the baby upright so the feet touch a flat surface—the legs move up and down as if walking
    2. By touching the side of the cheek, thus causing the baby's head to turn to the touched side
    3. By stroking the sole of the foot and observing the big toe rising and the other toes fanning out
    4. By placing an object just beneath the toes that causes the toes to curl around it
8. While working with a pediatric health care provider, a nurse is often questioned about when to begin toilet training. What is the appropriate response by the nurse that indicates when a toddler is ready for toilet training?
    1. The toddler stands and walks well and recognizes the need for elimination.
    2. The toddler cannot delay elimination consistently.
    3. The toddler is still crawling.
    4. The toddler is 12 months or older.
9. The nurse is caring for an adolescent client. Which statement would encourage the best communication for this age group?
    1. "We need to discuss this situation with your parents."
    2. "Read this article and it will answer all of your questions."
    3. "Watch this cartoon about your problem."
    4. "You are the fifth teenager this week to have these same issues."
10. Parents of a newborn boy insist that their son be circumcised on the 8th day after his birth. This is an example of a cultural religious ritual practiced in Judaism. What should the nurse do regarding the circumcision?
    1. Perform it on the second day of birth per routine orders.
    2. Notify the health care provider of the parents' request and obtain further orders.
    3. Take no action at this time.
    4. Inform the parents that circumcision is not allowed in the United States.

CHAPTER 22

PROMOTING HEALTH IN YOUNG AND MIDDLE-AGED ADULTS

KEY TERM REVIEW

Match each term with its appropriate definition.

1. _______ Baby boomers
2. _______ Boomerang kids
3. _______ Climacteric
4. _______ Generation X
5. _______ Generation Y
6. _______ Generativity
7. _______ Intimacy
8. _______ Maturity
9. _______ Menopause
10. _______ Papanicolaou (Pap) test

a. When menstruation ceases
b. Concern for establishing and guiding the next generation
c. Andropause
d. Born in years 1945–1964
e. Born in years 1965–1978
f. Screening examination of cells from the uterine cervical os
g. Born in years 1979–2000
h. Young adults who move back into their parents' homes after an initial period of independence
i. State of maximal function and integration
j. Very close friendship

KEY TOPIC REVIEW

1. How is adulthood categorized, and what are the age ranges?
2. What three distinct generations are included in adulthood?
   a.
   b.
   c.
3. Health risks for young adults are related to ______ and ______.
4. _____ is the state of maximal function and integration, or the state of being fully developed.
5. _____ is defined as the concern for establishing and guiding the next generation.
6. According to Havighurst, what are four developmental tasks for middle-aged adults?
   a.
   b.
   c.
   d.
7. What are two health threats that begin to affect persons in middle age?
   a.
   b.
8. The mystery of life, of faith, and of belief in God is explored actively by some young adults.
   a. True b. False
9. Erikson's developmental task for the middle adult is ______.
10. What are four psychosocial concerns for young adults?
    a.
    b.
    c.
    d.

FOCUSED STUDY TIPS

1. What are common health problems in young adults?
2. What sexually transmitted infections (STIs) are prevalent among young adults?
3. What is the definition of adulthood? What are the criteria to determine this state?
4. Define the following terms: baby boomers, Generation X, Generation Y, intimacy, maturity.
5. Compare and contrast menopause and andropause.
6. Compare and contrast the various generational groups.

CASE STUDY

1. Mary and Lou are both 29 years old, employed, and have been married for 2 years. Lou has been going out with friends several nights a week to drink alcohol.
   a. What health problem could Lou be at risk for, especially since Mary reported to you that he has been staying out late and arrives home with alcohol on his breath?
   b. How can the nurse help Mary, Lou, and their families in dealing with this concern?
   c. What other resources might help the couple resolve their other issues?

REVIEW QUESTIONS

1. What is the leading cause of death for individuals 1 to 44 years of age?
   1. Suicide
   2. Cancer
   3. STIs
   4. Unintentional injury
2. "Boomerang kids" are young adults who have moved back into their parents' homes. What are the associated factors that influence these moves?
   1. High divorce and unemployment rates
   2. Fear of intimacy
   3. Lack of supervision
   4. Request from parents that the children return
3. Which population group of young adults has the highest incidence of hypertension?
   1. Native American
   2. Hispanic American
   3. African American
   4. Caucasian American
4. While lecturing a group of young male adults, the nurse discusses the most common neoplasm in men ages 20 to 34. What type of cancer is the nurse instructing the group on?
   1. Testicular cancer
   2. Lung cancer
   3. Kidney cancer
   4. Prostate cancer
5. A 47-year-old female states that she is very hot and breaking out in a sweat, has insomnia, and seems to be gaining weight. What should the nurse consider as a contributory cause for the reported symptoms?
   1. Climacteric
   2. Menopause
   3. Breast cancer
   4. Poor diet

6. The nurse is caring for a 46-year-old female complaining of gaining weight. She wants to know why she has trouble losing weight now. What are leading causes of obesity in middle-aged adults?
   1. Decreased physical and metabolic activities
   2. Increase in caloric need
   3. Lack of time to exercise
   4. Unknown at this time
7. During an admission assessment, a client reports that she is very active in civic groups and works at a local homeless soup kitchen. This is an appropriate psychosocial developmental milestone for which group?
   1. Middle-aged adults
   2. Young adults
   3. Older adults
   4. Adolescents
8. What comment would be indicative of a young adult client meeting one of the psychosocial development tasks?
   1. "I go to my parents' house for lunch every day."
   2. "I am headed in the right direction; I am due for a promotion soon."
   3. "I never go out at night. I don't have any friends."
   4. "I never see my family."
9. If a client was born in 1963, which generation would that client be identified with?
   1. Generation X
   2. Generation Y
   3. Baby boomer
   4. Boomerang kid
10. What concept best describes generativity?
    1. The concern for establishing and guiding the next generation
    2. The discrimination against an individual based on the individual's age
    3. The differences of opinion among various generations
    4. The concern for one's own generation
11. What psychosocial developmental concepts are true regarding the middle-aged adult? (Select all that apply.)
    1. The adult is in the generativity versus stagnation phase of Erikson's stage of development.
    2. The adult has leisure activities as a central theme.
    3. The adult moves from the conventional level to the postconventional level according to Kohlberg.
    4. The adult feels the need to achieve adult civic and social responsibility.
    5. The adult is adjusting to aging parents.

CHAPTER 23

PROMOTING HEALTH IN OLDER ADULTS

KEY TERM REVIEW

Match each term with its appropriate definition.

1. _______ Activity theory
2. _______ Adult day care
3. _______ Ageism
4. _______ Alzheimer's disease
5. _______ Assisted living
6. _______ Cataracts
7. _______ Continuity theory
8. _______ Dementia
9. _______ Disengagement theory
10. _______ Dyspnea
11. _______ E-health
12. _______ Geriatrics
13. _______ Gerontology
14. _______ Hypothermia
15. _______ Kyphosis
16. _______ Long-term memory
17. _______ Osteoporosis
18. _______ Pathologic fractures
19. _______ Perception
20. _______ Presbycusis
21. _______ Presbyopia
22. _______ Recent memory
23. _______ Sarcopenia
24. _______ Sensory memory
25. _______ Short-term memory

a. Recent memory
b. Progressive loss of cognitive function
c. Spontaneous fractures
d. Associated with the medical care of older adults
e. Stooping posture
f. Daytime programs that provide health and social services to the older individual who lives at home
g. Lens opacity that impairs vision
h. A condition characterized by progressive dementia, memory loss, inability to care for self
i. Proposes that individuals maintain their values, habits, and behavior in old age
j. Momentary perception of stimuli from the environment
k. Steady decrease in muscle fibers
l. Repository for information stored for periods longer than 72 hours
m. Body temperature below normal
n. Difficulty breathing
o. Used to describe the use of technology in the delivery of health care and health information
p. Activities in the past few minutes to hours
q. The best way to age is to stay active physically and mentally, according to Havighurst
r. Inability to focus due to loss of flexibility of the lens, causing decreased near vision
s. A situation in which older adults who do not feel safe living on their own live in a facility that provides meals, activities, and opportunities for socialization
t. Term used to define the study of aging and older adults

u. Describes negative attitudes toward aging or older adults

v. Loss of hearing ability related to aging

w. Proposes that aging involves mutual withdrawal between older person and others in the older person's environment

x. Ability to interpret the environment

y. A pathologic decrease in bone density

KEY TOPIC REVIEW

1. Why are individuals living longer in today's world?
2. By the mid-21st century in the United States, the ________ ________ population is projected to outnumber ________ individuals.
3. What category of the aging population is the fastest growing of all the age groups in the country?
4. Fill in the correct data in the blanks.
   a. The young-old are ________ to ________ years old.
   b. Old-________ are ________ to ________ years old.
   c. Centenarians are over ________ years old.
5. What are the two new *Healthy People 2020* objectives for older adults?
   a.
   b.
6. Disease is an outcome of aging.
   a. True b. False
7. Ageism is a term that celebrates aging within a population or group.
   a. True b. False
8. Many older adults consider faith, and they display a high level of spirituality.
   a. True b. False
9. ________ is a term used to define the study of aging and older adults. ________ is associated with the medical care of older adults.
10. Describe gerontological nursing. How do gerontological nurses obtain certification? What degrees are needed to practice as a nurse in this field?
11. What is the objective of long-term care facilities? What types of care are included in long-term care facilities?
12. Describe Alzheimer's disease (AD) and explain why specialized units are necessary for patients with AD.
13. What are the three hypotheses of the wear-and-tear theory of aging?
    a.
    b.
    c.

FOCUSED STUDY TIPS

1. What are the physical changes to the integumentary system associated with aging?
2. What are the physical changes to the gastrointestinal system associated with aging?
3. What are positive health practices that can promote health and wellness for all adults?
4. What are the common biologic theories of aging? Which one do you agree with and why?

5. Review health problems associated with the older adults and list those concerns.

6. Differentiate between presbycusis and presbyopia. What are some nursing interventions that may be implemented when caring for clients with these conditions?

7. Describe how the normal aging process may affect the older adult's nutritional status. What are some nursing interventions that promote adequate nutrition in the older adult?

CASE STUDY

1. A retired 90-year-old client lives alone in a rural town. Her children live in various states nearby and lead busy lives. The client insists that she is satisfied with her life. The church that she attends drives her to and from services and her friends visit her daily. Her children believe that their mother is depressed and needs medication, so they take her to a geriatric nurse practitioner.

   a. What age category of the aging population is this client currently in?

   b. What is the myth of aging that the client's children are subscribing to? What is the reality?

   c. According to Erikson, what developmental task occurs at this phase?

REVIEW QUESTIONS

1. An 84-year-old client complains of reduced visual acuity and the presence of glaring around objects. On physical exam, the nurse notices lens opacity. What is the term for this common vision disturbance in the older adult?

   1. Presbyopia
   2. Cataracts
   3. Glaucoma
   4. Presbycusis

2. Identify the normal findings of an older adult client's cardiovascular system. (Select all that apply.)

   1. The working capacity of the heart diminishes with age.
   2. The heart rate at rest may increase with age.
   3. The response of the heart rate is slower when responding to stressors.
   4. Arterial elasticity is reduced.
   5. The client may have orthostatic hypotension whenever he or she stands up suddenly.

3. The client reports that she attends a knitting class at the senior citizen center at least three times a week. What psychosocial aging theory would explain this activity?

   1. Continuity theory
   2. Activity theory
   3. Disengagement theory
   4. Growth and developmental theory

4. A caregiver for a client with Alzheimer's disease states that she has to attend a conference in another state. She requests information about how arrangements could be made for her mother's care during that time. What place could the nurse suggest?

   1. Nursing home
   2. Assisted living facility
   3. Adult day care
   4. Home health care

5. What is the leading cause of morbidity and mortality among older adult clients?
   1. Motor vehicle crashes
   2. Drownings
   3. Falls
   4. Homicides
6. What is the largest-growing population in the United States today?
   1. Newborns
   2. Adolescents
   3. Middle-aged adults
   4. Older adults
7. Based on your knowledge of older adult mistreatment, which of the following statements are true? (Select all that apply.)
   1. It may affect either gender equally.
   2. The abuse may involve physical, psychological, or emotional abuse.
   3. Older adults may be beaten and raped by family members or health care workers.
   4. Older adult abuse rarely occurs in private settings.
8. The nurse is planning health care interventions for an older adult client who has a nursing diagnosis of "risk for constipation related to complete bed rest/administration of pain medication/sedatives." Which of the following is the priority nursing intervention?
   1. Include adequate roughage and liquids in the diet.
   2. Assess risk factors for older adult abuse.
   3. Obtain weight of the client daily.
   4. Keep side rails of the client's bed up at all times.
9. What does the endocrine theory of aging propose?
   1. The faster an organism lives, the quicker it dies.
   2. An organism is genetically programmed for a predetermined number of cell divisions, and then the cells die.
   3. The immune system declines with age.
   4. The hypothalamus and pituitary are responsible for changes in hormone production and response, then the organism's decline.
10. While caring for an older adult client with osteoporosis, the nurse is instructing the client and family on fall prevention measures to take at home. Which measures should the nurse include? (Select all that apply.)
    1. Remove throw rugs.
    2. Wear sturdy, rubber-soled shoes.
    3. Place safety bars in the bathroom.
    4. Remove all carpet and keep floors waxed.
    5. Change position slowly to prevent orthostatic hypotension.

CHAPTER 24

PROMOTING FAMILY HEALTH

KEY TERM REVIEW

Match each term with its appropriate definition.

1. _______ Ecomap
2. _______ Extended family
3. _______ Family
4. _______ Family-centered nursing
5. _______ Genogram
6. _______ Nuclear family

a. A basic unit of society
b. Family structure of parents and their offspring
c. Nursing that considers the health of the family unit in addition to the health of the individual family members
d. Relatives of the nuclear family
e. Provides visual representation of how the family unit interacts with the external community
f. Visual representations of gender and lines of birth descent through the generations

KEY TOPIC REVIEW

1. The _________ is a basic unit of society.
2. A _________ is a set of interacting, identifiable parts or components.
3. Nurses are increasingly using _________ _________ to understand not only biological systems but also systems in families, communities, and nursing and health care.
4. What is the purpose of a family assessment?
5. One of the greatest stressors on a two-career family is _________ _________ _________.
6. Employment of a ___________ will help the nurse visualize how all family members are genetically related to each other and to grasp how patterns of chronic conditions are present within a family unit.
7. Of all types of households, about _________ million are single-parent families, and this number continues to increase; _________ million of these families are headed by women and _________ million by men.
8. Describe four stressors of single parenthood:

   a.

   b.

   c.

   d.
9. _________ is the mechanism by which some of the output of a system is returned to the system as input.
10. The _________ _________ focuses on family structure and function. The structural component of the theory addresses the membership of the family and the relationships among family members.

FOCUSED STUDY TIPS

1. Define, compare, and contrast the following terms: nuclear family, extended family, traditional family.
2. Discuss how family communications influence families. What happens when that communication does not correctly flow among family members?
3. The incidence of family violence has increased in recent years. What factors have influenced this increase?
4. How do sociologic factors and poverty influence the different types of families?
5. Review the various theories used when dealing with family health.
6. Define cohabiting families. What are the reasons for cohabiting?

CASE STUDY

1. A client presents to the emergency department with injuries that are suspiciously related to common patterns of physical abuse. The client reports that she "fell down several stairs while going to the basement." The client's husband is present and seems unwilling to leave the client's bedside.
   a. What would be the best interventions by the nurse in this situation?
   b. What should the nurse be observing during the interactions between herself, the client, and the spouse?

REVIEW QUESTIONS

1. A nurse is reviewing data gathered from a family assessment. The single mother of two children has been treated several times for drug overdose and has a history of substance abuse. What nursing diagnoses would be appropriate for this family based on this information? (Select all that apply.)
   1. *Interrupted Family Processes*
   2. *Readiness for Enhanced Family Coping*
   3. *Impaired Parenting*
   4. *Caregiver Role Strain*
2. The client has a history of diabetes in her family as identified by a detailed nursing health history. This data is identified as what type of risk for health problems?
   1. Maturity factors
   2. Hereditary factors
   3. Gender or race factors
   4. Lifestyle factors
3. In an effort to try to minimize or prevent the causes of some diseases and disabilities, the nurse is instructing a client on the need for exercise, stress management, and rest. On which area is the nurse focusing his or her instruction?
   1. Maturity factors
   2. Hereditary factors
   3. Gender or race factors
   4. Lifestyle factors
4. A 6-year-old client has been living with her grandparents. The client's parents are unable to care for the client because of substance abuse. What type of family unit does this client belong to?
   1. Foster family
   2. Traditional family

   3. Intragenerational family
   4. Cohabiting family

5. Which concept is assessed when the nurse is observing the ways the family expresses affection, love, sorrow, and anger?
   1. Family structure
   2. Physical health status
   3. Interaction patterns
   4. Family roles and functions

6. Which concept is assessed when the nurse is evaluating how the family members handle stressful situations and conflicting goals?
   1. Coping resources
   2. Family values
   3. Interaction patterns
   4. Family roles and functions

7. What are the late manifestations of family violence?
   1. Depression, alcohol and substance abuse, and suicide attempts
   2. Burns, cuts, fractures, and death
   3. Alcohol and substance abuse and fractures
   4. No differentiation from early manifestations

8. The nurse who is committed to family-centered care will do which of the following while caring for a client who is being treated for cancer?
   1. Ensure that the client understands the disease and treatment, leaving details out to avoid upsetting the client.
   2. Ensure that the client and family members understand the disease, treatment, and other matters related to the diagnosis of cancer.
   3. Ensure assessment of how the radiation treatments are affecting the client's skin.
   4. Ensure that the primary care provider understands how the treatment is affecting the family unit.

9. Who does the nurse evaluate when planning health care for family care?
   1. Family and community
   2. Individual and family
   3. Communities, political values, and families
   4. Families, individuals, and community

10. The school nurse promotes health of the entire family by presenting what type of programs to the third-grade students? (Select all that apply.)
    1. Hand washing to prevent infection
    2. Impact of truancy on education
    3. Personal hygiene
    4. Treatment for head lice
    5. Need for maintaining immunization schedule

CHAPTER 25

CARING

KEY TERM REVIEW

Match each term with its appropriate definition.

1. _______ Aesthetic knowing
2. _______ Caring
3. _______ Caring practice
4. _______ Empirical knowing
5. _______ Ethical knowing
6. _______ Personal knowing
7. _______ Reflection

a. Involves connections, mutual recognition, and involvement between nurse and client
b. Moral awareness
c. Creative action
d. Therapeutic use of self
e. People, relationships, and things matter
f. Thinking from a critical point of view
g. Scientific competence

KEY TOPIC REVIEW

1. _________ means that people, relationships, and things matter and is _________ to nursing practice.
2. List the three concepts involved with a caring practice.
   a.
   b.
   c.
3. According to Roach, what are the six C's of caring?
   a.
   b.
   c.
   d.
   e.
   f.

4. A noted philosopher, Melton Mayeroff, proposes that to care for another person is to help him grow and actualize himself.

   a. True b. False

For questions 5–10, match each theorist to the correct perception of "caring" in the nursing process.

5. _________ Caring is the moral ideal of nursing whereby the end is protection, enhancement, and preservation of human dignity. The two individuals in a caring transaction are both in a process of being and becoming.
6. _________ Caring is a nurturing behavior that has been present throughout history and is critical in helping people maintain or regain health.
7. _________ Caring in nursing is contextual and is influenced by the organizational structure.
8. _________ The emphasis is on the nurse knowing self as a caring person. Caring is a lifetime process and respect for persons as caring individuals in nursing is necessary.
9. _________ A nurturing way of relating to a valued "other," toward whom one feels a personal sense of commitment and responsibility.
10. _________ Caring is the human mode of being, or the most common, authentic criterion of humanness. Caring is not unique to nursing.

a. Leininger—theory of cultural care diversity and universality
b. Ray—theory of bureaucratic caring
c. Roach—caring, the human mode of being
d. Boykin and Schoenhofer—nursing as caring
e. Watson—theory of human care
f. Swanson—theory of caring

11. _________ ______________ is the art of nursing and is expressed by the individual nurse through creativity and style in meeting the needs of client.
12. __________ ___________ promotes wholeness and integrity in the personal encounter, achieves engagement rather than detachment, and denies the manipulative or impersonal approach.
13. _________ is thinking from a critical point of view, analyzing why one acted in a certain way and assessing the results of one's actions.
14. Nursing school instructors can teach all nursing students how to care.

    a. True b. False

FOCUSED STUDY TIPS

1. Define the following terms used in caring: caring, caring practice, empirical knowing, ethical knowing, personal knowing.
2. What nursing theory of caring matches your own personal philosophy of caring? Why?
3. Think about your encounters with various nurses in your lifetime. How does the "caring" nurse differ from others? What made you remember that caring nurse?
4. How does caring relate to the concept of professionalism in nursing? Is it possible to have one without the other?

CASE STUDY

1. Mrs. Al Khalifa has been admitted to the hospital after experiencing a stroke. She is unable to support her right arm, so the nurse has applied a sling.
   a. What are two additional interventions the nurse may implement to provide comfort measures?
2. A child who was involved in a motor vehicle crash has been admitted to your unit. The parents and a younger brother of the child passed away as a result of injuries sustained in the crash.
   a. As a student nurse assigned to this client, which of the six C's of caring in nursing do you want to incorporate in your interventions?
   b. If you are using the caring processes from Swanson's theory of caring, on what five processes would you base your nursing interventions for this client?
   c. What type of knowing would you demonstrate if you are observing and documenting phenomena as they occur in this case?

REVIEW QUESTIONS

1. Which nursing theorist developed the theory of culture care diversity and universality that is based on the assumption that nurses must understand different cultures in order to function effectively?
   1. Watson
   2. Miller
   3. Leininger
   4. Swanson
2. When it became apparent that the chaplain might not arrive before the death of a client, the nurse prayed with the dying client who requested a chaplain to visit. This is an example of what type of caring?
   1. Nursing implementation
   2. Empowering the client
   3. Compassion from the nurse
   4. Nursing competence
3. Caring for self means taking time to nurture oneself. What are some ways that a nurse may care for him- or herself? (Select all that apply.)
   1. Eating a balanced diet
   2. Performing regular exercise
   3. Obtaining adequate rest and sleep
   4. Taking medications for sleep as needed
   5. Working part-time shifts
4. The nurse is instructing the client on ways to "self-care" for relief of stress. Identify ways in which the client can lead a healthier lifestyle and carve out enough time to care for herself. (Select all that apply.)
   1. Replace negative affirmations with positive affirmations.
   2. Delay exercising until stress level and job demands have lessened.
   3. Use guided imagery to promote relaxation several times a day.
   4. Begin a yoga class to unite the mind, body, and spirit.

5. Which question made by the nurse best demonstrates personal knowing when reflecting about the death of a client who died after suffering a myocardial infarction (MI)?
   1. "What are my thoughts and emotions?"
   2. "Did I act for the best?"
   3. "What additional information was needed?"
   4. "Why did I respond the way I did to the situation?"
6. A nurse quietly sits with a client who is recovering from a spontaneous abortion. This is an example of what type of caring?
   1. Knowing the client
   2. Nursing presence
   3. Empowerment
   4. Resting
7. While caring for an older client with left-sided paralysis, the nurse strongly encourages the client to participate in her activities of daily living. What type of caring is the nurse displaying?
   1. Knowing the client
   2. Nursing presence
   3. Empowering the client
   4. Compassion
8. The nurse repositions an immobile client every 2 hours. What type of caring is the nurse displaying? (Select all that apply.)
   1. Competence
   2. Caring for self
   3. Spiritual care
   4. Compassionate care
9. The nurse instructs the client on mind–body therapies. Which mind–body therapy is used when the client pictures himself lying on a beach with the sounds of the waves, the cries of the seagull, and the warmth of the sun during periods of stress?
   1. Music therapy
   2. Guided imagery
   3. Yoga
   4. Storytelling
10. The postpartum nurse demonstrates caring by which of the following actions?
    1. Holding and rocking an infant so the mother can rest quietly for a few hours after being up all night
    2. Administering pain medications according to schedule
    3. Enforcing the hospital's visitation hours
    4. Performing the newborn assessment in a timely manner

CHAPTER 26

COMMUNICATING

KEY TERM REVIEW

Match each term with its appropriate definition.

1. __R__ Attentive listening
2. __O__ Boundaries
3. __K__ Bullying
4. __H__ Communication
5. __U__ Congruent communication
6. __B__ Decode
7. __S__ Elderspeak
8. __C__ Electronic communication
9. __n__ E-mail
10. __a__ Emotional intelligence
11. __W__ Empathy
12. __Q__ Encoding
13. __C__ Feedback
14. __T__ Group
15. __F__ Group dynamics
16. __Y__ Helping relationships
17. __P__ Incivility
18. __M__ Lateral violence
19. __D__ Nonverbal communication
20. __i__ Personal space
21. __l__ Process recording
22. __G__ Proxemics
23. __X__ Territoriality
24. __J__ Therapeutic communication
25. __V__ Verbal communication

a. Ability to form work relationships with colleagues, display maturity, and resolve conflicts while taking into consideration the emotions of others

b. To relate the message perceived to the receiver's storehouse of knowledge and experience and to sort out the meaning of the message

c. The response to a message that is sent

d. Uses gestures, facial expressions, and touch

e. Communication that uses technology

f. Communication that takes place in any group

g. The study of distance between people in their interactions

h. The exchange of information among two or more people

i. The distance people prefer in interactions with others

j. Promotes understanding and can help establish a constructive relationship; is client and goal directed

k. Offensive, abusive, intimidating, insulting behavior, which makes the recipient feel, upset, threatened, humiliated, or vulnerable

l. Verbatim account of a conversation

m. Term used to describe physical, verbal, or emotional abuse or aggression directed at RN coworkers at the same organizational level

n. Message sent by computer to another person or group of people

o. Limits in which a person may act or refrain from acting within a designated time or place

p. Rude, discourteous, or disrespectful behavior that reflects a lack of regard for others

q. Selection of specific signs or symbols to transmit the message

r. Listening actively, using all senses

s. Speech style similar to baby talk that gives the message of dependence and incompetence to older adults

t. Two or more people who have shared needs and goals

u. Verbal and nonverbal aspects of the message match

v. Uses spoken or written words

w. The ability to experience, in the present, a situation as another did at some time in the past

x. Concept of space and things that an individual considers as belonging to the self

y. Nurse–client relationships that involve a growth-facilitating process

KEY TOPIC REVIEW

1. Why are good communication skills essential in nursing? Teach and Persuade

2. Which of the following apply to the nonverbal communication process? (Select all that apply.)

   a. Pace and intonation
   b. Adaptability
   c. Personal appearance
   d. Posture
   e. Gestures
   f. Timing and relevance

3. What are three barriers to communication?

   a. Failure to listen
   b. Improper decoding clients message
   c. Placing Nurses Needs above Clients

4. What are four ways in which the nurse can demonstrate the actions of "physical attending" when communicating?

   a. Face Client

   b. Lean in

   c. Eye contact

   d. Relax

5. Which of the following signs are components of genuineness in conversation. (Select all that apply.)

   a. The nurse displays respect.

   b. The nurse displays sympathy.

   c. The client is open and nondefensive.

   d. The client displays honesty.

   e. The nurse assists the client to be specific rather than general.

6. Elderspeak is a speech style similar to baby talk that gives the message of dependence and incompetence and is seen as patronizing by older adults.

7. In Congruent Communication, the verbal and nonverbal aspects of a message match.

8. When seeking clarification during an initial health assessment, what is the best question the nurse could ask?

   a. "Would you tell me more?"

   b. "You smoke one pack of cigarettes a day? Are you trying to kill yourself?"

   c. "Why did you come to the emergency department?"

   d. "What are you saying?"

9. What is the difference between teaching groups and self-help groups?

   Give Info / Share info

FOCUSED STUDY TIPS

1. What is the difference between assertive and nonassertive communication?

2. What are the advantages and disadvantages of electronic communication? When should e-mail not be used in health care?

3. Describe personal space and proxemics. How is communication altered in accordance with the four distances?

4. What are the four phases of helping relationships?

5. How does the situational briefing model work in communication?

CASE STUDY

1. An 18-year-old presents with painful urination and severe back pain. She is pale, running a 38.3°C (101°F) oral temperature, has chills, and is teary eyed. The client states that she has never been to a hospital or health care provider without her mother present.

   a. What could the nurse do in order to create a more positive environment for the health interview?
   Exelain whats going to Happen, Angewer Questions, Openended Questions

   b. If the nurse shares a similar experience with the client, then what communication technique is the nurse using? Empalhetic listening

   c. What are three therapeutic responses the nurse could employ in this situation?
   Give Info, Acknowledge Appeehension, therapeutic touch

REVIEW QUESTIONS

1. The nurse is observing the postsurgical wound of a client who has had abdominal surgery. According to proxemics, what type of distance is the nurse using?
   1. Intimate
   2. Personal
   3. Social
   4. Public

2. While assessing a postoperative client for pain, the nurse notices the client is holding the surgical site and making facial grimaces. However, the client states that she is not hurting. What part of the communication process is incongruent?
   1. Sender
   2. Receiver
   3. Message
   4. Feedback

3. Which example best describes personal distance, according to proxemics?
   1. The nurse who is positioning an immobile client
   2. The nurse who is establishing an intravenous infusion
   3. The nurse who is making rounds on all the clients in the unit
   4. The nurse who is speaking at a conference

4. The nurse makes direct eye contact and has a pleasant expression on her face when changing a client's colostomy bag. The nurse tells the client, "The colostomy looks good." What type of communication is the nurse demonstrating?
   1. Nonverbal communication
   2. Process recoding
   3. Congruent communication
   4. Incongruent communication

5. The nurse is caring for a client with a major mental illness. What action best demonstrates professional boundaries?
   1. Keeping the focus on the client
   2. Sharing personal information with the client
   3. Displaying sympathy toward the client
   4. Encouraging mutual nurse–client goals
6. A client expresses anxiety about a surgical procedure. What would be the most appropriate therapeutic communication technique to use in this situation? (Select all that apply.)
   1. Using open-ended questions
   2. Using closed questions
   3. Restating or paraphrasing comments made by the client
   4. Offering ordered antianxiety medication
   5. Giving common advice
7. In which of the following situations would using the therapeutic communication of "touch" be appropriate?
   1. When a family member is making inappropriate comments to the nurse, touch is appropriate.
   2. Touch is never appropriate in the nursing profession.
   3. When an upset spouse is alone and the client has just expired, touch is appropriate.
   4. When a young healthy male client asks a young student nurse for a hug, touch is appropriate.
8. During the introductory phase of the nurse–client relationship, what type of behavior is the client exhibiting when he states that he will not need assistance with any aspect of his personal care?
   1. Resistant
   2. Introductory
   3. Preinteraction
   4. Trusting
9. The nurse is caring for a client admitted to the hospital due to substance abuse. The nurse and client mutually agree on the overall purpose of the nurse–client relationship. Which phase of the helping relationship is demonstrated?
   1. Preinteraction
   2. Introductory
   3. Working
   4. Termination
10. An older client asks the nurse if she needs to move into an assisted living facility instead of living alone. The nurse responds by telling the client that if the client were his mother, he would tell her to go into the assisted living facility because her meals would be cooked for her and she would not have to clean anything. The nurse is demonstrating what type of barrier to communication?
    1. Stereotyping
    2. Being defensive
    3. Challenging
    4. Giving common advice

CHAPTER 27

TEACHING

KEY TERM REVIEW

Match each term with its appropriate definition.

1. _______ Adherence
2. _______ Affective domain
3. _______ Andragogy
4. _______ Behaviorist theory
5. _______ Cognitive domain
6. _______ Cognitive theory
7. _______ Compliance
8. _______ Geragogy
9. _______ Health literacy
10. _______ Humanistic learning theory
11. _______ Imitation
12. _______ Learning
13. _______ Learning need
14. _______ Modeling
15. _______ Motivation
16. _______ Pedagogy
17. _______ Positive reinforcement
18. _______ Psychomotor domain
19. _______ Readiness
20. _______ Teaching

a. Includes fine and gross motor skills
b. The desire to do something
c. A change in human disposition or capability that persists and cannot be solely accounted for by growth
d. Pleasant experience that fosters repetition of an action
e. A system of activities intended to produce learning
f. Recognize the developmental level of the learner and acknowledge learner's motivation and environment
g. The discipline concerned with helping children learn
h. Demonstration of behaviors or cues that reflect motivation at a specific time
i. The process by which individuals copy or reproduce what they have observed
j. Believes that attitude and responses respond to changes in the stimulus condition or what occurs after the response
k. Includes emotional and social goals
l. Commitment or attachment to a regimen
m. Learning is believed to be self-motivated, self-initiated, and self-evaluated
n. Following through with appropriate behaviors that reflect learning
o. The capacity to obtain, process, and understand basic health information and services needed to make appropriate health decisions
p. Process involved in helping older adults learn
q. The art and science of teaching adults
r. Includes six intellectual abilities and thinking processes
s. A desire or requirement to know something that is presently unknown to the learner
t. The process by which a person learns by observing the behavior of others

KEY TOPIC REVIEW

1. Physiological events such as a critical illness, pain, or sensory deficits inhibit learning.

   a. True b. False

2. Motivation is generally greatest when an individual recognizes a need and believes the need will be met through learning.

   a. True b. False

3. Developmental readiness and individual readiness are key factors associated with cognitive approaches to learning.

   a. True b. False

4. Active learning, such as listening to a lecture or watching a film, does not foster optimal learning.

   a. True b. False

5. Individuals learn best when they believe they are accepted and will not be judged.

   a. True b. False

6. __ - ________ is the application of the Internet and other related technologies in the health care industry to improve the access, efficiency, effectiveness, and quality of clinical and business processes utilized by health care organizations, practitioners, clients, and consumers in an effort to improve the health status of clients.

7. A high level of ____________ resulting in agitation and the inability to focus or concentrate can also inhibit learning.

8. Repetition of key ____________ and facts facilitates retention of newly learned material.

9. A client's learning style may be based on that client's ____________ background.

10. The individual who is not ready to learn is more likely to ____________ the subject or situation.

11. Match the following terms with the correct definition.

a. Teaching	______	The term used to describe the process involved in stimulating and helping elders to learn
b. Learning need	______	A system of activities intended to produce learning
c. Imitation	______	The art and science of teaching adults
d. Motivation	______	A desire or a requirement to know something that is presently unknown to the learner
e. Modeling	______	A change in human disposition or capability that persists and that cannot be solely accounted for by growth
f. Learning	______	A commitment or attachment to a regimen
g. Geragogy	______	The discipline concerned with helping children learn
h. Pedagogy	______	The process by which a person learns by observing the behavior of others
i. Andragogy	______	Means to learn is the desire to learn
j. Adherence	______	The process by which individuals copy or reproduce what they have observed

12. ____________ is the art and science of teaching adults.

13. ____________ depicts learning as a complex cognitive activity.

14. The ____________ domain, the "skill" domain, includes motor skills such as giving an injection.
15. Which guidelines will the nurse adhere to when teaching clients from various ethnic backgrounds? (Select all that apply.)
    a. Obtain teaching materials, pamphlets, and instructions in languages used by clients.
    b. Use visual aids, such as pictures, charts, or diagrams, to communicate meaning.
    c. Invite and encourages questions during teaching.
    d. Use medical terminology during teaching.
16. When a nurse is using demonstration as a teaching strategy, which major type of learning would it be?
    a. Psychomotor
    b. Cognitive
    c. Affective
    d. All types of learning

FOCUSED STUDY TIPS

1. How would a nurse know that a client is ready for patient education?
2. List the seven elements in the nursing history that provide clues to learning needs.
3. Explain computer-assisted instruction (CAI).
4. Discuss the evaluation tools for cognitive learning.
5. Describe all types of learning.
6. Identify the parts of the teaching process that should be documented in the client's chart.

CASE STUDY

1. Melba Whitman is an 86-year-old client who has recently been diagnosed with hypertension. Ms. Whitman's daughter tells you her mother only completed the sixth grade and gets very anxious when learning something new because of her poor reading skills.
    a. How will you be able to determine if Ms. Whitman is ready to learn?
    b. Identify three ways you could facilitate Ms. Whitman's learning.
    c. Describe various teaching aids to help foster Ms. Whitman's learning.

REVIEW QUESTIONS

1. Andragogy is
    1. The process involved in stimulating and helping elders to learn.
    2. The art and science of teaching adults.
    3. The discipline concerned with helping children learn.
    4. The commitment or attachment to a regimen.

2. What is the process by which an individual learns by observing the behavior of others?
   1. Modeling
   2. Imitation
   3. Trial and error
   4. Positive reinforcement
3. Which domain is used when teaching a client how to self-administer insulin?
   1. Sensorimotor
   2. Psychomotor
   3. Cognitive
   4. Affective
4. In which situation would the nurse be applying the humanistic theory?
   1. Encouraging the learner to establish goals and promote self-directed learning
   2. Encouraging a positive teacher–learner relationship
   3. Providing a social, emotional, and physical environment conducive to learning
   4. Selecting multisensory teaching strategies since perception is influenced by the senses
5. When teaching a client about heart disease, the client may need to know the effects of smoking before recognizing the need to stop smoking. In this situation, what factor best facilitates client learning?
   1. Readiness
   2. Active involvement
   3. Motivation
   4. Allotted time
6. Which of the following is a barrier to learning? (Select all that apply.)
   1. Fear
   2. Sensory deficits
   3. Muscle weakness
   4. Chronic illness
   5. Medication use
7. Which of the following client behaviors may cause a nurse to suspect a literacy problem? (Select all that apply.)
   1. The client displays a pattern of compliance.
   2. The client reads the instructions slowly.
   3. The client states that he or she does not know the information presented.
   4. The client displays a pattern of excuses for not reading the instructions.
   5. The client who reads the instructions but cannot explain them in medical terms.

8. Which of the following is a learning outcome for a teaching plan?
   1. The client knows the factors that affect blood sugar level.
   2. The client selects low-fat foods from a menu.
   3. The client knows about cardiac risk factors.
   4. The client understands a low-salt diet.
9. E-health includes all of the following EXCEPT
   1. A client making an online appointment.
   2. E-mail access between the client and health care provider.
   3. Online health information.
   4. C computer-generated billing statement sent to the client's home address.
10. Which of the following is NOT an element in the nursing history that provides clues to learning needs?
    1. Age
    2. Economic factors
    3. Support systems
    4. Sexual orientation
11. What concept was introduced by behavioral theorist Skinner?
    1. Positive reinforcement
    2. Imitation
    3. Modeling
    4. Behaviorism
12. To increase the chance of the client retaining education, what strategies should the nurse implement? (Select all that apply.)
    1. Ask the client to write down the information presented.
    2. Read the information to the client several times.
    3. Provide handouts when instructing the client.
    4. Speak very slow when instructing the client.
    5. Encourage the client to be an active participant in the process.

CHAPTER 28

LEADING, MANAGING, AND DELEGATING

KEY TERM REVIEW

Match each term with its appropriate definition.

1. _______ Accountability
2. _______ Authoritarian leader
3. _______ Autocratic leader
4. _______ Bureaucratic leader
5. _______ Change agents
6. _______ Charismatic leader
7. _______ Democratic leader
8. _______ First-level manager
9. _______ Formal leader
10. _______ Informal leader
11. _______ Laissez-faire leader
12. _______ Manager
13. _______ Middle-level manager
14. _______ Permissive leader
15. _______ Preceptor
16. _______ Productivity
17. _______ Risk management
18. _______ Role model
19. _______ Shared governance
20. _______ Shared leadership
21. _______ Situational leader
22. _______ Top-level managers
23. _______ Transactional leader
24. _______ Transformational leader
25. _______ Upper-level managers

a. Makes decisions for the group
b. Individual who initiates, motivates, and implements change
c. Assumes individuals are capable of making decisions
d. Flexes task and relationship behaviors, considers staff members' abilities
e. Authoritarian leader
f. Selected by the organization
g. Uses incentives to promote loyalty and performance
h. Set goals, make decisions, solve problems
i. Supervise a number of first-level managers
j. Thought to emerge in relation to the challenges that confront the work group
k. Measures effectiveness and efficiency of care
l. Having in place a system to reduce danger to clients and staff
m. Distributes decision making among a group of people
n. Characterized by an emotional relationship between the leader and the group members
o. Establish goals, develop strategic plans
p. Setting the example for others to follow
q. Ability and willingness to assume responsibility for one's actions and to accept the consequences of one's behavior
r. Primary responsibility is to motivate staff to accomplish the organization's goals
s. Laissez-faire leader
t. Relationship in which someone with more experience assists the "new" employee in improving skills and judgments, as well as instilling understanding of the institution's routines, policies, and procedures
u. Fosters independence, individual growth, and change
v. Assumes a hands-off approach, assuming group members are internally motivated
w. Top-level manager
x. Relies on organization's rules, policies, and procedures to direct the group's work efforts
y. Recognized by the group as its leader

KEY TOPIC REVIEW

1. A leader influences others to work together to accomplish a specific goal.

   a. True b. False

2. The informal leader, or appointed leader, is selected by an organization and given official authority to make decisions and take action.

   a. True b. False

3. Theories about leadership style describe traits, behaviors, motivations, and choices used by individuals to effectively influence others.

   a. True b. False

4. An autocratic (authoritarian) leader makes decisions for the group.

   a. True b. False

5. A leader is an employee of an organization who is given authority, power, and responsibility for planning, organizing, coordinating, and directing the work of others, and for establishing and evaluating standards.

   a. True b. False

6. A ____________ leader encourages group discussion and decision making.

7. A ____________ leader recognizes the group's need for autonomy and self-regulation.

8. A ____________ leader does not trust self or others to make decisions and instead relies on the organization's rules, policies, and procedures to direct the group's work efforts.
9. A ____________ leader flexes task and relationship behaviors, considers the staff members' abilities, knows the nature of the task to be done, and is sensitive to the context or environment in which the task takes place.
10. A ____________ leader is rare and is characterized by an emotional relationship with the group members.
11. ____________ involves determining responsibilities, communicating expectations, and establishing the chain of command for authority and communication.
12. ____________ is defined as the legitimate right to direct the work of others.
13. ____________ is a process whereby professional links are established through which people can share ideas, knowledge, and information, offer support and direction to each other, and facilitate accomplishment of professional goals.
14. ____________ is a measure of the resources used in the provision of nursing services.
15. ____________ is the transference of responsibility and authority for an activity to a competent individual.

FOCUSED STUDY TIPS

1. Discuss the classic work of Lewin, who developed a model of change that involves three stages: unfreezing, moving, and refreezing.
2. Compare and contrast authoritarian, democratic, and laissez-faire leadership styles.
3. List several characteristics of effective leaders.
4. Describe the role of the leader/manager in planning for and implementing change.
5. List the five rights of delegation.
6. Describe the characteristics of tasks appropriate to delegate to unlicensed and licensed assistive personnel.
7. Identify the skills and competencies needed by a nurse manager.
8. Discuss the roles and functions of nurse managers.
9. Describe the four functions of management.

CASE STUDY

1. Nathaniel Thomas is a nursing director who influences others to work together to accomplish a specific goal. Mr. Thomas also has initiative and the ability and confidence to innovate change, motivate, facilitate, and mentor others. Mr. Thomas actively guides the group toward achieving group goals and assumes that individuals are internally motivated and capable of making decisions, and Mr. Thomas values their independence.
   a. Is Mr. Thomas assuming the role of a leader or manager?
   b. Compare and contrast the role of a leader and manager.
   c. What particular leadership style has Mr. Thomas developed?

REVIEW QUESTIONS

1. A nurse is planning a seminar on leadership styles. Which of the following statements describes a democratic leadership style?
   1. The leader assumes a "hands-off" approach.
   2. Under this leadership style, the group may feel secure because procedures are well defined and activities are predictable.
   3. This leadership style demands that the leader have faith in the group members to accomplish the goals.
   4. This leadership style does not trust self or others to make decisions and instead relies on the organization's rules, policies, and procedures to direct the group's work efforts.
2. A nursing director who fosters creativity, risk taking, commitment, and collaboration by empowering the group to share in the organization's vision is which type of leader?
   1. Charismatic
   2. Transactional
   3. Transformational
   4. Shared
3. The organizational executives who are primarily responsible for establishing goals and developing strategic plans are considered to be
   1. First-level managers.
   2. Middle-level managers.
   3. Upper-level managers.
   4. Supervising managers.
4. The nursing director who has the ability and willingness to assume responsibility for one's actions and to accept the consequences of one's behavior is demonstrating what management principle?
   1. Accountability
   2. Authority
   3. Responsibility
   4. Coordinating
5. The type of change that is an intended, purposeful attempt by an individual, group, organization, or larger social system to influence its own current status is referred to as
   1. Natural.
   2. Situational.
   3. Unplanned.
   4. Planned.
6. A nurse is planning a seminar on the comparison of leader and manager roles. Which of the following characteristics describes a leader role?
   1. Influences others toward goal setting, either formally or informally.
   2. Maintains an orderly, controlled, rational, and equitable structure.
   3. Relates to people according to their roles.
   4. Feels rewarded when fulfilling the organizational mission or goals.

7. Which role is the nurse assuming when initiating, motivating, and implementing change?
   1. Advocate
   2. Change agent
   3. Teacher
   4. Change role model
8. Which of the following is considered a driving force?
   1. Low tolerance for change related to intellectual or emotional insecurity
   2. Misunderstanding of the change and its implications
   3. Perception that the change will improve the situation
   4. Lack of time or energy
9. A nurse is planning a seminar on guidelines for dealing with resistance to change. Which of the following would NOT be an appropriate guideline for dealing with resistance to change?
   1. Clarify information and provide accurate information.
   2. Explain the positive and negative consequences of the change and how the individual or group will get the change done.
   3. Maintain a climate of trust, support, and confidence.
   4. Communicate with those who oppose the change. Get to the root of their reasons for opposition.
10. Which actions are true of a situational leader? (Select all that apply.)
    1. Flexes task and relationship behaviors.
    2. Considers the staff members' abilities.
    3. Knows the nature of the task to be done.
    4. Is sensitive to the context or environment in which the task takes place.
    5. Has a relationship with followers based on an exchange for some resource valued by the follower.

CHAPTER 29

VITAL SIGNS

KEY TERM REVIEW

Match each term with its appropriate definition.

1. _______ Apical pulse
2. _______ Apnea
3. _______ Arterial bloodpressure
4. _______ Bradycardia
5. _______ Bradypnea
6. _______ Cardiac output
7. _______ Compliance
8. _______ Diastolic pressure
9. _______ Dysrhythmia
10. _______ Expiration
11. _______ Hyperpyrexia
12. _______ Hypotension
13. _______ Hypoventilation
14. _______ Inspiration
15. _______ Orthostatic hypotension
16. _______ Oxygen satura-tion (SaO_2)
17. _______ Peripheral pulse
18. _______ Point of maximal impulse (PMI)
19. _______ Pulse deficit
20. _______ Pulse pressure
21. _______ Respiration
22. _______ Systolic pressure
23. _______ Tachycardia
24. _______ Tachypnea
25. _______ Ventilation

a. The movement of air in and out of the lungs

b. Measure of the pressure exerted by the blood as it flows through the arteries

c. Volume of blood pumped into the arteries by the heart

d. Intake of air into the lungs

e. A very high fever

f. Pressure when the ventricles are at rest

g. A central pulse

h. The percentage of all hemoglobin binding sites that are occupied by oxygen

i. Absence of breathing

j. Excessively fast heart rate

k. Act of breathing out air from the lungs

l. The ability of arteries to contract and expand

m. A heart rate in an adult less than 60 beats/min

n. Abnormally slow respirations

o. The pressure of the blood as a result of the contraction of the ventricles

p. Abnormally fast respirations

q. The act of breathing

r. Very shallow respirations

s. A blood pressure that falls when the client sits or stands

t. Any discrepancy between the apical and radial pulses

u. A pulse located away from the heart

v. Abnormal cardiac rhythm

w. A blood pressure that is below normal

x. The difference between the diastolic and systolic blood pressures

y. The location where the cardiac impulse can be best palpated on the chest wall.

KEY TOPIC REVIEW

1. Core temperature reflects the balance between the heat produced and the heat lost from the body, and is measured in heat units called degrees.

   a. True   b. False

2. Surface temperature is the temperature of the skin, the subcutaneous tissue, and fat.

   a. True   b. False

3. Cardiac output is the volume of blood pumped into the arteries by the heart and equals the result of the stroke volume (SV) times the heart rate (HR) per minute.

   a. True   b. False

4. The apical pulse is a pulse located away from the heart, for example, in the foot or wrist.

   a. True   b. False

5. Body temperature is the temperature of the deep tissues of the body, such as the abdominal cavity and pelvic cavity.

   a. True   b. False

6. Diastolic pressure is the pressure of the blood as a result of the contraction of the ventricles.

   a. True   b. False

7. ____________ are body temperature, pulse, respirations, and blood pressure.

8. Heat ____________ is a result of excessive heat and dehydration.

9. ____________ of the arteries is their ability to contract and expand.

10. A pulse ____________ is any discrepancy between the two pulse rates.

11. ____________ is a core body temperature below the lower limit of normal.

12. Match the following terms with the correct definition.

a. Radiation	______	When the amount of heat produced by the body equals the amount of heat lost
b. Conduction	______	The rate of energy utilization in the body required to maintain essential activities such as breathing
c. Convection	______	The transfer of heat from the surface of one object to the surface of another without contact between the two objects, mostly in the form of infrared rays
d. Pulse volume	______	The dispersion of heat by air currents
e. Basal metabolic rate (BMR)	______	When a wide range of temperature fluctuations (more than 2°C [3.6°F]) occurs over a 24-hour period, all of which are above normal
f. Tachycardia	______	A wave of blood created by contraction of the left ventricle of the heart
g. Pulse	______	An excessively fast heart rate.
h. Remittent fever	______	Also called the pulse strength or amplitude, refers to the force of blood with each beat
i. Heat balance	______	The transfer of heat from one molecule to a molecule of lower temperature

13. ____________ is the act of breathing.

a. Inhalation

b. Exhalation

c. Ventilation

d. Respiration

14. ____________ is the absence of breathing.

a. Bradypnea

b. Apnea

c. Tachypnea

d. Polypnea

15. ____________ refers to very deep, rapid respirations.

a. Hypoventilation

b. Respiratory rhythm

c. Hyperventilation

d. Respiratory quality/character

16. ____________ pressure is the pressure when the ventricles are at rest.

a. Diastolic

b. Arterial blood

c. Systolic

d. Pulse

17. ____________ is a blood pressure that is persistently above normal.

    a. Hypotension

    b. Orthostatic hypotension

    c. Hypertension

    d. Pulse oximeter

FOCUSED STUDY TIPS

1. List and explain the various vital signs.
2. Identify when it is appropriate to delegate measurement of vital signs to unlicensed assistive personnel.
3. Discuss measurement of blood oxygenation using pulse oximetry.
4. Describe methods and sites used to measure blood pressure.
5. Describe five phases of Korotkoff's sounds.
6. Differentiate systolic from diastolic blood pressure.
7. Identify the components of a respiratory assessment.
8. Describe the mechanics of breathing and the mechanisms that control respirations.
9. Explain how to measure the apical pulse and the apical-radial pulse.
10. List the characteristics that should be included when assessing pulses.
11. Identify nine sites used to assess the pulse and state the reasons for their use.
12. Describe appropriate nursing care for alterations in body temperature.
13. Compare methods of measuring body temperature.
14. Identify the variations in normal body temperature, pulse, respirations, and blood pressure that occur from infancy to old age.
15. Describe factors that affect the vital signs and accurate measurement of them.
16. Differentiate between ventilation and respiration.

CASE STUDY

A 20-year-old client is brought into the clinic with complaints of fever, chills, and fatigue. His vital signs upon admission are BP 120/70 mmHg, P 116 beats/min, RR 20/min, T (oral) 38.9°C (102.1°F). His mother reports that his temperature rises to fever level rapidly and then returns to normal within a few hours. The doctor who examines him orders blood work.

1. What are the normal vital signs for a 20-year-old male client?
2. What type of fever is the client most likely experiencing?
3. Why has the doctor ordered blood work?

REVIEW QUESTIONS

1. Conduction is:
    1. the transfer of heat from one molecule to a molecule of lower temperature.
    2. the transfer of heat from the surface of one object to the surface of another without contact between the two objects, mostly in the form of infrared rays.
    3. the continuous evaporation of moisture from the respiratory tract and from the mucosa of the mouth and from the skin.
    4. the dispersion of heat by air currents.
2. Which type of fever is a client experiencing when the body temperature alternates at regular intervals between periods of fever and periods of normal or subnormal temperatures?
    1. Intermittent
    2. Remittent
    3. Relapsing
    4. Constant
3. A client reports that he has been exercising in hot weather; he feels warm, is flushed, and is not sweating. His temperature is 41°C (106°F) and he just experienced a seizure. What condition is the client most likely experiencing?
    1. Hypothermia
    2. Heat exhaustion
    3. Heatstroke
    4. Hypertension
4. The body temperature is measured in degrees on two scales: Celsius (centigrade) and Fahrenheit. When the Celsius reading is 40, the Fahrenheit reading is:
    1. 100.
    2. 101.
    3. 103.
    4. 104.
5. The posterior tibial pulse site is on the medial surface of the ankle where the posterior tibial artery passes behind the:
    1. medial malleolus.
    2. knee.
    3. inguinal ligament.
    4. wrist.
6. Which of the following can cause an erroneously low blood pressure result?
    1. Cuff wrapped too loosely or unevenly
    2. Bladder cuff too narrow
    3. Arm above level of the heart
    4. Assessing immediately after a meal or while client smokes or has pain

7. Which of the following actions by a nurse would be incorrect when taking an adult's temperature using a tympanic thermometer?
   1. Inserting the probe slowly using a circular motion until snug
   2. Pointing the probe slightly anteriorly, toward the eardrum
   3. Pulling the pinna straight back and upward
   4. Not inserting the tympanic thermometer into the client's ear when cerumen is present
8. A nurse is evaluating a nursing student's understanding of altered breathing patterns and sounds. Which of the following statements demonstrates a need for further teaching?
   1. Stertor is a snoring or sonorous respiration, usually due to a partial obstruction of the upper airway.
   2. A wheeze is a continuous, high-pitched musical squeak or whistling sound occurring on expiration and sometimes on inspiration when air moves through a narrowed or partially obstructed airway.
   3. Bubbling is a gurgling sound heard as air passes through moist secretions in the respiratory tract.
   4. Stridor is difficult and labored breathing during which the individual has a persistent, unsatisfied need for air and feels distressed.
9. A nurse is planning a seminar on secretions and coughing. Which of the following describes a condition in which blood is present in the sputum?
   1. Hemoptysis
   2. Productive cough
   3. Nonproductive cough
   4. Orthopnea
10. A nurse is evaluating a nursing student's understanding of Korotkoff's sounds. Which of the following statements demonstrates a need for further teaching?
    1. Phase 1 is the pressure level at which the first faint, clear tapping or thumping sounds are heard. These sounds gradually become more intense.
    2. Phase 2 is the period during deflation when the sounds have a muffled, whooshing, or swishing quality.
    3. Phase 4 is the time when the sounds become muffled and have a soft, blowing quality.
    4. Phase 5 is the first tapping sound heard during deflation of the cuff and is the systolic blood pressure.

CHAPTER 30

HEALTH ASSESSMENT

KEY TERM REVIEW

Match each term with its appropriate definition.

1. _______ Angle of Louis
2. _______ Aphasia
3. _______ Astigmatism
4. _______ Bruit
5. _______ Cataracts
6. _______ Conductive hearing loss
7. _______ Cyanosis
8. _______ Diastole
9. _______ Erythema
10. _______ Exophthalmos
11. _______ Fasciculation
12. _______ Fremitus
13. _______ Glaucoma
14. _______ Miosis
15. _______ Mixed hearing loss
16. _______ Mydriasis
17. _______ Nystagmus
18. _______ Pallor
19. _______ Percussion
20. _______ Precordium
21. _______ Resonance
22. _______ Sensorineural hearing loss
23. _______ Stereognosis
24. _______ Systole
25. _______ Thrill

a. Result of inadequate circulating blood and subsequent reduction in tissue oxygen

b. An uneven curvature of the cornea

c. Combination of conduction and sensorineural loss

d. Rapid involuntary rhythmic eye movement

e. A vibrating sensation like the purring of a cat or water running through a hose

f. Skin redness

g. Protrusion of the eyeballs with elevation of the upper eyelids

h. A bluish tinge

i. Hollow sound elicited by percussion

j. Opacity of the lens or its capsule

k. The junction between the body of the sternum and the manubrium

l. Period in which the ventricles contract

m. An abnormal contraction of a bundle of muscle fibers that appears as a twitch

n. The act of recognizing objects by touching and manipulating them

o. Results from damage to the inner ear, auditory nerve, or the hearing center of the brain

p. Result of interrupted transmission of sound waves through the outer and middle ear structures

q. Constricted pupils

r. A blowing or swishing sound

s. A disturbance in the circulation of aqueous fluid, which increases intraocular pressure

t. Any defect in or loss of the power to express oneself by speech, writing, or signs, or to comprehend spoken or written language

u. The act of striking the body surface to elicit sounds or vibrations

v. Period in which the ventricle relaxes

w. Faintly perceptible vibration

x. Enlarged pupils

y. Area of the chest overlaying the heart

KEY TOPIC REVIEW

1. Inspection is the visual examination—that is, assessing by using the sense of sight.

   a. True b. False

2. Percussion is the examination of the body using the sense of touch.

   a. True b. False

3. The middle finger of the nondominant hand is referred to as the pleximeter.

   a. True b. False

4. Tympany is a musical or drumlike sound produced from an air-filled stomach.

   a. True b. False

5. Palpation is the act of striking the body surface to elicit sounds that can be heard or vibrations that can be felt.

   a. True b. False

6. ______ is a sound created by turbulence of blood flow due to either a narrowed arterial lumen or a condition, such as anemia or hyperthyroidism, that elevates cardiac output.

7. Any defects in or loss of the power to express oneself by speech, writing, or signs, or to comprehend spoken or written language due to disease or injury of the cerebral cortex is called _______.

8. A _______ is an automatic response of the body to a stimulus.

9. A ______ is a protrusion of the intestine through the inguinal wall or canal.

10. ______ is the ability to sense whether one or two areas of the skin are being stimulated by pressure.

11. Match the following terms with the correct definitions.

a. Hyperopia	______	The process of listening to sounds produced within the body
b. Otoscope	______	Nearsightedness
c. Cerumen	______	Loss of elasticity of the lens and thus loss of ability to see close objects
d. Astigmatism	______	An uneven curvature of the cornea that prevents horizontal and vertical rays from focusing on the retina; is a common problem that may occur in conjunction with myopia and hyperopia
e. Eustachian tube	______	A disturbance in the circulation of aqueous fluid, which causes an increase in intraocular pressure; is the most frequent cause of blindness in people over age 40
f. Glaucoma	______	Constricted pupils that may indicate an inflammation of the iris or result from such drugs as morphine or pilocarpine
g. Miosis	______	An instrument for examining the interior of the ear, especially the eardrum, consisting essentially of a magnifying lens and a light
h. Myopia	______	A part of the middle ear that connects the middle ear to the nasopharynx
i. Auscultation	______	Earwax that lubricates and protects the canal
j. Presbyopia	______	Farsightedness

12. ______ is an extremely dull sound produced by very dense tissue, such as muscle or bone.

    a. Dullness
    b. Flatness
    c. Resonance
    d. Hyperresonance

13. ______ refers to the loudness or softness of a sound.

    a. Pitch
    b. Quality
    c. Duration
    d. Intensity

14. ______ is the result of inadequate circulating blood or hemoglobin and subsequent reduction in tissue oxygenation.

    a. Cyanosis
    b. Erythema
    c. Jaundice
    d. Pallor

15. ______ is the presence of excess interstitial fluid.

a. Vitiligo
b. Alopecia
c. Edema
d. Clubbing

16. ______ is what a normal head size is referred to.

a. Exophthalmos
b. Visual acuity
c. Normocephalic
d. Visual fields

FOCUSED STUDY TIPS

1. Define dullness, flatness, and resonance.
2. List the common refractive errors of the lens of the eye.
3. Explain the process of air-conducted transmission of sound.
4. Define thrill and bruit.
5. Describe common inflammatory visual problems.
6. Identify the client positions that are frequently required during the physical assessment.
7. Define clubbing and describe two clinical examples of when clubbing may be present.
8. Discuss variations in examination techniques appropriate for clients of different ages.
9. Describe suggested sequencing to conduct a physical health examination in an orderly fashion.
10. Identify the steps in selected examination procedures.
11. Identify expected outcomes of health assessment.
12. Explain the significance of alterations in normal skin color. Describe two clinical examples when this may occur.
13. Explain the four methods used in physical examination.
14. Identify the purposes of the physical examination.
15. Summarize auscultated sounds that are described according to their pitch, intensity, duration, and quality.

CASE STUDY

1. A nursing student is preparing for her clinical rotation at a clinic. She has been told that she will be responsible for preparing clients for physical examinations.
   a. Discuss the purposes of the physical examination.
   b. Several client positions are frequently required during the physical assessment. List six client positions used during the physical assessment and provide a description of each one.
   c. List the equipment and supplies used for a health examination.

REVIEW QUESTIONS

1. A client asks the nurse "What is the purpose of a physical examination?" What is the nurse's best response? (Select all that apply.)
   1. "To obtain data at any given time about a client's functional abilities."
   2. "To obtain data that will help establish nursing diagnoses and plans of care."
   3. "To identify areas for health promotion and disease prevention."
   4. "To supplement, confirm, or refute data obtained in the nursing history."
   5. "To implement appropriate, individualized care."
2. Auscultation is the:
   1. Visual examination—that is, assessing by using the sense of sight.
   2. Examination of the body using the sense of touch.
   3. Act of striking the body surface to elicit sounds that can be heard or vibrations that can be felt.
   4. Process of listening to sounds produced within the body.
3. Jaundice is:
   1. The result of inadequate circulating blood or hemoglobin and a subsequent reduction in tissue oxygenation.
   2. A bluish tinge and is most evident in the nail beds, lips, and buccal mucosa.
   3. A yellowish tinge that may first be evident in the sclera of the eyes and then in the mucous membranes and the skin.
   4. A redness associated with a variety of rashes.
4. Which of the following terms means nearsightedness?
   1. Myopia
   2. Hyperopia
   3. Presbyopia
   4. Astigmatism
5. A nurse is evaluating a nursing student's understanding of the air-conducted sound transmission process. Which of the following statements demonstrates a need for further teaching?
   1. A sound stimulus enters the external canal and reaches the tympanic membrane.
   2. The sound waves vibrate the tragus and reach the ossicles.
   3. The sound waves travel from the ossicles to the opening in the inner ear (oval window).
   4. The cochlea receives the sound vibrations.

6. A nurse is planning a seminar on the organs in the nine abdominal regions. Which of the following information is incorrect?
   1. The epigastric region includes the aorta, the pyloric end of the stomach, part of the duodenum, and the pancreas.
   2. The umbilical region includes the omentum, the mesentery, the lower part of the duodenum, and part of the jejunum and ileum.
   3. The right lumbar region includes the ascending colon, the lower half of the right kidney, and part of the duodenum and jejunum.
   4. The left lumbar region includes the stomach, the spleen, the tail of the pancreas, the splenic flexure of the colon, the upper half of the left kidney, and the suprarenal gland.
7. A nurse is evaluating a nursing student's understanding of cranial nerves. Which of the following statements demonstrates a need for further teaching?
   1. Cranial nerve I is assessed by asking the client to close his or her eyes and identify different mild aromas, such as coffee, vanilla, peanut butter, orange/lemon, or chocolate.
   2. Cranial nerve IV is assessed by asking the client to read a Snellen-type chart.
   3. Cranial nerve VI is assessed by observing the client's directions of gaze.
   4. Cranial nerve VII is assessed by asking the client to smile, raise the eyebrows, frown, puff out cheeks, close eyes tightly.
8. Which adventitious breath sound is a superficial grating or creaking sound heard during inspiration and expiration?
   1. Friction rub
   2. Crackles
   3. Wheeze
   4. Gurgles
9. A nurse is preparing to complete a physical examination on a client's pelvis and vagina. The position the client is placed in for this examination is:
   1. Prone.
   2. Supine.
   3. Lithotomy.
   4. Sitting.
10. Which of the following actions is most correct for the nurse assessing a client who has just had a cast applied to the lower leg?
    1. Assess tissue turgor, fluid intake and output, and vital signs.
    2. Assess peripheral perfusion of toes, capillary blanch test, pedal pulse if able, and vital signs.
    3. Assess apical pulse and compare with baseline data.
    4. Assess level of consciousness using Glasgow Coma Scale; assess pupils for reaction to light and accommodation; assess vital signs.

CHAPTER 31

ASEPSIS

KEY TERM REVIEW

Match each term with its appropriate definition

1. S Acquired immunity
2. N Active immunity
3. A Antibodies
4. B Antigen
5. V Asepsis
6. F Bacteremia
7. H Cell-mediated defenses
8. I Cellular immunity
9. E Circulating immunity
10. C Exudate
11. J Granulation tissue
12. K Humoral immunity
13. M Immunoglobulins
14. Y Leukocytosis
15. W Local infection
16. O Medical asepsis
17. P Nosocomial infections
18. Q Passive immunity
19. R Resident flora
20. G Sepsis
21. L Septicemia
22. T Sterile technique
23. D Sterilization
24. U Surgical asepsis
25. X Virulence

a. Part of body's plasma proteins, produced by B cell

b. Substance that induces a state of sensitivity or immunity

c. Consisting of fluid that escaped from the blood vessels, dead phagocytic cells, and dead tissue cells and products that they release

d. Process that destroys all microorganisms, including spores and viruses

e. Host receives natural or artificial antibodies from another source

f. Condition in which microorganisms are found in a person's blood

g. The state of infection

h. On exposure to an antigen, the lymphoid tissues release large numbers of activated T cells into the lymph system

i. Cell-mediated defenses

j. A fragile gelatinous tissue, appearing pink or red

k. Also known as circulating immunity

l. When bacteremia results in a systemic infection

m. Antibodies

n. Host produces antibodies in response to natural or artificial antigens

o. Includes all practices intended to confine a specific microorganism to a specific area

p. Infections that originate in the hospital

q. Also known as acquired immunity

r. Normal bacteria in one part of the body, yet produce infection in another

s. Immunity a newborn baby is born with

t. Surgical asepsis

u. Practices that keep an area or object free of all microorganisms

v. Freedom from disease-causing microorganisms

w. Limited to the specific part of the body where the microorganisms remain

x. Ability to produce diseases

y. The production and release of large numbers of leukocytes into the bloodstream

KEY TOPIC REVIEW

1. A disease is an invasion of body tissue by microorganisms and their growth within that tissue.

   a. True　　b. False

2. Virulence is the ability to produce disease.

   a. True　　b. False

3. Pathogenicity is the ability to produce disease; thus a pathogen is a microorganism that causes disease.

   a. True　　b. False

4. Surgical asepsis, or sterile technique, includes all practices intended to confine a specific microorganism to a specific area, limiting the number, growth, and transmission of microorganisms.

   a. True　　b. False

5. Sepsis is a state of infection and can take many forms, including septic shock.

   a. True　　b. False

6. If the infectious agent can be transmitted to an individual by direct or indirect contact or as an airborne infection, the resulting condition is called a ______ disease. Communicable

7. A(An) ______ pathogen causes disease only in a susceptible individual. Opportunistic

8. ______ is the freedom from disease-causing microorganisms. Asepsis

9. Bacteria are by far the most common infection-causing microorganisms.

10. In medical asepsis, objects are considered clean or Dirty

11. Match the following terms with the correct definition.

Term	Answer	Definition
a. Vehicle	J	Consist primarily of nucleic acid and therefore must enter living cells in order to reproduce
b. Iatrogenic infections	H	Include yeasts and molds
c. Compromised host	F	Live on other living organisms
d. Colonization	D	The process by which strains of microorganisms become resident flora
e. Nonspecific defenses	B	The direct result of diagnostic or therapeutic procedures
f. Parasites	I	A person or animal reservoir of a specific infectious agent that usually does not manifest any clinical signs of disease
g. Vector	A	Any substance that serves as an intermediate means to transport and introduces an infectious agent into a susceptible host through a suitable portal of entry
h. Fungi	G	An animal or flying or crawling insect that serves as an intermediate means of transporting the infectious agent
i. Carrier	C	A person at increased risk, an individual who for one or more reasons is more likely than others to acquire an infection
j. Viruses	E	Protect the person against all microorganisms, regardless of prior exposure

12. ______ is limited to the specific part of the body where the microorganisms remain.

a. Bacteremia

b. Systemic infection

c. Septicemia

(d) Local infection

13. ______ infections are classified as infections that are associated with the delivery of health care services in a health care facility.

a. Acute

(b) Nosocomial

c. Chronic

d. Endogenous

14. ______ is a local and nonspecific defensive response of the tissues to an injurious or infectious agent.

a. Hyperemia

b. Leukocytes

(c) Inflammation

d. Leukocytosis

15. ______ is the replacement of destroyed tissue cells by cells that are identical or similar in structure and function.

a. Regeneration

b. Antigen

c. Immunity

d. Antibodies

16. ______ are agents that inhibit the growth of some microorganisms.

a. Sterilization

b. Antiseptics

c. Airborne precautions

d. Disinfectants

FOCUSED STUDY TIPS

1. Discuss the relationship between hygiene, rest, activity, and nutrition in the chain of infection.
2. Discuss the use of antimicrobial soaps and effective disinfectants.
3. Describe the steps to take in the event of a bloodborne pathogen exposure.
4. Explain aseptic practices, including hand washing; donning and removing a face mask, gown, and disposable gloves; managing equipment used for isolation clients; and maintaining a sterile field.
5. Compare and contrast category-specific, disease-specific, universal, body substance, standard, and transmission-based isolation precaution systems.
6. Identify measures that break each link in the chain of infection.
7. Identify interventions used to reduce risks for infection.
8. Identify relevant nursing diagnoses and contributing factors for clients at risk for infection, and for clients who have an infection.
9. Identify signs of localized and systemic infections.
10. Identify factors influencing a microorganism's capability to produce an infectious process.
11. Differentiate active from passive immunity.
12. Identify anatomic and physiologic barriers that defend the body against microorganisms.
13. Identify risks for nosocomial infections.
14. Explain the concepts of medical and surgical asepsis.
15. Define virulence. What is its relationship to infection?
16. Describe variances in immunity across the life span.

CASE STUDY

1. Brent is a new nursing student. You will be his preceptor for the next 3 days. On the first day, Brent asks you the following questions:
   a. What is the difference between asepsis and sepsis, and between medical asepsis and surgical asepsis?
   b. What four major categories of microorganisms cause infection in humans?
   c. Explain the difference between standard precautions and transmission-based precautions.

REVIEW QUESTIONS

1. Which of the following means freedom from disease-causing microorganisms?
   1. Medical asepsis
   2. Asepsis
   3. Surgical asepsis
   4. Sepsis
2. Which of the following consists primarily of nucleic acid and therefore must enter living cells in order to reproduce?
   1. Fungi
   2. Bacteria
   3. Viruses
   4. Parasites
3. Inflammation is a local and nonspecific defensive response of the tissues to an injurious or infectious agent. Which of the following is NOT a sign of inflammation?
   1. Pain
   2. Swelling
   3. Redness
   4. Fatigue
4. Four commonly used methods of sterilization are moist heat, gas, boiling water, and radiation. Which of the following is the most practical and inexpensive method for sterilizing in the home?
   1. Gas
   2. Moist heat
   3. Radiation
   4. Boiling water
5. A nurse is evaluating a nursing student's understanding of the various types of infections. Which of the following statements demonstrates a need for further teaching?
   1. A local infection is limited to the specific part of the body where the microorganisms remain.
   2. If the microorganisms spread and damage different parts of the body, it is a systemic infection.
   3. Acute infections may occur slowly, over a very long period, and may last months or years.
   4. Nosocomial infections are classified as infections that are associated with the delivery of health care services in a health care facility.

6. A nurse is planning a seminar on the chain of infection. Which of the following is NOT one of the six links?
   1. Etiologic agent
   2. Reservoir
   3. Hand hygiene
   4. Mode of transmission
7. An antigen is a:
   1. Host that produces antibodies in response to natural antigens (e.g., infectious microorganisms) or artificial antigens (e.g., vaccines).
   2. Substance that induces a state of sensitivity or immune responsiveness (immunity).
   3. Host that receives natural (e.g., from a nursing mother) or artificial (e.g., from an injection of immune serum) antibodies produced by another source.
   4. Part of the body's plasma proteins.
8. The CDC recommends antimicrobial hand cleansing agents in all of the following situations EXCEPT:
   1. When there are unknown multiple nonresistant bacteria.
   2. Before invasive procedures.
   3. In special care units, such as nurseries and ICUs.
   4. Before caring for severely immunocompromised clients.
9. Which of the following statements about disinfectants is incorrect?
   1. A disinfectant is a chemical preparation, such as a phenol or iodine compound, used on inanimate objects.
   2. Disinfectants are frequently caustic and toxic to tissues.
   3. Disinfectants and antiseptics often have similar chemical components, but the disinfectant is a less concentrated solution.
   4. A disinfectant is an agent that destroys pathogens other than spores.
10. Which types of precautions are used for clients known or suspected to have serious illnesses transmitted by particle droplets larger than 5 microns?
    1. Airborne
    2. Droplet
    3. Contact
    4. Connection

CHAPTER 32

SAFETY

KEY TERM REVIEW

Match each term with its appropriate definition.

1. _______ Asphyxiation
2. _______ Bioterrorism
3. _______ Burn
4. _______ Carbon monoxide
5. _______ Chemical restraints
6. _______ Electric shock
7. _______ Heimlich maneuver
8. _______ Physical restraints
9. _______ Restraints
10. _______ Safety monitoring devices
11. _______ Scald
12. _______ Seizure
13. _______ Seizure precautions

a. Medications used to control socially disruptive behavior

b. Any manual method or physical or mechanical device attached to the client's body that restricts movement

c. Occurs when a current travels through the body to the ground rather than through electric wiring

d. Safety measures taken to protect clients from injury should they have a seizure

e. Procedure that can dislodge foreign objects lodged in the throat

f. Used to detect when clients are attempting to move or get out of bed

g. Suffocation

h. A burn from a hot liquid or vapor

i. Results from excessive exposure to thermal, electric, chemical, or radioactive agents

j. A single temporary event that consists of uncontrolled electrical neuronal discharge of the brain resulting in an interruption of normal brain function

k. The use of biologic agents as a weapon that poses a pathogenic risk to a large number of people, and poses a risk to national security

l. An odorless, colorless, tasteless gas that is very toxic

m. Protective devices used to limit the physical activity of the client or a part of the body

KEY TOPIC REVIEW

1. Individuals with impaired touch perception, hearing, taste, smell, and vision are highly susceptible to injury.
   a. True b. False
2. Restraints are used for staff convenience or client punishment.
   a. True b. False
3. The universal sign of distress is the victim's grasping the anterior neck and being unable to speak or cough.
   a. True b. False
4. Generalized seizures (also called focal) involve electrical discharges from one area of the brain.
   a. True b. False
5. People of any age can fall, but infants and elders are particularly prone to falling and causing serious injury.
   a. True b. False
6. ______ can include chemical, biological, or nuclear weapons.
7. Suicide and ______ are two leading causes of death among teenagers.
8. A ______ is a burn from a hot liquid or vapor, such as steam.
9. ______ injury can occur from overexposure to radioactive materials used in diagnostic and therapeutic procedures.
10. ______ assessment tools are available to determine clients at risk both for specific kinds of injury, such as falls, or for the general safety of the home and health care setting.
11. Match the following terms with the correct definition.

Term		Definition
a. Seizure	______	An intentional attack using weapons of viruses, bacteria, and other infectious agents
b. Asphyxiation	______	A bed or chair ______ has a position-sensitive switch that triggers an audio alarm when the client attempts to get out of the bed or chair
c. Electric shock	______	A sudden onset of excessive electrical discharges in one or more areas of the brain
d. Chemical restraints	______	Safety measures taken by the nurse to protect clients from injury should they have a seizure
e. Restraints	______	An odorless, colorless, tasteless gas that is very toxic
f. Safety monitoring device	______	Suffocation, or ______, is lack of oxygen due to interrupted breathing
g. Heimlich maneuver	______	The emergency response is the ______, or abdominal thrust, which can dislodge the foreign object and reestablish an airway
h. Bioterrorism	______	Protective devices used to limit the physical activity of the client or a part of the body
i. Seizure precautions	______	Occurs when a current travels through the body to the ground rather than through electric wiring, or from static electricity that builds up on the body
j. Carbon monoxide (CO)	______	Medications such as neuroleptics, anxiolytics, sedatives, and psychotropic agents used to control socially disruptive behavior

12. Which of the following is NOT a type of restraint?

    a. Jacket

    b. Mitt

    c. Foot

    d. Limb

13. ______ restraints are any manual method or physical or mechanical device, material, or equipment attached to the client's body; they cannot be removed easily and they restrict the client's movement.

    a. Chemical

    b. Physical

    c. Medical

    d. Standard

14. Health care organizations are now expected to address which of the four specific phases of disaster planning?

    a. Preparedness

    b. Recovery

    c. Response

    d. Migration

15. Which of the following is NOT a basic firearm safety rule?

    a. Store the bullets in a different location from the guns.

    b. Ensure the firearm is unloaded and the action is open when handing it to someone else.

    c. Tell children never to touch a gun or stay in a friend's house where a gun is accessible.

    d. Have firearms that are regularly used inspected by a qualified gunsmith at least every 5 years.

16. Excessive noise is a health hazard that can cause hearing loss, depending on all of the following EXCEPT:

    a. The overall level of noise.

    b. The frequency range of the noise.

    c. The individual family history.

    d. The duration of exposure.

FOCUSED STUDY TIPS

1. How is excessive noise a health hazard?
2. List the types of restraints.
3. Explain how to promote safety across the life span.
4. Discuss the factors affecting safety.
5. Describe the five criteria a nurse should use when selecting a restraint.
6. Identify the four sequential priorities a nurse should follow during a fire.
7. Summarize the legal implications of restraints.

8. Compare and contrast a scald and a burn.

9. Define electric shock.

10. Recall the common home hazards causing scalds.

11. Discuss risk factors and preventive measures for falls.

12. Describe alternatives to restraints.

13. Explain the home hazard appraisal.

14. Define seizure and seizure precautions.

15. List the 2014 National Patient Safety Goals.

16. Describe the key risk factors for suicide among older adults.

CASE STUDY

1. A couple just purchased a new home last week. During your assessment, the couple tells you they do not have a fire plan, fire extinguishers, carbon monoxide alarms, or working smoke alarms in their home.
   a. What preventive measures do you need to teach the couple?
   b. Explain the three categories of fires.

REVIEW QUESTIONS

1. According to the 2014 National Patient Safety Goals (NPSGs), what are the ways to improve accuracy of patient information? (Select all that apply.)
   1. Use at least two patient identifiers when providing care, treatment, and services.
   2. Report critical results of tests and diagnostic procedures on a timely basis.
   3. Eliminate transfusion errors related to patient misidentification.
   4. Maintain and communicate accurate patient medication information.
   5. Label all medications, medication containers, and other solutions on and off the sterile field in perioperative and other procedural settings.
2. When evaluating a parent's understanding of safety measures for an infant, which of the following statements indicates a need for further teaching?
   1. "I will store all household chemicals in the garage."
   2. "I will make sure my infant is in his car seat before starting the car."
   3. "I will keep small crafting beads locked in the cabinet."
   4. "I will keep the trash bags in the kitchen on the bottom shelf by the sink."
3. A nurse planning a safety instruction class for parents of adolescents knows that the focus of the class should be on:
   1. Teaching adolescents to sleep on a low bed.
   2. Teaching adolescents about driver safety.
   3. Teaching adolescents not to ingest lead paint chips.
   4. Teaching adolescents not to run or ride a tricycle into the street.

4. Suicide and homicide are two leading causes of death among teenagers. When planning a workshop on adolescent suicide and homicide, the nurse knows that which of the following is NOT among the most common factors influencing the high suicide and homicide rates?

   1. Economic deprivation
   2. Strong emotions toward friendships
   3. Availability of firearms
   4. Family breakup

5. A nurse teaching a safety class for parents identifies the main causes of death for school-age children. Which of the following is NOT one of the leading causes?

   1. Natural disasters
   2. Fires
   3. Drownings
   4. Firearms

6. When planning a safety in-service program for an independent living community for older adults, the nurse will include information on which of the following as the leading causes of injury among older adults? (Select all that apply.)

   1. Firearms
   2. Drownings
   3. Suicide
   4. Falls
   5. Natural disasters

7. Which of the following actions by the nurse indicates that the nurse needs further instruction on the nursing assessment prior to applying restraints on a client?

   1. The nurse checks the status of skin to which a restraint is to be applied.
   2. The nurse checks the circulatory status proximal to restraints.
   3. The nurse takes consideration of other protective measures that may be implemented before applying a restraint.
   4. The nurse determines underlying cause for assessed behavior.

8. When evaluating a parent's understanding of poisoning prevention, which of the following statements indicates a need for further teaching?

   1. "We'll store toxic liquids or solids in food containers, such as soft drink bottles, peanut butter jars, or milk cartons."
   2. "We'll display the phone number of the poison control center near or on all telephones in our home so that it is available to babysitters, family, and friends."
   3. "We'll teach our children never to eat any part of an unknown plant or mushroom and not to put leaves, stems, bark, seeds, nuts, or berries from any plant into their mouths."
   4. "We'll not refer to medicine as candy or pretend false enjoyment when taking medications in front of our children."

9. A nurse who is planning care for a client requiring seizure precautions should plan to include which of the following?
    1. Provide education to the client and family regarding the need to wear a medical identification tag.
    2. Assist the client in alerting all persons in the community about their seizure disorder.
    3. Provide education regarding safety precautions for inside of the home only.
    4. Discuss with the client, family, and persons in the community factors that may precipitate a seizure.
10. Which of the following would NOT be a preventive measure for an older client with poor vision?
    1. Ensure eyeglasses are functional.
    2. Ensure appropriate lighting.
    3. Mark doorways only.
    4. Keep the environment tidy.

CHAPTER 33

HYGIENE

KEY TERM REVIEW

Match each term with its appropriate definition.

1. _______ Alopecia
2. _______ Apocrine glands
3. _______ Bactericidal
4. _______ Callus
5. _______ Cerumen
6. _______ Cleansing baths
7. _______ Corn
8. _______ Dandruff
9. _______ Dental caries
10. _______ Eccrine glands
11. _______ Fissures
12. _______ Gingiva
13. _______ Gingivitis
14. _______ Hirsutism
15. _______ Hygiene
16. _______ Ingrown toenail
17. _______ Lanugo
18. _______ Pediculosis
19. _______ Periodontal disease
20. _______ Plaque
21. _______ Plantar warts
22. _______ Pyorrhea
23. _______ Scabies
24. _______ Sebum
25. _______ Sudoriferous glands

a. Advanced periodontal disease with loose teeth; pus expresses when gums are pressed

b. Appears as a diffuse scaling of the scalp

c. Growth of excessive body hair

d. Sweat glands located in the axillae and anogenital areas; they begin to function at puberty

e. Given chiefly for hygiene purposes

f. Parasitic insects that infest mammals

g. Characterized by a lesion that is short, wavy, brown or black, threadlike

h. A keratosis caused by friction and pressure from a shoe, usually on a bony prominence

i. Growth of nail into the lateral corners of the nail bed

j. Produce sweat that cools body through evaporation

k. Oily substance secreted by the skin that softens and lubricates the hair and skin

l. Gums

m. Bacteria killing

n. Deep grooves

o. Red, swollen gums

p. Science of health and its maintenance

q. Invisible soft film that adheres to the enamel surface of teeth

r. Appear on sole of the foot, caused by papovavirus hominis

s. Earwax

t. Fine hair on the body of the fetus

u. Thickened portion of epidermis

v. Cavities

w. Characterized by gingivitis, bleeding, formation of pockets between teeth and gums

x. Produce sweat from almost all body surfaces

y. Hair loss

KEY TOPIC REVIEW

1. A dry mouth can be aggravated by poor fluid intake, heavy smoking, alcohol use, high salt intake, anxiety, and many medications.

   a. True b. False

2. Most dentists recommend that dental hygiene should begin after the fifth tooth erupts.

   a. True b. False

3. Fluoride toothpaste is often recommended because of its antibacterial protection.

   a. True b. False

4. An initial dental visit for a child should be at about 2 or 3 years of age, as soon as all 20 primary teeth have erupted.

   a. True b. False

5. Water used for the shampoo should be 46.1°C (115°F) for an adult or child to be comfortable and not injure the scalp.

   a. True b. False

6. ______ is the condition of infestation of lice.

7. ______ is a contagious skin infestation by the itch mite.

8. The growth of excessive body hair is called ______.

9. ______ is the fine hair on the body of the fetus, also referred to as *down* or *woolly hair*.

10. ______ is an *invisible* soft film that adheres to the enamel surface of teeth; it consists of bacteria, molecules of saliva, and remnants of epithelial cells and leukocytes.

11. Match the following terms with the correct definition.

a. Tinea pedis	______	Personal ______ is the self-care by which people attend to such functions as bathing, toileting, general body hygiene, and grooming
b. Ingrown toe nail	______	Are on all body surfaces except the lips and parts of the genitals
c. Therapeutic baths	______	The ______, located largely in the axillae and anogenital areas, begin to function at puberty under the influence of androgens.
d. Apocrine glands	______	Given for physical effects, such as to soothe irritated skin or to treat an area (e.g., the perineum)
e. Callus	______	Thickened portion of epidermis, a mass of keratotic material
f. Fissures	______	A keratosis caused by friction and pressure from a shoe
g. Tartar	______	Deep grooves that frequently occur between the toes as a result of dryness and cracking of the skin
h. Hygiene	______	Athlete's foot, or ______ (ringworm of the foot), is caused by a fungus
i. Sudoriferous (sweat) glands	______	The growing inward of the nail into the soft tissues around it; most often results from improper nail trimming
j. Corn	______	A visible, hard deposit of plaque and dead bacteria that forms at the gum lines

12. ______ tends to cling to clothing, so that when a client undresses, the lice may not be in evidence on the body; these lice suck blood from the person and lay their eggs on the clothing.

    a. *Pediculus corporis*

    b. *Pediculus pubis*

    c. *Pediculus capitis*

    d. Scabies

13. Dry mouth, also called ______, occurs when the supply of saliva is reduced.

    a. Xeroma

    b. Xerostomia

    c. Xerosis

    d. Xerotic

14. Dental caries occur frequently during the ______ period, often as a result of the excessive intake of sweets or a prolonged use of the bottle during naps and at bedtime.

    a. Infant

    b. Toddler

    c. School-age

    d. Newborn

15. ______ are usually conical (circular and raised).

    a. Plantar warts
    b. Calluses
    c. Corns
    d. Fissures

16. The ______ is the most widely used type because it fits snugly behind the ear. The hearing aid case, which holds the microphone, amplifier, and receiver, is attached to the earmold by a plastic tube.

    a. In-the-canal (ITC) aid
    b. Body hearing aid
    c. Behind-the-ear (BTE, or postaural) aid
    d. In-the-ear aid (ITE, or intra-aural)

FOCUSED STUDY TIPS

1. What is the proper way to make a hospital bed?
2. List the six different types of baths that could be given to a client.
3. Explain the factors affecting client hygiene practices.
4. Discuss the importance of brushing and combing a client's hair.
5. Describe *Pediculus capitis*, *Pediculus corporis*, and *Pediculus pubis*.
6. Identify the diseases that ticks can transmit.
7. Summarize a variety of ways to shampoo a client's hair.
8. Compare and contrast sudoriferous glands, eccrine glands, and apocrine glands.
9. Define plaque, tartar, and gingivitis.
10. List the elements of contact lens care.
11. Discuss eyeglass care.
12. Describe general hearing aid care.
13. Explain how to insert a contact lens.
14. Define dental caries and periodontal disease.
15. Describe a method of correct dental hygiene.

CASE STUDY

1. You are assigned to give a bath to an 83-year-old man who has cognitive problems.
   a. What is the proper water temperature for the client's bath?
   b. List two reasons why a nurse should check the temperature of the bath water.
   c. Why is it important to verify the temperature of the water for this client?

REVIEW QUESTIONS

1. A nurse is making the client's bed. Which of the following actions should the nurse perform? (Select all that apply.)
   1. Hold the soiled linen close to his or her uniform to conserve energy.
   2. Avoid shaking soiled linen in the air because shaking can disseminate secretions and excretions and the microorganisms they contain.
   3. When stripping and making a bed, conserve time and energy by stripping and making up one side as much as possible before working on the other side.
   4. Place the clean linens on another client's bed if needed, in order to strip the client's dirty linens.
   5. Raise the bed to a comfortable working height when stripping and making the bed.
2. What is the correct bath water temperature for an adult client?
   1. 110°F to 125°F
   2. 90°F to 100°F
   3. 100°F to 115°F
   4. 125°F to 135°F
3. The parent of a toddler is cleaning the child's teeth. Which of the following statements indicates a need for further teaching?
   1. "I'll brush my child's teeth with a hard toothbrush."
   2. "I'll give a fluoride supplement daily or as recommended by the physician or dentist, unless the drinking water is fluoridated."
   3. "I'll schedule an initial dental visit for my child at about 2 or 3 years of age or as soon as all 20 primary teeth have erupted."
   4. "I'll seek professional dental attention for any problems such as discoloring of the teeth, chipping, or signs of infection such as redness and swelling."
4. During discharge planning, the nurse is teaching a client how to prevent dry skin. Which of the following statements by the client indicates the need for further teaching?
   1. "Bathe using soap or detergent only."
   2. "Use bath oils, but take precautions to prevent falls caused by slippery tub surfaces."
   3. "Humidify the air with a humidifier or by keeping a tub or sink full of water."
   4. "Use moisturizing or emollient creams that contain lanolin, petroleum jelly, or cocoa butter to retain skin moisture."

5. When providing foot care for a client, the nurse would perform which of the following?
   1. When washing, inspect the skin of the feet for breaks or red or swollen areas.
   2. Do not cover the feet and between the toes with creams or lotions to moisten the skin.
   3. Do not check the water temperature before immersing the feet.
   4. Wash the feet every other day, and dry them well, especially between the toes.
6. A nurse is evaluating a client's understanding of nail hygiene. Which of the following statements indicates a need for further teaching?
   1. "I should have clean, short nails with smooth edges."
   2. "I should have intact cuticles."
   3. "I will avoid trimming or digging into nails at the lateral corners."
   4. "I'll cut or file around the end of the fingernail or toenail."
7. A nurse is evaluating a client's understanding of dental care. Which of the following statements indicates a need for further teaching?
   1. Brush the teeth thoroughly after meals and at bedtime.
   2. Floss the teeth daily.
   3. Avoid sweet foods and drinks between meals.
   4. Have a checkup by a dentist every year.
8. A male client is having his facial hair shaved with a razor. Which action by the student nurse is NOT correct?
   1. The student nurse holds the skin taut, particularly around creases, to prevent cutting the skin.
   2. The student nurse wears gloves in case facial nicks occur and she comes in contact with blood.
   3. The student nurse applies shaving cream or soap and water to soften the bristles and make the skin more pliable.
   4. The student nurse holds the razor so that the blade is at a 90° angle to the skin, and shaves in short, firm strokes in the direction of hair growth.
9. Which of the following actions is NOT appropriate for the nurse bathing a person with dementia?
   1. Move quickly and let the person know when you are going to move him or her.
   2. Use a supportive, calm approach and praise the person often.
   3. Gather everything that you will need for the bath (e.g., towels, washcloths, clothes) before approaching the person.
   4. Help the person feel in control.
10. The nurse needs to insert a hearing aid into a client's ear. Which of the following actions is NOT correct?
    1. Determine from the client if the earmold is for the left or the right ear.
    2. Gently press the earmold into the ear while rotating it forward.
    3. Inspect the earmold to identify the ear canal portion.
    4. Check that the earmold fits snugly by asking the client if it feels secure and comfortable.

CHAPTER 34

DIAGNOSTIC TESTING

KEY TERM REVIEW

Match each term with its appropriate definition.

1. _______ Abdominal paracentesis
2. _______ Angiography
3. _______ Anoscopy
4. _______ Arterial blood gases
5. _______ Blood urea nitrogen (BUN)
6. _______ Colonoscopy
7. _______ Computed to mography (CT)
8. _______ Creatinine
9. _______ Cystoscopy
10. _______ Echocardiogram
11. _______ Electrocardiogram (ECG)
12. _______ Guaiac test
13. _______ Hemoglobin A_{1C} (HbA_{1C})
14. _______ Intravenous pyelography (IVP)
15. _______ Lumbar puncture
16. _______ Magnetic resonance imaging (MRI)
17. _______ Occult blood
18. _______ Peak level
19. _______ Positive emission tomography (PET)
20. _______ Proctoscopy
21. _______ Retrograde pyelography
22. _______ Serum osmolality
23. _______ Stress electrocardiography
24. _______ Thoracentesis
25. _______ Trough level

a. A test for occult blood

b. A procedure performed to obtain a specimen of cerebrospinal fluid through a needle inserted into the subarachnoid space of the spinal canal

c. Procedure during which the bladder, ureteral orifices, and urethra can be directly visualized

d. Viewing of the large intestine

e. Uses ECGs to assess the client's response to an increased cardiac workload during exercise

f. A measure of the solute concentration of the blood used to evaluate fluid balance

g. Radiographic studies used to evaluate the urinary tract during which contrast medium is instilled directly into the renal pelvis via the urethra, bladder, and ureters

h. A radiopaque dye is injected into the vessels to be examined, and flow through the vessels is assessed and areas of narrowing or blockage can be observed

i. Produced by the muscles, excreted by the kidneys, and related to renal excretory function

j. Viewing of the rectum

k. A noninvasive test that uses ultrasound to visualize structures of the heart and evaluate left ventricular function

l. Indicates the highest concentration of a drug in the blood serum

m. Measurement of blood glucose that is bound to hemoglobin; is a reflection of how well blood glucose levels have been controlled during the prior 3 to 4 months

n. A noninvasive radiologic study that involves injection or inhalation of a radioisotope

o. Procedure used to remove excess fluid or air to ease breathing

p. Hidden blood; a test performed on stool

q. The recorded waveforms of the electrical impulses of the heart to detect dysrhythmias and alterations in conduction

r. Measurement of the end product of protein metabolism

s. A painless, noninvasive x-ray procedure that produces a three-dimensional image of the organ or structure; has the capability of distinguishing minor differences in the density of tissues

t. Radiographic studies used to evaluate the urinary tract during which contrast medium is injected intravenously

u. Procedure during which ascites is removed for laboratory study from the abdominal cavity to relieve pressure or obtain a fluid specimen

v. Taking of arterial blood specimen from the radial, brachial, or femoral artery

w. Viewing of the anal canal

x. Noninvasive diagnostic scanning technique in which the client is placed in a magnetic field

y. Represents the lowest concentration of a drug in the blood serum

KEY TOPIC REVIEW

1. Prior to radiologic studies, it is important to ask female clients if pregnancy is possible.

   a. True b. False

2. Blood tests are one of the most commonly used diagnostic tests and can provide valuable information about the hematologic system and many other body systems.

   a. True b. False

3. Elevated RBC counts are indicative of anemia.

   a. True b. False

4. The leukocyte or white blood cell (WBC) count determines the number of circulating WBCs per cubic millimeter of whole blood.

   a. True b. False

5. Serum electrolytes are often routinely ordered for any client admitted to a hospital as a screening test for electrolyte and acid–base imbalances.

   a. True b. False

6. Sputum and throat culture specimens help determine the presence of disease-producing ______.

7. A liver ______ is a short procedure, generally performed at the client's bedside, in which a sample of liver tissue is aspirated.

8. During a lumbar puncture, the physician frequently takes CSF pressure readings using a ______, a glass or plastic tube calibrated in millimeters.

9. ______ is the withdrawal of fluid that has abnormally collected (e.g., pleural cavity, abdominal cavity) or to obtain a specimen (e.g., cerebral spinal fluid).

10. ______ is the concentration of RBCs in the blood, expressed as a percentage (%).

11. Match the following terms with the correct definitions.

a. Phlebotomist	______	A person from a laboratory who performs venipuncture to collect a blood specimen for tests ordered by a physician
b. Complete blood count (CBC)	______	The number of RBCs per cubic millimeter of whole blood
c. Hemoglobin	______	The main intracellular protein of erythrocytes
d. Hematocrit	______	Produced in relatively constant quantities by the muscles and is excreted by the kidneys
e. Red blood cell (RBC) count	______	Substance used in a chemical reaction to detect a specific substance
f. Creatinine	______	A measure of the solute concentration of urine and a more exact measurement of urine concentration than specific gravity
g. Serum osmolality	______	An indicator of urine concentration, or the amount of solutes (metabolic wastes and electrolytes) present in the urine
h. Reagent	______	A measure of the solute concentration of the blood
i. Urine osmolality	______	Measures the percentage of red blood cells in the total blood volume
j. Specific gravity	______	Includes hemoglobin and hematocrit measurements, erythrocyte (RBC) count, leukocyte (WBC) count, red blood cell (RBC) indices, and a differential white cell count

12. ______ are basic elements in the blood that promote coagulation.

a. Hemoglobin

b. Neutrophils

c. Platelets

d. Leukocytes

13. Which of the following is the viewing of the rectum and sigmoid colon?

a. Proctosigmoidoscopy

b. Anoscopy

c. Proctoscopy

d. Sigmoidoscopy

14. ______ is a noninvasive test that uses ultrasound to visualize structures of the heart and evaluate left ventricular function.

a. Angiography

b. Echocardiogram

c. Electrocardiography

d. Electrocardiogram

15. ______ is a painless, noninvasive x-ray procedure that has the unique capability of distinguishing minor differences in the density of tissues.

    a. Magnetic resonance imaging

    b. Positron emission tomography

    c. Aspiration

    d. Computed tomography

16. The ______, a person from a laboratory who performs venipuncture, collects a blood specimen for tests ordered by a physician.

    a. Venipuncturist

    b. Erotologist

    c. Phlebotomist

    d. Physician

FOCUSED STUDY TIPS

1. Discuss some of the environments in which diagnostic testing occurs.
2. Give some examples of aspiration/biopsy tests.
3. Explain some of the reasons/tests for which nurses collect urine specimens.
4. Discuss the three phases of diagnostic testing.
5. What are some of the nursing responsibilities associated with specimen collection?
6. List several blood chemistry tests that may be performed on blood serum (the liquid portion of the blood).
7. Summarize the measurement of arterial blood gases as an important diagnostic procedure.
8. Discuss what occult blood is and how it is tested for.
9. Discuss some tests performed and the purpose for timed urine specimens.
10. List some examples of indirect and direct visualization procedures.
11. Discuss how to collect a stool specimen correctly.
12. What is a clean-catch or midstream voided specimen?
13. Explain what may cause inaccurate test results.
14. List and describe several of the different urine tests.
15. List some examples of aspiration/biopsy tests.

CASE STUDY

1. A 73-year-old female was brought into the hospital by her son. The son tells you, "My mother has lost weight and has been having night sweats. She is also spitting up blood." The health care provider orders the client to have three sputum samples for acid-fast bacillus (AFB).
   a. Why did the health care provider order sputum specimens?
   b. How will you collect the sputum specimens?
   c. What PPE should you wear when you collect the sputum specimens?
   d. What information should you document in the client medical record after collecting the sputum specimens?
   e. How should the specimens be stored until they are transported to the laboratory?

REVIEW QUESTIONS

1. The nurse is assessing an admitted female client's serum laboratory values. Which of the following is abnormal and should be reported immediately?
   1. Hemoglobin 13 g/dL
   2. RBC 5.1 million/mm^3
   3. Hematocrit 25%
   4. MCV 102 μm^3
2. Which serum laboratory value is abnormal and would require the nurse to report immediately?
   1. Sodium 137 mEq/L
   2. Potassium 2.5 mEq/L
   3. Chloride 97 mEq/L
   4. Magnesium 1.9 mEq/L
3. The nurse assessing a client's serum laboratory values recognizes that the normal hematocrit level for an adult male is:
   1. 37%–49%.
   2. 13%–18%.
   3. 13.8–18 g/dL.
   4. 37–49 g/dL.
4. Which technique is NOT correct when collecting a urine specimen for culture and sensitivity by clean catch?
   1. Explain to the client that a urine specimen is required, give the reason, and explain the method to be used to collect it.
   2. Perform hand hygiene and observe other appropriate infection control procedures.
   3. Explain to female clients that a circular motion should be used to clean the urinary meatus.
   4. Ensure that the specimen label is attached to the specimen cup, not the lid, and that the laboratory requisition provides the correct information.

5. Which of the following is the correct position for a client during a bone marrow biopsy?
   1. Knee–chest
   2. Prone
   3. Lithotomy
   4. Dorsal recumbent
6. Which is the correct position for a client after a lumbar puncture?
   1. Knee–chest
   2. Prone
   3. Lithotomy
   4. Dorsal recumbent
7. After a client returns from a thoracentesis, the nurse should have the client lie on the unaffected side with the head of the bed elevated ______ degrees for at least 30 minutes.
   1. 10
   2. 15
   3. 30
   4. 90
8. Which of the following situations during an abdominal paracentesis is correct?
   1. The maximum amount of fluid, 1,500 mL, was drained at one time.
   2. The fluid was drained at several time intervals.
   3. The fluid was drained quickly.
   4. Sterile technique is not necessary.
9. The nurse is providing patient education about a fecal occult blood test. Which of the following statements is correct?
   1. "Take the sample from the center of a formed stool to ensure a uniform sample."
   2. "Use a pencil to label the specimens with your name, address, age, and date of specimen."
   3. "Urine or toilet tissue will not contaminate the specimen."
   4. "You can collect the specimens during your menstrual period."
10. The nurse needs to obtain a throat culture from a child client. Which of following techniques is correct?
    1. The nurse wears sterile gloves during the procedure.
    2. The nurse wears clean gloves during the procedure.
    3. The nurse inserts the swab into the oropharynx and runs the swab along the adenoids and areas on the larynx that are reddened or contain exudate.
    4. The nurse has the client say "ugh" to relax the throat muscles and to help minimize dilation of the constrictor muscle of the larynx.

CHAPTER 35

MEDICATIONS

KEY TERM REVIEW

Match each term with its appropriate definition.

1. _______ Anaphylactic reaction
2. _______ Antagonist
3. _______ Buccal
4. _______ Drug allergy
5. _______ Drug dependence
6. _______ Drug half-life
7. _______ Drug tolerance
8. _______ Drug toxicity
9. _______ Elimination half-life
10. _______ Epidural
11. _______ Iatrogenic disease
12. _______ Idiosyncratic effect
13. _______ Inhibiting effect
14. _______ Intradermal (ID)
15. _______ Intramuscular (IM)
16. _______ Intraspinal
17. _______ Intrathecal
18. _______ Metered-dose inhaler (MDI)
19. _______ Ophthalmic
20. _______ Otic
21. _______ Peak plasma level
22. _______ Percutaneous
23. _______ Physiological dependence
24. _______ Potentiating effect
25. _______ Psychological dependence

a. A drug that inhibits cell function by occupying receptor sites; it blocks the effect of a natural body substance or other drugs

b. A person's reliance on or need to take a drug or substance

c. Time required for the elimination process to reduce the concentration of the drug to one half of what it was at initial administration

d. Deleterious effects of a drug on an organism or tissue

e. Parenteral administration into the epidural space

f. Disease caused unintentionally by medical therapy

g. Medication held in the mouth against the mucous membranes of the cheek until the drug dissolves

h. An unusually low physiological response to a drug; increases in the dosage are required to maintain a given therapeutic effect

i. Effect that is unexpected; may be individual to a client

j. A severe allergic reaction usually occurring immediately after the administration of a drug

k. A drug interaction in which the effect of one or both drugs is decreased

l. Drug half-life

m. Under the epidermis

n. Into a muscle

o. Intraspinal administration of medication

p. A handheld nebulizer that releases medication through a mouthpiece

q. Medications for the eyes

r. Intrathecal parenteral administration

s. These biochemical changes in body tissues come to require a substance for normal functioning

t. Immunologic reaction to a drug

u. Instillations or irrigations of the external auditory canal

v. Highest plasma level achieved by a single dose when the elimination rate of a drug equals the absorption rate

w. Absorption through the skin

x. A drug interaction in which the effect of one or both drugs is increased

y. Emotional reliance on a drug to maintain a sense of well-being accompanied by feelings of need or cravings for that drug

KEY TOPIC REVIEW

1. Medications cannot have natural (e.g., plant, mineral, and animal) sources; they must be synthesized in the laboratory.

   a. True

   b. False

2. Medications vary in strength and activity.

   a. True

   b. False

3. Medications must be pure and of uniform strength if drug dosages are to be predictable in their effect.

   a. True

   b. False

4. The action of a drug in the body can be described in terms of its half-life, the time interval required for the body's elimination processes to reduce the concentration of the drug in the body by 25%.

   a. True

   b. False

5. Parenteral administration is the most common, least expensive, and most convenient route for most clients.

   a. True

   b. False

6. Medications for the ___________, called ophthalmic medications, are instilled in the form of liquids or ointments.

7. A major consideration in the administration of ___________ injections is the selection of a safe site located away from large blood vessels, nerves, and bone.

8. A ___________ is a small glass bottle with a sealed rubber cap.

9. A needle has three discernible parts: the hub, which fits onto the syringe; the cannula, or shaft, which is attached to the hub; and the ___________, which is the slanted part at the tip of the needle.

10. Syringes have three parts: the tip, which connects with the needle; the barrel, or outside part, on which the scales are printed; and the ___________, which fits inside the barrel.

11. Match the following terms with the correct definition.

a. Prescription	______	The written direction for the preparation and administration of a drug
b. Medication	______	A drug's name given by the drug manufacturer
c. Generic name	______	The study of the effect of drugs on living organisms
d. Trade name	______	A book containing a list of products used in medicine, with descriptions of the product, chemical tests for determining identity and purity, and formulas and prescriptions
e. Pharmacology	______	A secondary effect of a drug, one that is unintended
f. Pharmacy	______	Deleterious effects of a drug on an organism or tissue that results from overdosage, ingestion of a drug intended for external use, and buildup of the drug in the blood because of impaired metabolism or excretion (cumulative effect)
g. Pharmacopoeia	______	The ___________ of a drug, also referred to as the desired effect, is the primary effect intended, that is, the reason the drug is prescribed.
h. Therapeutic effect	______	The art of preparing, compounding, and dispensing drugs
i. Side effect	______	Given before a drug officially becomes an approved medication
j. Drug toxicity	______	A substance administered for the diagnosis, cure, treatment, or relief of a symptom or for prevention of disease.

12. ___________ is the process by which a drug changes the body (e.g., alters cell physiology).

   a. Receptor

   b. Pharmacodynamics

   c. Agonist

   d. Antagonist

13. A ___________ order indicates that the medication is to be given immediately and only once.

   a. prn

   b. Standing

   c. Single

   d. Stat

14. The study of the effect of drugs on living organisms is called:
    a. Pharmacopoeia.
    b. Pharmacist.
    c. Pharmacy.
    d. Pharmacology.
15. When two different drugs increase the action of one or another drug, this effect is termed:
    a. Synergistic.
    b. Drug tolerance.
    c. Drug interaction.
    d. Cumulative effect.
16. A(An) __________ syringe comes in 1-,3-, and 5-mL sizes. This syringe may have two scales marked on it: the minim and the milliliter. The milliliter scale is the one normally used; the minim scale is used for very small dosages.
    a. Insulin
    b. Tuberculin
    c. Hypodermic
    d. None of the above

FOCUSED STUDY TIPS

1. Discuss the medication ordering process.
2. List three places hospitals correctly keep controlled substances.
3. Explain how to properly handle controlled substances wasted during preparation.
4. Discuss how the client's environment can affect the action of drugs.
5. Describe how the time of administration of oral medications affects the relative speed with which they act.
6. Identify and list three factors that indicate the size and length of the needle to be used.
7. Summarize the absorption process by which a drug passes into the bloodstream.
8. Compare and contrast the three systems of measurements used in North America.
9. .List three routes for parenteral administration.
10. Define and discuss the types of topical applications.
11. List and describe the essential parts of a drug order.
12. Describe how to instruct a client on taking a sublingual medication.
13. Describe how to correctly insert a rectal suppository and describe its advantages.
14. List and describe the different kinds syringes used for irrigations.

CASE STUDY

1. The health care provider has ordered Compazine 10 mg IM every 4 hours prn for a 37-year-old male client who is awake and alert. The client tells you that he is not currently taking any other medications or natural supplements.
   a. What are the 10 "rights" of medication administration?
   b. The Compazine is available in an ampule. How will you properly prepare the Compazine from the ampule?
   c. Describe the process of administering Compazine by intramuscular injection.

REVIEW QUESTIONS

1. The nurse is preparing a subcutaneous injection for a client. Which of the following statements is correct?
   1. A 45° angle is used when 1 inch of tissue can be grasped at the site.
   2. A 90° angle is used when 1 inch of tissue can be grasped at the site.
   3. Generally a 3- to 5-mL syringe is used for most subcutaneous injections.
   4. A #28-gauge, 1/2-inch needle is used for adults of normal weight.
2. The nurse knows and understands that a drug that produces the same type of response as the physiological or endogenous substance is called a(an):
   1. Agonist.
   2. Antagonist.
   3. Receptor.
   4. Biotransformation.
3. A nurse is preparing a seminar on drug misuse. Which of the following terms describes a mild form of psychological dependence, where the individual develops the habit of taking the substance and feels better after taking it, and the individual tends to continue the habit even though it may be injurious to health?
   1. Drug dependence
   2. Drug habituation
   3. Physiological dependence
   4. Psychological dependence
4. A client weighs 110 lb. What is the correct kilogram amount a nurse should calculate if he or she understands how to convert pounds to kilograms?
   1. 25 kg
   2. 50 kg
   3. 75 kg
   4. 100 kg
5. Erythromycin 500 mg is ordered. It is supplied in a liquid form containing 250 mg in 5 mL. How many milliliters would the nurse administer?
   1. 10
   2. 20
   3. 30
   4. 40

6. The nurse is preparing a Compazine injection to be given to a client. Which of the following statements is correct?

   1. When handling a syringe, the nurse may touch the outside of the barrel and the handle of the plunger.
   2. The nurse may touch the tip of the barrel with an unsterile object.
   3. The nurse may touch the shaft of the plunger with an unsterilized object.
   4. The nurse may touch the tip of the needle with an unsterilized object.

7. A client in the emergency department is to receive a rectal suppository. Which of the following nursing actions is NOT correct for administering a rectal suppository?

   1. The client can be placed in a left Sims' position.
   2. The smooth, rounded end of the rectal suppository is lubricated.
   3. After inserting the rectal suppository, press the client's buttocks together for a few minutes.
   4. Have the client remain in the left lateral position for 1 minute to help retain the suppository.

8. The nurse is performing an ear irrigation. Which nursing action is correct?

   1. The nurse explains that the client may experience a feeling of fullness, warmth, and, occasionally, discomfort when the fluid comes in contact with the tympanic membrane.
   2. The nurse angles the ear canal prior to inserting the tip of the syringe into the auditory meatus.
   3. The nurse pushes the solution gently downward against the bottom of the canal.
   4. The nurse places a cotton-tipped applicator in the auditory meatus to absorb the excess fluid after the procedure.

9. When evaluating a client's understanding of administering a vaginal foam, which of the following statements indicates a need for further teaching?

   1. "I will gently insert the applicator into the vagina about 5 cm (2 in.)."
   2. "I will remain lying in the supine position for 2 minutes following the insertion of the vaginal foam."
   3. "I will slowly push the plunger of the applicator until the applicator is empty."
   4. "I will discard the applicator if it is a disposable type."

10. A nurse is evaluating a nursing student's transdermal patch application to a comatose client. Which of the following actions demonstrates a need for further teaching? The student:

    1. Selects a clean, dry area that is free of hair.
    2. Removes the patch from its protective covering.
    3. Holds the patch by touching the adhesive edges.
    4. Applies the patch by pressing firmly with the palm of the hand for about 10 seconds.

CHAPTER 36

SKIN INTEGRITY AND WOUND CARE

KEY TERM REVIEW

Match each term with its appropriate definition.

1. _______ Aerobic
2. _______ Anaerobic
3. _______ Approximated
4. _______ Debridement
5. _______ Dehiscence
6. _______ Eschar
7. _______ Evisceration
8. _______ Excoriation
9. _______ Exudate
10. _______ Fibrin
11. _______ Granulation tissue
12. _______ Hematoma
13. _______ Hemorrhage
14. _______ Hemostasis
15. _______ Keloid
16. _______ Maceration
17. _______ Phagocytosis
18. _______ Primary intention healing
19. _______ Purulent exudate
20. _______ Reactive hyperemia
21. _______ Sanguineous exudate
22. _______ Secondary intention healing
23. _______ Serosanguineous
24. _______ Suppuration
25. _______ Tertiary intention

a. A wound covering of dried plasma proteins and dead cells that occurs if the wound does not close by epithelialization

b. The initial translucent, fragile tissue that forms during the proliferative phase of wound healing

c. Protrusion of the internal viscera through an incision

d. The process of pus formation

e. Material that has escaped from blood vessels during the inflammatory process and is deposited in the tissue or on tissue surfaces

f. Hypertrophic scar

g. Bloody

h. Growing only in the presence of oxygen

i. Removal of necrotic material

j. The process during which macrophages engulf cellular debris and microorganisms

k. Occurs where the tissue surfaces have been approximated, and there is minimal or no tissue loss

l. Red flush of skin that occurs when pressure is relieved from an area

m. Occurs in a wound that is extensive, and the edges cannot be approximated

n. Growing only in the absence of oxygen

o. Cessation of bleeding

p. Massive bleeding

q. Tissue softened by prolonged wetting or soaking

r. A localized collection of blood underneath the skin that may appear as reddish-blue swelling

s. Connective tissue

t. Thicker, yellow-, blue-, or green-tinged exudate

u. Closed

v. Partial or total rupturing of a sutured wound

w. Wounds left open for 3 to 5 days, then surgically closed

x. Area of loss of the superficial layers of the skin

y. Mixed drainage consisting of clear and blood-tinged material

KEY TOPIC REVIEW

1. The skin is the largest organ in the body and serves a variety of important functions in maintaining health and protecting the individual from injury.

   a. True

   b. False

2. Hypoproteinemia is an abnormally high protein content in the blood.

   a. True

   b. False

3. Wound beds that are too dry or disturbed too often fail to heal.

   a. True

   b. False

4. Although an inadequate intake of calories, protein, vitamins, and iron is believed to be a risk factor for pressure ulcer development, nutritional supplements should not be considered for nutritionally compromised clients.

   a. True

   b. False

5. Any at-risk client confined to bed, even when a special support mattress is used, should be repositioned at least every 2 hours, depending on the client's need, to allow another body surface to bear the weight.

   a. True

   b. False

6. The appearance of the skin and skin integrity are influenced by internal factors such as genetics, age, and the underlying ______ of the individual as well as external factors such as activity.

7. Moisture from incontinence promotes skin ______ (tissue softened by prolonged wetting or soaking) and makes the epidermis more easily eroded and susceptible to injury.

8. Wound ______ involves the removal of debris (i.e., foreign materials, excess slough, necrotic tissue, bacteria, and other microorganisms).

9. Using ______ syringes instead of bulb syringes to irrigate a wound reduces the risk of aspirating drainage and provides safe, effective pressure.

10. The ______ is the largest organ in the body and serves a variety of important functions in maintaining health and protecting the individual from injury.

11. Match the following terms with the correct definitions.

a. Regeneration	______	A force acting parallel to the skin surface
b. Hemostasis	______	A reduction in the amount and control of movement a person has
c. Exudate	______	Renewal of tissues
d. Bandage	______	The cessation of bleeding that results from vasoconstriction of the larger blood vessels in the affected area, retraction (drawing back) of injured blood vessels, the deposition of fibrin (connective tissue), and the formation of blood clots in the area
e. Ischemia	______	A whitish protein substance that adds tensile strength to the wound
f. Irrigation (lavage)	______	A material, such as fluid and cells, that has escaped from blood vessels during the inflammatory process and is deposited in tissue or on tissue surfaces
g. Pressure ulcer	______	The washing or flushing out of an area
h. Collagen	______	A strip of cloth used to wrap some part of the body
i. Friction	______	Any lesion caused by unrelieved pressure (a compressing downward force on a body area) that results in damage to underlying tissue, as defined by the U.S. Public Health Service's Panel for the Prediction and Prevention of Pressure Ulcers in Adults
j. Immobility	______	A deficiency in the blood supply to the tissue

12. The ______ phase, the second phase in healing, extends from day 3 or 4 to about day 21 postinjury.

a. Maturation

b. Proliferative

c. Inflammatory

d. Remodeling

13. ______ is a process in which extra blood flows to the area to compensate for the preceding period of impeded blood flow.

a. Vasodilation

b. Friction

c. Shearing force

d. Immobility

14. If a wound does not close by epithelialization, the area becomes covered with dried plasma proteins and dead cells. This is called ______.

a. Keloid

b. Eschar

c. Exudate

d. Suppuration

15. The risk of hemorrhage is greatest during the first ______ hours after surgery.
    a. 48
    b. 72
    c. 96
    d. 120
16. ______ is the partial or total rupturing of a sutured wound.
    a. Evisceration
    b. Debridement
    c. Dehiscence
    d. Protein

FOCUSED STUDY TIPS

1. Describe the phases of healing.
2. List the four recognized stages of pressure ulcers related to observable tissue damage.
3. Discuss some of the chronic illnesses and their treatments and how they can affect skin integrity.
4. Discuss some of the factors contributing to the formation of pressure ulcers.
5. Discuss some changes in the skin and its supporting structures associated with the aging process.
6. List the three phases into which the wound healing process can be broken down.
7. Discuss the four different ways debridement may be achieved.
8. Compare and contrast the proper procedures for untreated wounds versus treated wounds.
9. List some of the purposes for which wound dressings would be applied.
10. Discuss gauze packing using the wet-to-moist technique.
11. Discuss some of the items that may cause hemorrhage from a wound.
12. Describe what the nurse notes when a pressure ulcer is present.
13. Discuss some of the different types of dressings.
14. List the type of heat and cold applications.
15. Discuss basic turns for roller bandages.
16. Describe the differences between friction and shearing forces, and list an example of each.
17. Differentiate between maceration and excoriation.

CASE STUDY

1. A 17-year-old high school senior sustained a left ankle injury during a soccer game 1 hour ago. The health care provider has ordered an ice pack to be applied to the injured area for 20 minutes.

   a. Explain the local effects of cold.

   b. Explain the systemic effects of cold.

   c. List some indications for applying ice to the injured ankle.

   d. Summarize the guidelines a nurse should follow for all local cold applications.

REVIEW QUESTIONS

1. The nurse is assessing a wound and notes that the exudate is purulent. What would you expect the exudate to look like?

   1. The exudate is thick with the presence of pus and is yellow in color.
   2. The exudate is clear and appears blood tinged.
   3. The exudate is red to pink and watery.
   4. The exudate is bright red and bloody.

2. During discharge planning, the nurse is teaching a client how to apply an electric heat pad to his back. Which of the following statements indicates that the patient requires further teaching?

   1. "I will not insert any sharp objects into the electric heating pad because the pin could damage a wire and cause an electric shock."
   2. "I will ensure that my back is dry unless there is a waterproof cover on the electric heating pad because electricity in the presence of water can cause a shock."
   3. "I do not need to use an electric heating pad with a preset heating switch."
   4. "I will not lie on top of the electric heating pad because the heat will not dissipate, and I may be burned."

3. Which of the following actions taken by a client self-administering a hot water bottle to his back indicates to the nurse the need for further teaching?

   1. The client fills the bag two thirds full with water.
   2. After filling the bag with water, the client dries the bag and holds it upside down to test it for leakage.
   3. The client expels the remaining air out of the bag before securing the top.
   4. The client fills the bag with water at a temperature of 135°F.

4. The nurse is assessing a student nurse's knowledge of bandages. Which of the following statements from the student nurse indicates a need for further teaching?

   1. "Bandages can be used to support a wound."
   2. "Bandages can be used to immobilize a wound."
   3. "Bandages can be used to apply pressure to a wound."
   4. "Bandages can be firm and tight."

5. A nurse is planning a seminar on dressing wounds. Which of the following is NOT correct information about the purpose of dressing wounds? Dressings are applied to:
   1. Protect the wound from mechanical injury.
   2. Prevent hemorrhage.
   3. Prevent thermal insulation.
   4. Protect the wound from microbial contamination.
6. During a discharge teaching session with a client, which statement by the client indicates a need for further teaching?
   1. "Transparent dressings act as temporary skin."
   2. "Transparent dressings are nonporous, nonabsorbent, and self-adhesive."
   3. "Transparent dressings cannot be placed over a joint without disrupting mobility."
   4. "Transparent dressings adhere only to the skin area around the wound and not to the wound itself because they keep the wound moist."
7. The nurse is caring for a client who has a wound covered with thick necrotic tissue, or eschar, and it requires debridement. What color would this wound most likely be?
   1. Red
   2. Yellow
   3. Black
   4. Blue
8. Any at-risk client confined to bed, even when a special support mattress is used, should be repositioned at least every 2 hours, depending on the client's need, to allow another body surface to bear the weight. The nurse should NOT place the client in which position?
   1. Prone
   2. Knee–chest
   3. Supine
   4. Sims'
9. The nurse knows albumin is an important indicator of nutritional status. The nurse understands that a value below ______ g/dL indicates poor nutrition and may increase the risk of poor healing and infection.
   1. 3.5
   2. 3.6
   3. 3.8
   4. 3.9
10. The nurse is preparing to obtain a wound drainage specimen for culture from a client. Which of the following is part of the preparation?
    1. Check the progress notes to determine if the specimen is to be collected for an aerobic (growing only in the presence of oxygen) culture.
    2. Check the medical orders to determine if the specimen is to be collected for an anaerobic (growing only in the absence of oxygen) culture.
    3. Administer an analgesic 90 minutes before the procedure if the client is complaining of pain at the wound site.
    4. Administer an analgesic 5 minutes before the procedure if the client is complaining of pain at the wound site.

CHAPTER 37

PERIOPERATIVE NURSING

KEY TERM REVIEW

Match each term with its appropriate definition.

1. _______ Atelectasis
2. _______ Circulating nurse
3. _______ Closed-wound drainage system
4. _______ Conscious sedation
5. _______ Elective surgery
6. _______ Emboli
7. _______ Emergency surgery
8. _______ Epidural anesthesia
9. _______ General anesthesia
10. _______ Intraoperative phase
11. _______ Local anesthesia
12. _______ Major surgery
13. _______ Minor surgery
14. _______ Nerve block
15. _______ Penrose drain
16. _______ Peridural anesthesia
17. _______ Perioperative period
18. _______ Postoperative phase
19. _______ Preoperative phase
20. _______ Regional anesthesia
21. _______ Scrub person
22. _______ Spinal anesthesia
23. _______ Subarachnoid block (SAB)
24. _______ Surface anesthesia
25. _______ Suture

a. Injection of anesthetic agent into the epidural space, the area inside the spinal column but outside the dura mater

b. Role is to assist the surgeons; often a UAP

c. Epidural anesthesia

d. Infiltration; injected into a specific area and used for minor surgical procedures

e. Begins when the decision to have surgery is made; ends when the client is transferred to the operating table

f. Coordinates activities and manages client care

g. A thread used to sew body tissues together

h. Involves a high degree of risk

i. The delivery of nursing care through the framework of the nursing process

j. Topical anesthesia

k. Refers to minimal depression of the level of consciousness; client retains the ability to maintain a patent airway and respond appropriately to commands

l. Temporary interruption of the transmission of nerve impulses to and from a specific area or region of the body

m. A technique in which the anesthetic agent is injected into and around a nerve or small nerve group

n. Performed when surgical intervention is the preferred treatment for a condition that is not imminently life threatening

o. Requires lumbar puncture through one of the interspaces between lumbar disc 2 and the sacrum

p. Performed immediately to preserve function or the life of the client

q. The loss of all sensation and consciousness

r. Normally involves little risk, produces few complications, and is often performed in an outpatient setting

s. Begins with the admission of the client to the postanesthesia area and ends when healing is complete

t. Collapse of the alveoli

u. A drain that has an open end that drains onto a dressing

v. Blood clot that has moved

w. Consists of a drain connected to either an electric suction or a portable drainage suction

x. Spinal anesthesia

y. Phase begins when the client is transferred to the operating table and ends when the client is admitted to the postanesthesia care unit

KEY TOPIC REVIEW

1. The intraoperative phase begins when the decision to have surgery is made and ends when the client is transferred to the operating table.
   a. True
   b. False
2. An embolus is a blood clot that has moved.
   a. True
   b. False
3. Adequate nutrition is not necessarily required for normal tissue repair.
   a. True
   b. False
4. Prior to any surgical procedure, informed consent is required from the client or legal guardian.
   a. True
   b. False
5. Surgery is least risky when the client's general health is good.
   a. True
   b. False
6. Pale, cyanotic, cool, and moist skin may be a sign of ______ problems.
7. A ______ is a thread used to sew body tissues together.
8. Conscious ______ refers to minimal depression of the level of consciousness in which the client retains the ability to maintain a patent airway and respond appropriately to commands.
9. A thrombus is a stationary ______ adhered to the wall of a vessel.
10. A ______-wound drainage system consists of a drain connected to either an electric suction or a portable drainage suction.

11. Match the following terms with the correct definition.

a. Preoperative phase	______	Begins with the admission of the client to the postanesthesia area and ends when healing is complete
b. Intraoperative phase	______	A technique in which the anesthetic agent is injected into and around a nerve or small nerve group that supplies sensation to a small area of the body
c. Postoperative phase	______	Used most often for procedures involving the arm, wrist, and hand
d. Regional anesthesia	______	An injection of an anesthetic agent into the epidural space, the area inside the spinal column but outside the dura mater
e. Local anesthesia	______	The passage of blood through the vessels
f. Tissue perfusion	______	Begins when the decision to have surgery is made and ends when the client is transferred to the operating table
g. Intravenous block (Bier block)	______	(Infiltration) is injected into a specific area and is used for minor surgical procedures such as suturing a small wound or performing a biopsy
h. Epidural (peridural) anesthesia	______	Applied directly to the skin and mucous membranes, open skin surfaces, wounds, and burns
i. Nerve block	______	The temporary interruption of the transmission of nerve impulses to and from a specific area or region of the body
j. Topical (surface) anesthesia	______	Begins when the client is transferred to the operating table and ends when the client is admitted to the postanesthesia care unit (PACU), also called the postanesthetic room or recovery room

12. ______ anesthesia is the loss of all sensation and consciousness.

   a. Regional
   b. Local
   c. Topical
   d. General

13. Which of the following routine preoperative tests is given to evaluate fluid and electrolyte status?

   a. Complete blood count (CBC)
   b. Blood grouping and cross-matching
   c. Serum electrolytes
   d. Fasting blood glucose

14. Which of the following routine preoperative tests is given to evaluate liver function?

   a. Blood urea nitrogen (BUN) and creatinine
   b. ALT, AST, LDH, and bilirubin
   c. Serum albumin and total protein
   d. Urinalysis

15. Which of the following routine preoperative tests is given to evaluate respiratory status and heart size?
    a. Chest x-ray
    b. Electrocardiogram
    c. Pregnancy test
    d. Complete blood count (CBC)
16. The ______ phase begins with the admission of the client to the postanesthesia area and ends when healing is complete.
    a. Intraoperative
    b. Preoperative
    c. Postoperative
    d. None of the above

FOCUSED STUDY TIPS

1. Discuss some of the risks involved with surgery.
2. List some factors affecting the degree of risk involved in a surgical procedure.
3. Explain the three different types/classifications of anesthesia.
4. What is preoperative consent?
5. Describe how to properly give a physical assessment.
6. Identify three commonly used preoperative medications and their uses.
7. List some of the different types of antiembolic stockings and what they are used for.
8. Compare and contrast elective surgery and emergency surgery.
9. State the overall goal during the preoperative period.
10. Discuss the fluid and nutrition requirements before surgery.
11. Discuss elimination requirements before surgery.
12. Describe how to properly prepare for ongoing care of the postoperative client.
13. Discuss proper client hygiene before a surgery.
14. List the three steps involved in the Joint Commission's Universal Protocol for Preventing Wrong Site, Wrong Procedure, Wrong Person Surgery.
15. Compare and contrast major surgery and minor surgery.
16. Define atelectasis and describe methods to prevent this condition.
17. List two types of closed-wound drainage systems and describe their purpose.

CASE STUDY

1. A 58-year-old client has been admitted for abdominal surgery. After you have taken his vital signs, he asks, "What is the difference between a major surgery and a minor surgery?" He then states "I have a lot of hair on my belly. Will I have that hair shaved off before the surgery?"
   a. Define major surgery and minor surgery.
   b. Give two examples of major surgery and two examples of minor surgery.
   c. Why would you need to remove the hair on the client's abdomen before surgery?

REVIEW QUESTIONS

1. Surgery is a unique experience of a planned physical alteration encompassing three phases. Which phase begins when the client is transferred to the operating table and ends when the client is admitted to the postanesthesia care unit (PACU)?
   1. Preoperative
   2. Intraoperative
   3. Postoperative
   4. Perioperative
2. The regular use of certain medications can increase surgical risk. Which of the following would NOT increase surgical risk as much as the others?
   1. Anticoagulants
   2. Tranquilizers
   3. Diuretics
   4. Antibiotics
3. Which of the following is NOT a correct action to reduce the risk of postoperative wound infection?
   1. Clean the surgical site only.
   2. Remove hair from the surgical site only when necessary.
   3. Document surgical skin preparation in the client's record.
   4. Prepare the surgical site with an antimicrobial agent.
4. Which of the following actions is appropriate for the nurse removing skin sutures?
   1. The nurse puts on exam gloves.
   2. The nurse removes the skin sutures without an order.
   3. The nurse grasps the suture at the knot with a pair of clamps.
   4. The nurse cuts the suture as close to the skin as possible.

5. During discharge planning, the nurse is teaching the client how to maintain comfort, promote healing, and restore wellness. Which of the following actions is NOT correct?

   1. Instruct the client to use pain medications as ordered, not allowing pain to become severe before taking the prescribed dose.
   2. Teach the client to avoid using alcohol or other central nervous system depressants while taking narcotic analgesics.
   3. Instruct the client to report promptly to the primary care practitioner any decreased redness, swelling, pain, or discharge from the incision or drain sites.
   4. Emphasize the importance of adequate rest for healing and immune function.

6. The spouse of a client is preparing to apply a sterile dressing. Which of the following indicates a need for further teaching? The spouse:

   1. Puts on sterile gloves.
   2. Places the bulk of the dressing along the edges of the wound.
   3. Secures the dressing with tape or ties.
   4. Applies the sterile dressings one at a time over the drain and the incision.

7. A nurse is evaluating a client's understanding of performing deep-breathing exercises. Which of the following statements indicates a need for further teaching?

   1. "I will hold my breath for 6 to 8 seconds."
   2. "I will exhale slowly through the mouth."
   3. "I will always be in a sitting position."
   4. "I will inhale slowly and evenly through the nose until the greatest chest expansion is achieved."

8. When irrigating a gastrointestinal tube for a client, which of the following would be appropriate? The nurse:

   1. Attaches the syringe to the nasogastric tube.
   2. Aspirates the solution harshly.
   3. Draws up 90 mL of irrigating solution into the syringe.
   4. Quickly injects the solution.

9. A nurse is evaluating a nursing student who is applying antiembolic stockings to a client. Which of the following actions demonstrates a need for further teaching?

   1. Assists the client to a sitting position in bed.
   2. Reaches inside the stocking from the top and, grasping the heel, turns the upper portion of the stocking inside out so the foot portion is inside the stocking leg.
   3. Has the client point his or her toes, then positions the stocking on the client's foot.
   4. Eases the stocking over the toes, taking care to place the toe and heel portions of the stocking appropriately.

10. A nurse is planning a seminar on potential postoperative problems. Which of the following describes a condition in which alveoli collapse and are not ventilated?

    1. Thrombophlebitis
    2. Pulmonary embolism
    3. Pneumonia
    4. Atelectasis

CHAPTER 38

SENSORY PERCEPTION

KEY TERM REVIEW

Match each term with its appropriate definition.

1. _______ Acute confusion
2. _______ Auditory
3. _______ Awareness
4. _______ Cultural care deprivation
5. _______ Cultural deprivation
6. _______ Delirium
7. _______ Gustatory
8. _______ Kinesthetic
9. _______ Olfactory
10. _______ Sensoristasis
11. _______ Sensory deficit
12. _______ Sensory deprivation
13. _______ Sensory overload
14. _______ Sensory perception
15. _______ Sensory reception
16. _______ Stereognosis
17. _______ Tactile
18. _______ Visceral
19. _______ Visual

a. The lack of culturally assistive, supportive, or facilitative acts
b. Impaired reception, perception, or both of one or more of the senses
c. Touch
d. Acute confusion
e. Taste
f. Any large organ within the body
g. Ability to perceive and understand an object through touch by its size, shape, and texture
h. Occurs when a person is unable to process or manage the amount or intensity of sensory stimuli
i. Hearing
j. The state in which a person is in optimal arousal
k. Involves conscious organization and translation of the data or stimuli into meaningful information
l. Sight
m. Cultural care deprivation
n. Has an abrupt onset, and a cause that, when treated, reverses the condition
o. The ability to perceive internal and external stimuli, and to respond appropriately through thought and action
p. The process of receiving stimuli or data
q. Smell
r. Decrease in or lack of meaningful stimuli
s. Awareness of the position and movement of body parts

KEY TOPIC REVIEW

1. Sensory reception is the process of receiving stimuli or data.

   a. True

   b. False

2. Visceral refers to the ability to perceive and understand an object through touch by its size, shape, and texture.

   a. True

   b. False

3. Glaucoma is a group of diseases of the eye caused by increased intraocular pressure that can lead to optic nerve damage and eventual vision loss.

   a. True

   b. False

4. Confusion can occur in clients of all ages, but is most commonly seen in older people.

   a. True

   b. False

5. Sensory overload is generally thought of as a decrease in or lack of meaningful stimuli.

   a. True

   b. False

6. For an individual to be aware of the surroundings, four aspects of the sensory process must be present: a stimulus, a receptor, impulse conduction, and ____________.

7. During times of increased ____________, people may find their senses overloaded and thus seek to decrease sensory stimulation.

8. An individual's ____________ often determines the amount of stimulation that an individual considers usual or "normal."

9. Gaining the ____________ of a client with a hearing impairment is an essential first step toward effective communication.

10. Sensory ____________ can prevent the brain from ignoring or responding to specific stimuli.

11. ________% of individuals ages 62 to 88 have mild hearing impairment.

    a. 10

    b. 23

    c. 26

    d. 30

12. Which of the following states of awareness would be best described as extreme drowsiness but will respond to stimuli?

    a. Confused

    b. Somnolent

    c. Semicomatose

    d. Coma

13. All of the following would be correctly categorized as an affective change EXCEPT:
    a. Hallucinations.
    b. Rapid mood swings.
    c. Depression.
    d. Anxiety.
14. Which of the following states of awareness would be best described as reduced awareness, easily bewildered; poor memory, misinterprets stimuli; impaired judgment?
    a. Full consciousness
    b. Disoriented
    c. Confused
    d. Somnolent
15. Age-related macular degeneration (ARMD) is the leading cause of blindness in adults ages ______ and older.
    a. 50
    b. 55
    c. 60
    d. 65

FOCUSED STUDY TIPS

1. Explain how the client's environment can affect the senses.
2. Discuss some of the techniques used to help prevent sensory deprivation.
3. Discuss sensory deprivation.
4. Describe some of the tasks nurses need to perform in a health care setting for clients with visual impairments.
5. Explain how physical assessment determines whether the senses are impaired.
6. Discuss the importance of communication, particularly with clients who have sensory deficits.
7. Explain some of the sensory aids that are available for clients who have visual and hearing deficits.
8. Discuss sensory overload.
9. Describe some of the techniques used to help prevent sensory overload.
10. Discuss some of the techniques used in promoting healthy sensory function.
11. List the four aspects of the sensory process that must be present for an individual to be aware of the surroundings.
12. Explain some of the techniques used when one sense is lost to promote the use of the other senses.
13. Discuss some considerations for clients with impaired tactile senses.
14. Discuss some considerations for clients with impaired olfactory senses.

15. Describe some of the tasks nurses need to perform in a health care setting for clients with hearing impairments.

16. Compare and contrast stereognosis and sensory perception.

17. Describe the various states of awareness.

CASE STUDY

1. An 87-year-old client was admitted to your floor yesterday. During report you are told that the client has visual and hearing impairments.
   a. What actions should you take to help with the client's visual impairment?
   b. What actions should you take to help with the client's hearing impairments?
   c. How can environmental stimuli be adjusted for this client?

REVIEW QUESTIONS

1. A nurse is evaluating a nursing student who is assisting a client who has a visual deficit. Which of the following actions demonstrates a need for further teaching? The student nurse:
   1. Announces her presence when entering the client's room and identifies herself by name.
   2. Speaks in a louder voice than necessary.
   3. Speaks in a warm and pleasant tone of voice.
   4. Always explains what she is about to do before touching the client.
2. A nurse planning a seminar on delirium and dementia plans to explain the characteristics differentiating the two. Which of the following describes an alertness that fluctuates—that is, the client may be alert and oriented during the day, but becomes confused and disoriented at night?
   1. Dementia
   2. Delirium
   3. Hallucinations
   4. Delusions
3. During discharge planning, the nurse is teaching the client how to prevent sensory disturbances. Which of the following actions is correct?
   1. Wear protective eye goggles when using power tools.
   2. Wear ear protectors when working in an environment with low noise levels.
   3. When wearing sunglasses, it is acceptable to look directly into the sun.
   4. Have health examinations every 5 to 10 years.
4. Which of the following actions is NOT appropriate for the nurse who is promoting a therapeutic environment for a client with acute confusion?
   1. "Good morning, Mr. Richards. I am Betty Brown. I will be your nurse today."
   2. "Today is December 5, and it is 8:00 in the morning."
   3. "Can you tell me where you are right now?"
   4. "I'm going to turn on the radio while you read the newspaper, and I'll leave the window open for you."

5. The spouse of a client is preparing sensory aids for the visual and hearing deficits of the client. Which of the following indicates a need for further teaching? The spouse:
   1. Gets a phone dialer with large numbers.
   2. Gets reading material with cursive print.
   3. Gets amplified telephones.
   4. Gets a magnifying glass.
6. The nurse is providing care to an unconscious client. Which of the following actions by the nurse is correct? (Select all that apply.)
   1. Provides nose care.
   2. Performs range-of-motion exercises.
   3. Provides a lot of environmental stimuli.
   4. Informs client of the care prior to it being provided.
   5. Assists client to bedside commode.
7. Stereognosis is:
   1. The process of receiving stimuli or data.
   2. The ability to perceive and understand an object through touch by its size, shape, and texture.
   3. The conscious organization and translation of data or stimuli into meaningful information.
   4. The term used to describe when a person is in optimal arousal.
8. When planning interventions to prevent sensory deprivation, which of the following would NOT be included in the client's plan of care?
   1. Encourage the client to use eyeglasses and hearing aids only when interacting with someone.
   2. Address the client by name and touch the client while speaking if this is not culturally offensive.
   3. Provide a telephone, radio and/or TV, clock, and calendar.
   4. Encourage the use of self-stimulation techniques such as singing, humming, whistling, or reciting.
9. Which of the following questions by the nurse assesses the gustatory sensory reception?
   1. "When did you last visit an eye doctor?"
   2. "Have you experienced any dizziness or vertigo?"
   3. "Have you experienced any changes in taste?"
   4. "Can you distinguish foods by their odors and tell when something is burning?"
10. The nurse is assessing for sensory function. Using a Snellen chart or other reading material, such as a newspaper, and visual fields assesses which of the following?
    1. Hearing acuity
    2. Visual acuity
    3. Olfactory senses
    4. Tactile senses

CHAPTER 39

SELF-CONCEPT

KEY TERM REVIEW

Match each term with its appropriate definition.

1. _______ Body image
2. _______ Core self-concept
3. _______ Global self
4. _______ Global self-esteem
5. _______ Ideal self
6. _______ Role
7. _______ Role ambiguity
8. _______ Role conflicts
9. _______ Role development
10. _______ Role mastery
11. _______ Role performance
12. _______ Role strain
13. _______ Self-awareness
14. _______ Self-concept
15. _______ Self-esteem
16. _______ Specific self-esteem

a. A set of expectations about how the individual occupying one position behaves
b. Arise from opposing or incompatible expectations
c. How an individual in a particular role acts in comparison to the behaviors expected of that role
d. One's judgment of one's own worth, how that individual's standards and performances compare to others, and ideal self
e. Refers to the relationship between one's perception of self and others' perceptions of him or her
f. When expectations are unclear, individuals do not know what to do or how to do it
g. The beliefs and images that are most vital to an individual's identity
h. How much one likes oneself as a whole
i. One's mental image of oneself
j. An individual's behaviors meet social expectations for a role
k. How an individual perceives the size, appearance, and functioning of the body and its parts
l. Socialization into a particular role
m. Collective beliefs and images one holds about oneself; most complete descriptions that individuals can give of themselves
n. How we should or would prefer to be
o. How much one approves of a certain part of oneself
p. Occurs when one is frustrated because the individual feels or is made to feel inadequate or unsuited to a role

KEY TOPIC REVIEW

1. Self-concept is one's mental image of oneself.
   a. True
   b. False
2. A client's attitude to a newly acquired disability is rarely the determining factor in successful rehabilitation.
   a. True
   b. False
3. Individuals who grow up in families whose members value each other are likely to feel good about themselves.
   a. True
   b. False
4. The weavings that form the patterns in one's life are experiences, knowledge, and dreams.
   a. True
   b. False
5. Self-awareness refers to the relationship between one's perception of himself or herself and others' perceptions of him or her.
   a. True
   b. False
6. A ____________ self-concept is essential to an individual's physical and psychological well-being.
7. Self-esteem is derived from ____________ and others.
8. ____________ self-esteem is how much one approves of a certain part of oneself.
9. Nursing interventions to promote a positive self-concept include helping a client to identify areas of ____________.
10. An individual's self-perception can differ from the individual's perception of how others see him or her and from the ____________ self, that is, how the individual would like to be.
11. Which of the following would NOT be considered a self-esteem stressor that affects self-concept?
    a. Loss of body parts
    b. Lack of positive feedback from significant others
    c. Abusive relationship
    d. Loss of financial security
12. Which of the following is NOT one of Erikson's stages of psychosocial development?
    a. Infancy: trust vs. mistrust
    b. Toddlerhood: autonomy vs. shame and doubt
    c. Early childhood: initiative vs. guilt
    d. Early adulthood: segregation vs. separation

13. ___________ is one's judgment of one's own worth, that is, how that individual's standards and performances compare to others and to one's ideal self.

    a. Self-esteem

    b. Self-knowledge

    c. Self-expectation

    d. Self-concept

14. All of the following would be considered an identity stressor EXCEPT:

    a. A change in physical appearance.

    b. The inability to achieve goals.

    c. Sexuality concerns.

    d. Ambiguous or conflicting role expectations.

15. Which one of the following is NOT one of the four dimensions of self-concept?

    a. Self-knowledge

    b. Social evaluation

    c. Self-expectation

    d. Self-evaluation

FOCUSED STUDY TIPS

1. List some strategies nurses can employ to reinforce strengths.

2. Discuss the stage of development as a factor that can affect self-concept.

3. Discuss the concept of body image, including how and when it develops.

4. List some of the guidelines for conducting a psychosocial assessment.

5. Discuss family and culture and how they can affect self-concept.

6. Define and discuss personal identity.

7. Discuss the formation of self-concept according to Erikson.

8. List three of the NANDA nursing diagnostic labels relating specifically to the domain of self-perception and the classes of self-concept, self-esteem, and body image.

9. Discuss stressors as a factor that can affect self-concept.

10. Individuals are thought to base their self-concept on how they perceive and evaluate themselves in several areas. List some of these areas.

11. Discuss resources and how they can affect self-concept.

12. Discuss illness and how it can affect self-concept.

13. Give some examples of questions a nurse can ask to determine a client's self-esteem.

14. List some nursing techniques that may help clients analyze the problem and enhance the self-concept.

15. Compare and contrast role ambiguity and role strain.

16. Discuss how family and culture influence values.

CASE STUDY

1. You are working in a psychiatric facility and caring for an older adult client.. The client tells you she has low self-esteem.

   a. What nursing techniques may help clients analyze the problem and enhance self-concept?

   b. List five stressors that affect self-concept.

   c. During your assessment, what questions should you ask the client?

REVIEW QUESTIONS

1. When planning interventions to reinforce a client's strengths, which of the following would NOT be included in the client's plan of care?

   1. Stress self-negation rather than positive thinking.
   2. Notice and verbally reinforce client strengths.
   3. Provide honest, positive feedback.
   4. Encourage the setting of attainable goals.

2. The nurse is conducting a psychosocial assessment. Which of the following actions by the nurse is correct?

   1. Create a quiet, private environment.
   2. Do not limit interruptions.
   3. Use intermittent eye contact.
   4. Sit above the eye level of the client.

3. A nurse is planning a seminar on conducting a psychosocial assessment. Which of the following guidelines is appropriate for conducting a psychosocial assessment?

   1. Indicate acceptance of the client by not criticizing, frowning, or demonstrating shock.
   2. Ask close-ended questions.
   3. Maximize the writing of detailed notes during the interview.
   4. Ask more personal questions than what are actually needed.

4. A nurse is evaluating a nursing student who is asking a client questions to determine the client's self-esteem. Which of the following statements demonstrates a need for further teaching?

   1. "Are you satisfied with your life?"
   2. "How do you feel about yourself?"
   3. "Are you accomplishing what you want?"
   4. "What are your responsibilities in the family?"

5. During discharge planning, the nurse is teaching the client how to enhance her son's self-esteem. Which of the following actions is correct?
   1. Give him opportunities to "practice" who he is.
   2. Do not allow him to explore and experiment with the world around him.
   3. Do not allow him to express himself as a unique individual.
   4. Encourage him to stay connected with all memories.
6. Which of the following questions is NOT appropriate for the nurse assessing body image?
   1. Is there any part of your body you would like to change?
   2. What are your relationships like with your other relatives?
   3. Are you comfortable discussing your surgery?
   4. How do you feel about your appearance?
7. Ideal self is:
   1. The collective beliefs and images one holds about oneself.
   2. How a person perceives the size, appearance, and functioning of the body and its parts.
   3. The individual's perception of how one should behave based on certain personal standards, aspirations, goals, and values.
   4. One's mental image of oneself.
8. According to Erikson's stages of psychosocial development, the middle adulthood stage is:
   1. Identity vs. role confusion.
   2. Intimacy vs. isolation.
   3. Integrity vs. despair.
   4. Generativity vs. stagnation.
9. When a client feels or is made to feel inadequate or unsuited to a role, he or she is experiencing which of the following?
   1. Role conflict
   2. Role strain
   3. Role ambiguity
   4. Role development
10. Which of the following is considered to be a stressor affecting self-concept?
    1. Change or loss of job or other significant role
    2. Financial security
    3. Stable relationship
    4. Realistic expectations

CHAPTER 40

SEXUALITY

KEY TERM REVIEW

Match each term with its appropriate definition.

1. _______ Anal stimulation
2. _______ Androgyny
3. _______ Cross-dressing
4. _______ Desire phase
5. _______ Dysmenorrhea
6. _______ Dyspareunia
7. _______ Excitement phase
8. _______ Female orgasmic disorder
9. _______ Female sexual arousal disorder
10. _______ Gender identity
11. _______ Gender-role behavior
12. _______ Genital inter-course
13. _______ Hypoactive sexual desire disorder
14. _______ Intersex
15. _______ Male erectile disorder
16. _______ Male orgasmic disorder
17. _______ Oral–genital sex
18. _______ Orgasmic phase
19. _______ Resolution phase
20. _______ Sexual aversion disorder
21. _______ Sexual self-concept
22. _______ Transgender
23. _______ Vaginismus
24. _______ Vestibulitis
25. _______ Vulvodynia

a. Involuntary climax of sexual tension, accompanied by physiological and psychological release

b. Sexual response stops before orgasm occurs

c. Characterized by two physiological changes, vasocongestion and myotonia

d. Flexibility in gender roles; belief that most characteristics and behaviors are human qualities and should not be limited to a specific gender

e. Outward expression of a person's sense of maleness or femaleness and what is perceived as gender-appropriate behavior

f. Period of return to unaroused state

g. Lack of vaginal lubrication causes discomfort or pain during sexual intercourse

h. Severe pain only on touch or attempted vaginal entry

i. Painful menstruation

j. Constant, unremitting burning that is localized to the vulva with an acute onset

k. Contradictions among chromosomal sex, gonadal sex, internal organs, and external genital appearance

l. Dressing in the clothing of the other gender; makes outward appearance consistent with inner identity and gender role; increases their comfort with themselves

m. How one values oneself as a sexual being

n. One's self-image as a female or male

o. A person whose sexual anatomy is not consistent with gender identity

p. The response cycle starts in the brain, with conscious sexual desires

q. Persistently low or lack of interest in sexual activity

r. Diagnosis when man has erection problems during 25% or more of his sexual interactions

s. Pain during or immediately after intercourse

t. Penile–vaginal intercourse (for heterosexual couples)

u. Kissing, licking, or sucking male or female genitals

v. Can be a source of sexual pleasure because of the rich nerve supply in the anus

w. A severe distaste for sexual activity, or the thought of sexual activity, which leads to a phobic avoidance of sex

x. Erection can be attained and maintained, but ejaculation is extremely difficult

y. Involuntary spasm of the outer one third of the vaginal muscles, making penetration of the vagina painful, and sometimes impossible

KEY TOPIC REVIEW

1. The development of sexuality begins with conception and ends with puberty.

   a. True

   b. False

2. The ability of the human body to experience a sexual response is present before birth.

   a. True

   b. False

3. An individual's gender identity may be easily changed once established.

   a. True

   b. False

4. Sexually transmitted infections (STIs) are the most common bacterial infections among adolescents.

   a. True

   b. False

5. Older women remain capable of multiple orgasms and may, in fact, experience an increase in sexual desire after menopause.

   a. True

   b. False

6. Sexual health includes both freedoms and ___________.

7. Current practice dictates the use of a ___________ in all forms of intercourse to prevent the transmission of disease.

8. The sexual response cycle starts in the ___________.

9. Sexual ___________ refers to the physiological responses and subjective sense of excitement experienced during sexual activity.

10. ___________ is the belief that most characteristics and behaviors are human qualities that should not be limited to one specific gender or the other.

11. Match the following terms with the correct definition.

a. Sexual self-concept	_____	Painful menstruation
b. Gender-role behavior	_____	How one values oneself as a sexual being
c. Masturbation	_____	One's self-image as a female or male
d. Sexual aversion disorder	_____	The outward expression of a person's sense of maleness or femaleness as well as the expression of what is perceived as gender-appropriate behavior
e. Orgasmic phase	_____	Flexibility in gender roles, the belief that most characteristics and behaviors are human qualities that should not be limited to one specific gender or the other
f. Resolution phase	_____	One's attraction to people of the same sex, other sex, or both sexes
g. Dysmenorrhea	_____	The ongoing love affair that each of us has with ourselves throughout our lifetime
h. Sexual orientation	_____	The involuntary climax of sexual tension, accompanied by physiological and psychological release
i. Androgyny	_____	The period of return to the unaroused state; may last 10 to 15 minutes after orgasm, or longer if there is no orgasm
j. Gender identity	_____	A severe distaste for sexual activity or the thought of sexual activity, which then leads to a phobic avoidance of sex

12. ___________ is the involuntary spasm of the outer one third of the vaginal muscles, making penetration of the vagina painful and sometimes impossible.

   a. Vestibulitis

   b. Vaginismus

   c. Vulvodynia

   d. Dyspareunia

13. ___________ is oral stimulation of the penis by licking and sucking.

    a. Masturbation
    b. Fellatio
    c. Genital intercourse
    d. Intersex

14. Which of the following is NOT one of the five critical components of sexual health?

    a. Freedoms and responsibilities
    b. Gender-role behavior
    c. Mental image
    d. Body image

FOCUSED STUDY TIPS

1. Discuss how older adults may define sexuality.
2. List some of the common sexual messages children get from their families.
3. Discuss how family influences a person's sexuality.
4. Discuss the desire phase of the sexual response cycle.
5. What are some of the health factors that can interfere with people's expression of sexuality?
6. Discuss how culture influences a person's sexuality.
7. Identify the forms of male and female sexual dysfunction.
8. Discuss the orgasmic phase of the sexual response cycle.
9. What is rapid ejaculation?
10. Summarize how religion influences a person's sexuality.
11. Explain sexual pain disorders.
12. Describe physiological changes in males and females during the sexual response cycle.
13. Discuss some of the problems with attaining sexual satisfaction.
14. Discuss the resolution phase of the sexual response cycle.
15. Describe how to correctly perform a breast self-examination and explain its importance.

CASE STUDY

1. A 21-year-old man is in the clinic today to get an employment physical. The health care provider has asked you to provide the client with education about testicular cancer and STIs. After you are done providing this education, the client makes a sexual advance toward you.
   a. Explain how to provide client teaching for testicular self-examination.
   b. Explain how to prevent the transmission of STIs and HIV.
   c. Summarize the nursing strategies to deal with the client's inappropriate sexual behavior.

REVIEW QUESTIONS

1. During discharge planning, the nurse is teaching the client how to prevent transmission of STIs and HIV. Which of the following actions is correct?
   1. Use condoms in monogamous relationships only.
   2. Follow safe sex practices only during intercourse.
   3. Report to a health care facility for examination only when there are signs of an STI.
   4. Notify all partners and encourage them to seek treatment when an STI is diagnosed.
2. A nurse is evaluating a client's understanding of performing breast self-examination. Which of the following statements indicates a need for further teaching?
   1. Use the finger pads (tips) of the three middle fingers (held together) on your left hand to feel for lumps.
   2. Press the breast tissue against the chest wall firmly enough to know how your breast feels. A ridge of firm tissue in the lower curve of each breast is abnormal.
   3. Use small circular motions systematically all the way around the breast as many times as necessary until the entire breast is covered.
   4. Look for any change in size or shape; lumps or thickenings; any rashes or other skin irritations; dimpled or puckered skin; any discharge or change in the nipples.
3. A nurse is evaluating a nursing student who is discussing nursing strategies for inappropriate sexual behavior from a client. Which of the following actions demonstrates a need for further teaching?
   1. "I will communicate that the behavior is not acceptable."
   2. "I will identify the client behaviors that are acceptable."
   3. "I will set firm limits with the client."
   4. "I will not report the incident to my nursing instructor, charge nurse, or clinical nurse specialist."
4. A nurse is planning a seminar on methods of contraception. Which of the following is NOT a correct method of contraception?
   1. Chemical barriers including vaginal diaphragm, cervical cap, and condom
   2. Abstinence
   3. Surgical sterilization
   4. Intrauterine devices (IUDs)

5. The nurse is providing education to a client about effects of medications on sexual function. Which of the following statements by the nurse is correct?
   1. "Antipsychotics increase sexual desire."
   2. "Diuretics decrease vaginal lubrication."
   3. "Narcotics increase sexual desire and response."
   4. "Barbiturates in large doses increase sexual desire."
6. The spouse of a client is verbalizing understanding of common conceptions of sex. Which of the following indicates a need for further teaching? The spouse states:
   1. "Sexual ability is not lost due to age."
   2. "There is no evidence that sexual activity weakens a person."
   3. "Chronic alcoholism is associated with erectile dysfunction."
   4. "Alcohol is a sexual stimulant."
7. The orgasmic phase is:
   1. The response cycle that starts in the brain, with conscious sexual desires.
   2. The involuntary climax of sexual tension, accompanied by physiological and psychological release.
   3. The period of return to the unaroused state, may last 10 to 15 minutes after orgasm, or longer if there is no orgasm.
   4. An increase of tension in muscles; may increase until released by orgasm, or it may also simply fade away.
8. Body image is:
   1. A central part of the sense of self, and is constantly changing.
   2. One's self-image as a female or male.
   3. The outward expression of a person's sense of maleness or femaleness as well as the expression of what is perceived as gender-appropriate behavior.
   4. The belief that most characteristics and behaviors are human qualities that should not be limited to one specific gender or the other.
9. The nurse who is evaluating a sexual health class recognizes that further teaching is necessary when which of the following statements is made by a participant?
   1. "Rapid ejaculation is one of the most common sexual dysfunctions among men."
   2. "Preorgasmic women have experienced an orgasm."
   3. "Vulvodynia is constant, unremitting burning that is localized to the vulva with an acute onset."
   4. "Vestibulitis causes severe pain only on touch or attempted vaginal entry."
10. One technique nurses can use to help clients with altered sexual function is the ____________ model.
    1. PLISSIT
    2. PLIISIT
    3. PLLISSIT
    4. PLISIT

CHAPTER 41

SPIRITUALITY

KEY TERM REVIEW

Match each term with its appropriate definition.

1. _______ Agnostic
2. _______ Atheist
3. _______ Holy day
4. _______ Kosher
5. _______ Meditation
6. _______ Prayer
7. _______ Presencing
8. _______ Religion
9. _______ Spiritual care
10. _______ Spiritual development
11. _______ Spiritual distress
12. _______ Spiritual health
13. _______ Spiritual well-being
14. _______ Spirituality

a. Being with a client, listening with full awareness of the privilege of doing so

b. Food prepared according to Jewish law

c. An intuitive, interpersonal, altruistic, and integrative expression that reflects the client's reality

d. Disturbance in the belief or value system that provides strength, hope, meaning to life

e. Spiritual health

f. A person who doubts the existence of God or a supreme being

g. The human experience that seeks to transcend self and find meaning and purpose through connection with others, nature, and/or a supreme being

h. Human communication with divine and spiritual entities

i. An organized system of beliefs and practices

j. A person who is without belief in a deity

k. Manifested by a feeling of being generally alive, purposeful, and fulfilled

l. The act of focusing one's thoughts or engaging in self-reflection or contemplation

m. A day set aside for special religious observance

n. Specific stages through which individuals may progress while maturing spiritually

KEY TOPIC REVIEW

1. Religion generally involves a belief in a relationship with some higher power, creative force, divine being, or infinite source of energy.

   a. True

   b. False

2. A holy day is a day set aside for special religious observance.

   a. True

   b. False

3. Prayer is human communication with divine and spiritual entities.

   a. True

   b. False

4. Meditation is the act of focusing one's thoughts or engaging in self-reflection or contemplation.

   a. True

   b. False

5. Nursing care that supports clients' spiritual health will help promote other dimensions of health.

   a. True

   b. False

6. Religious law may dictate how food is prepared; for example, many Jewish people require ___________ food, which is food prepared according to Jewish law.

7. ___________, which is defined as being present, being there, or just being with a client, is a term that identifies one of the competencies incorporated by expert nurses.

8. In the ___________ phase, the nurse identifies interventions to help the client achieve the overall goal of maintaining or restoring spiritual well-being so that spiritual strength, serenity, and satisfaction are realized.

9. ___________ symbols include jewelry, medals, amulets, icons, totems, or body ornamentation (e.g., tattoos) that carry religious or spiritual significance.

10. Clients facing imminent death may seek ___________ from others as well as from God.

11. Match the following terms with the correct definitions.

a. Spiritual distress	______	To believe in or be committed to something or someone
b. Religion	______	A concept that incorporates spirituality
c. Atheist	______	The belief in more than one God
d. Polytheism	______	The belief in the existence of one God
e. Spirituality	______	One without belief in a God
f. Faith	______	A person who doubts the existence of God or a supreme being or believes the existence of God has not been proved
g. Hope	______	An organized system of beliefs and practices
h. Monotheism	______	A challenge to the spiritual well-being or to the belief system that provides strength, hope, and meaning to life
i. Agnostic	______	Is manifested by a feeling of being "generally alive, purposeful, and fulfilled"
j. Spiritual health/well-being	______	Refers to that part of being human that seeks meaningfulness through intra-, inter-, and transpersonal connection

12. Which of the following is NOT one of the aspects of spirituality?
    a. Meaning
    b. Value
    c. Connection
    d. Religion

13. ____________ will most likely not have insurance coverage and rely on the religious community for support.
    a. Amish, Mennonites
    b. Buddhists
    c. Christian Scientists
    d. Hindus

14. ____________ avoid alcohol, caffeine, and smoking. They prefer to wear temple undergarments. Arrange for priestly blessing if requested.
    a. Jehovah's Witnesses
    b. Jews
    c. Latter-Day Saints/Mormons
    d. Muslims

15. According to Vardey, organized religions offer all of the following EXCEPT:
    a. A sense of community bound by common beliefs.
    b. A place of aversion.
    c. The collective study of scripture.
    d. The performance of ritual.

16. Spiritual ____________ refers to a challenge to the spiritual well-being or to the belief system that provides strength, hope, and meaning to life.

    a. Duress

    b. Interest

    c. Guidance

    d. Distress

FOCUSED STUDY TIPS

1. Describe nursing interventions to support clients' spiritual beliefs and religious practices.
2. Identify the desired outcomes for evaluating the client's spiritual health.
3. List some of the factors associated with spiritual distress and the manifestations of that stress.
4. Discuss the influence of spiritual and religious beliefs about diet on health care.
5. What are some of the ways people nurture or enhance their spirituality?
6. Describe the spiritual development of the individual across the life span.
7. Discuss the influence of spiritual and religious beliefs about birth and death on health care.
8. Explain the concept of forgiveness.
9. Describe the influence of spiritual and religious beliefs about prayer and meditation on health care.
10. Discuss the concept of hope.
11. Describe the concept of spirituality.
12. List some of the characteristics of spiritual health.
13. Discuss the influence of spiritual and religious beliefs about dress on health care.
14. Briefly explain some of the varying religious beliefs related to birth.
15. What does the acronym FICA stand for?

CASE STUDY

1. A 37-year-old male client has been admitted to the hospital with terminal cancer. His condition is rapidly deteriorating. He has been living at home with his mother and father for the past 6 months. He is expressing fear and anger about his condition and states that he does not believe he will be alive much longer.

    a. The client asks you to pray with him. Describe some of the guidelines you should follow.

    b. Summarize the practice guidelines you should follow to support the client's religious practices.

    c. Give some examples of spiritual needs that would be related to others.

REVIEW QUESTIONS

1. Which religion avoids unnecessary treatments on the Sabbath?
   1. Buddhism
   2. Jehovah's Witness
   3. Latter-Day Saints (LDS or Mormon)
   4. Seventh-Day Adventist
2. Religion is:
   1. An organized system of beliefs and practices. It offers a way of spiritual expression that provides guidance for believers in responding to life's questions and challenges.
   2. A challenge to the spiritual well-being or to the belief system that provides strength, hope, and meaning to life.
   3. Manifested by a feeling of being "generally alive, purposeful, and fulfilled."
   4. Part of being human that seeks meaningfulness through intra-, inter-, and transpersonal connection.
3. A client tells you he is an atheist. You know this to mean:
   1. He is an individual who doubts the existence of God or a supreme being or believes the existence of God has not been proved.
   2. He is an individual without a belief in a God.
   3. He is an individual who believes in the existence of one God.
   4. He is an individual who believes in more than one God.
4. A client's religion may have rules about which foods and beverages are allowed and which are prohibited. Clients of which religion do not eat shellfish or pork?
   1. Buddhism
   2. Orthodox Jew
   3. Hindu
   4. Mormon
5. A nurse is evaluating a nursing student's understanding of presencing. Which of the following statements demonstrates a need for further teaching? A distinguishing feature of presencing is:
   1. "Giving of self in the present moment."
   2. "Being there in a way that is meaningful to yourself."
   3. "Listening, with full awareness of the privilege of doing so."
   4. "Being available with all of the self."
6. The nurse who is evaluating a supporting religious practices class recognizes that further teaching is necessary when which of the following statements is made by a participant?
   1. "Create a trusting relationship with the client so that any religious concerns or practices can be openly discussed and addressed."
   2. "If unsure of client religious needs, ask how nurses can assist in having these needs met."
   3. "Always discuss personal spiritual beliefs with a client."
   4. "Acquaint yourself with the religions, spiritual practices, and cultures of the area in which you are working."

7. A nurse is evaluating a nursing student who is just about to pray with a client. Which of the following actions demonstrates a need for further teaching? The student nurse tells the nurse:

   1. "Clients' preferences for prayer reflect their personalities."
   2. "Before praying, assess what clients would like you to pray for."
   3. "Prayer may be the springboard to further discussion or catharsis."
   4. "Prayers should never be personalized."

8. A nurse caring for a Muslim client recognizes that the client practices prayer ____________ times a day and that the Muslim client may need assistance to maintain this commitment.

   1. Three
   2. Four
   3. Five
   4. Six

9. When a nurse is planning in relation to a client's spiritual needs, plans should NOT be designed to do which of the following?

   1. Help the client fulfill religious obligations.
   2. Help the client draw on and use inner resources more effectively to meet the present situation.
   3. Help the client find meaning in existence and the present situation.
   4. Promote a sense of hopelessness.

10. A nurse is planning a seminar on spiritual needs. Which of the following is NOT an example of spiritual needs related to the self?

    1. Need for meaning and purpose
    2. Need to express creativity
    3. Need for hope
    4. Need to cope with loss of loved ones

CHAPTER 42

STRESS AND COPING

KEY TERM REVIEW

Match each term with its appropriate definition.

1. _______ Alarm reaction
2. _______ Anger
3. _______ Anxiety
4. _______ Burnout
5. _______ Caregiver burden
6. _______ Coping
7. _______ Coping mechanism
8. _______ Coping strategy
9. _______ Countershock phase
10. _______ Crisis intervention
11. _______ Depression
12. _______ Ego defense mechanisms
13. _______ Fear
14. _______ General adaptation syndrome (GAS)
15. _______ Local adaptation syndrome (LAS)
16. _______ Shock phase
17. _______ Stage of exhaustion
18. _______ Stage of resistance
19. _______ Stimulus-based stress models
20. _______ Stress
21. _______ Stressor
22. _______ Transactional stress theory

a. An extreme feeling of sadness, despair, dejection, lack of worth

b. Reaction to long-term stress in family members who take care of a person in the home

c. Natural or learned way of responding to a changing environment

d. The changes produced in the body during shock

e. Any event or stimulus that causes an individual to experience stress

f. Defines stress as a stimulus, life event, or a set of circumstances that arouses physiological and/or psychological reactions that may increase the individual's vulnerability to illness

g. Initial reaction of the body to stress

h. A condition in which a person experiences changes in the normal balanced state

i. Stressor may be perceived consciously or unconsciously; stressors stimulate the sympathetic nervous system

j. Dealing with change

k. Encompasses a set of cognitive, affective, and adaptive responses that arise out of person–environment transactions

l. Characterized by a chain or pattern of physiological events

m. Short-term helping process of assisting clients to work through a crisis to its resolution

n. At the end of this stage, the body may either rest and return to normal, or death may be the ultimate consequence

o. Emotional state consisting of a subjective feeling of animosity or strong displeasure

p. A complex system of behaviors that can be likened to the exhaustion stage of GAS

q. Coping mechanism

r. Body can react locally; one organ or a part of the body reacts alone

s. Stage during which the body attempts to cope with a stressor, and to limit stressor to smallest area of the body that can deal with it

t. Unconscious psychological adaptive mechanisms that develop as the personality attempts to defend itself, establish compromises, and calm inner tensions

u. A state of mental uneasiness apprehension, dread, or foreboding

v. Emotion or feeling of apprehension aroused by impending or seeming danger, pain, or another perceived threat

KEY TOPIC REVIEW

1. A stressor is a condition in which the person experiences changes in the normal balanced state.

   a. True

   b. False

2. In stimulus-based stress models, stress is defined as a stimulus, a life event, or a set of circumstances that arouses physiological and/or psychological reactions that may increase the individual's vulnerability to illness.

   a. True

   b. False

3. Problem solving involves thinking through a threatening situation, using specific steps to arrive at a solution.

   a. True

   b. False

4. Structuring (discipline) is assuming a manner and facial expression that convey a sense of being in control or in charge.

   a. True

   b. False

5. Self-control is the arrangement or manipulation of a situation so that threatening events do not occur.
   a. True
   b. False
6. ____________ is consciously and willfully putting a thought or feeling out of mind: “I won’t deal with that today. I’ll do it tomorrow.”
7. ____________, or daydreaming, is likened to make-believe.
8. ____________ may be described as dealing with change—successfully or unsuccessfully.
9. Crisis ____________ is a short-term helping process of assisting clients to work through a crisis to its resolution and restore their precrisis level of functioning.
10. A coping ____________ (coping mechanism) is a natural or learned way of responding to a changing environment or specific problem or situation.
11. Match the following terms with the correct definition.

a. Shock phase	______	Unconscious psychological adaptive mechanisms or, according to Sigmund Freud (1946), mental mechanisms that develop as the personality attempts to defend itself, establish compromises among conflicting impulses, and calm inner tensions
b. Stage of resistance	______	An extreme feeling of sadness, despair, dejection, lack of worth, or emptiness; affects millions of Americans a year
c. Anger	______	An emotional state consisting of a subjective feeling of animosity or strong displeasure
d. Stressor	______	An emotion or feeling of apprehension aroused by impending or seeming danger, pain, or other perceived threat
e. Ego defense mechanisms	______	A state of mental uneasiness, apprehension, dread, or foreboding or a feeling of helplessness related to an impending or anticipated unidentified threat to self or significant relationships
f. Depression	______	When the body’s adaptation takes place
g. Local adaptation syndrome	______	When the changes produced in the body during the shock phase are reversed
h. Anxiety	______	The stressor may be perceived consciously or unconsciously by the person
i. Countershock phase	______	One organ or a part of the body reacts alone
j. Fear	______	Any event or stimulus that causes an individual to experience stress

12. ____________ focuses on solving immediate problems and involves individuals, groups, or families.
    a. Crisis intervention
    b. Caregiver burden
    c. Crisis counseling
    d. Burnout

13. What concept refers to efforts to improve a situation by making changes or taking action?

    a. Problem-focused coping

    b. Emotion-focused coping

    c. Long-term coping

    d. Short-term coping

14. ___________ is resorting to an earlier, more comfortable level of functioning that is characteristically less demanding and responsible.

    a. Reaction formation

    b. Projection

    c. Minimization

    d. Regression

15. ___________ is displacement of energy associated with more primitive sexual or aggressive drives into socially acceptable activities.

    a. Sublimation

    b. Substitution

    c. Undoing

    d. Repression

16. Which of the following is NOT a cognitive indicator or thinking response to stress?

    a. Structuring

    b. Suppression

    c. Anxiety

    d. Problem solving

FOCUSED STUDY TIPS

1. Compare and contrast anxiety and fear.
2. List and define 10 defense mechanisms.
3. Explain burnout.
4. Summarize ways to mediate anger.
5. Recall the concepts and sources of stress.
6. Define general adaptation syndrome (GAS) and local adaptation syndrome (LAS).
7. Describe interventions to help clients minimize and manage stress.
8. Identify nursing diagnoses related to stress.
9. Identify essential aspects of assessing a client's stress and coping patterns.
10. Discuss types of coping and coping strategies.
11. Identify behaviors related to specific ego defense mechanisms.

12. Differentiate four levels of anxiety.

13. Identify physiological, psychological, and cognitive indicators of stress.

14. Describe the three stages of Selye's general adaptation syndrome.

15. Differentiate the concepts of stress as a stimulus, as a response, and as a transaction.

16. Describe the key difference between effective and ineffective coping.

CASE STUDY

1. A 37-year-old client has an inability to relax, concentrate, and focus. She also complains of a headache, dizziness, and nausea. The health care provider has asked for you to provide the client with information about anxiety.
   a. What level of anxiety is the client most likely experiencing?
   b. Describe various methods you could teach the client to minimize stress and anxiety.
   c. Explain the difference between anxiety and fear.

REVIEW QUESTIONS

1. A client comes into the clinic with tremors and pitch changes in her voice. She also has facial twitches and shakiness. Her respiratory and heart rates are slightly elevated. At the end of her assessment she tells you, "I feel like I have butterflies in my stomach." Which level of anxiety is this client experiencing?
   1. Mild
   2. Moderate
   3. Severe
   4. Panic
2. The spouse of a client is discussing the difference between anxiety and fear. Which of the following statements indicates a need for further teaching?
   1. "The source of anxiety is identifiable and the source of fear may not be identifiable."
   2. "Anxiety is related to the future, that is, to an anticipated event. Fear is related to the present."
   3. "Anxiety is vague, whereas fear is definite."
   4. "Anxiety is the result of psychological or emotional conflict; fear is the result of a discrete physical or psychological entity."
3. Which of the following is an appropriate strategy for dealing with a client's anger?
   1. Try to understand the meaning of the client's anger.
   2. Do not let clients talk about their anger until you are ready.
   3. After the interaction is completed, avoid processing your feelings and responses to the client with your colleagues.
   4. Listen to the client, and act just like the client.
4. Which of the following techniques prevents burnout for nurses?
   1. Avoid collegial support groups.
   2. Avoid involvement in constructive change efforts.
   3. Learn to say no.
   4. Engage in exercise when you can to direct energy inward.

5. At which developmental stage would a client experience getting married, leaving home, managing a home, getting started in an occupation, continuing one's education, and having children?
   1. Adolescent
   2. Young adult
   3. Middle adult
   4. Older adult
6. Which of the following is an example of the defense mechanism of displacement?
   1. A husband and wife have an argument, and the husband becomes so angry he hits a door instead of his wife.
   2. A woman, though told her father has metastatic cancer, continues to plan a family reunion 18 months in advance.
   3. A mother is told her child must repeat a grade in school, and the mother blames this on the teacher's poor instruction.
   4. A woman wants to marry a man exactly like her deceased father, and settles for someone whose appearance resembles her father..
7. A nurse is taking care of an adult client when he throws a temper tantrum because he does not get his own way. Which defense mechanism is the adult client displaying?
   1. Repression
   2. Regression
   3. Reaction formation
   4. Rationalization
8. A nurse is planning a seminar on minimizing stress and anxiety. Which of the following statements is NOT correct?
   1. Provide an atmosphere of warmth and trust; convey a sense of caring and empathy.
   2. Listen attentively; try to understand the client's perspective on the situation.
   3. Control the environment to minimize additional stressors, such as by reducing noise, limiting the number of individuals in the room, and providing care by the same nurse as much as possible.
   4. Communicate in long, detailed sentences.
9. During discharge planning, the nurse is teaching the client common characteristics of crises. Which of the following statements is NOT correct?
   1. The person is not aware of a warning signal and does not "see it coming."
   2. The crisis is often experienced as ultimately life threatening, whether this perception is realistic or not.
   3. Communication with significant others is often increased.
   4. There may be a perceived or real displacement from familiar surroundings or loved ones.
10. A nurse is evaluating a nursing student's understanding of the clinical manifestations of stress. Which of the following statements by the nursing student demonstrates a need for further teaching?
    1. "Pupils constrict to decrease visual perception when serious threats to the body arise."
    2. "Sweat production (diaphoresis) increases to control elevated body heat due to increased metabolism."
    3. "Heart rate and cardiac output increase to transport nutrients and by-products of metabolism more efficiently."
    4. "Skin is pallid because of constriction of peripheral blood vessels, an effect of norepinephrine."

CHAPTER 43

LOSS, GRIEVING, AND DEATH

KEY TERM REVIEW

Match each term with its appropriate definition.

1. _______ Actual loss
2. _______ Algor mortis
3. _______ Anticipatory grief
4. _______ Anticipatory loss
5. _______ Bereavement
6. _______ Cerebral death
7. _______ Closed awareness
8. _______ Complicated grief
9. _______ End-of-life care
10. _______ Grief
11. _______ Heart–lung death
12. _______ Higher brain death
13. _______ Hospice
14. _______ Livor mortis
15. _______ Loss
16. _______ Mortician
17. _______ Mourning
18. _______ Mutual pretense
19. _______ Open awareness
20. _______ Palliative care
21. _______ Perceived loss
22. _______ Rigor mortis
23. _______ Shroud
24. _______ Undertaker

a. Client is not made aware of impending death
b. Mortician
c. Approach that improves quality of life of clients and their families facing life-threatening illness, through prevention and relief of suffering
d. Gradual decrease of the body's temperature after death
e. A large piece of plastic or cotton material used to enclose a body after death
f. Mottling discoloration that occurs in the lowermost or dependent areas of the body
g. Behavioral process through which grief is eventually resolved or altered
h. Client and others know about impending death and feel comfortable talking about it
i. Exists when the strategies to cope with the loss are maladaptive; usually lasts more than 6 months
j. Cessation of apical pulse, respirations, and blood pressure
k. Experienced by one individual but cannot be verified by others
l. Occurs when the cerebral cortex is irreversibly destroyed
m. Client, family, and health personnel know that the prognosis is terminal but do not talk about it
n. The subjective response experienced by the surviving loved ones
o. An actual or potential situation in which something that is valued is changed or no longer available
p. Cerebral death
q. Stiffening of the body that occurs about 2 to 4 hours after death
r. Can be recognized by others

s. Total response to the emotional experience related to loss

t. Focuses on support and care of the dying person and family; goal is facilitating a peaceful and dignified death

u. Experienced before the loss actually occurs

v. Care provided in the final weeks before death

w. Experienced in advance of the event

x. An individual trained in care of the dead

KEY TOPIC REVIEW

1. Everyone experiences loss, grieving, and death at some time.
   a. True
   b. False
2. Actual loss is experienced before the loss actually occurs.
   a. True
   b. False
3. Higher brain death occurs when the higher brain center, the cerebral cortex, is irreversibly destroyed.
   a. True
   b. False
4. In closed awareness, the client is not made aware of impending death.
   a. True
   b. False
5. With mutual pretense, the client, family, and health personnel know that the prognosis is terminal but do not talk about it and make an effort not to raise the subject.
   a. True
   b. False
6. Rigor ____________ is the stiffening of the body that occurs about 2 to 4 hours after death.
7. ____________ mortis is the gradual decrease of the body's temperature after death.
8. A ____________ is an individual trained in care of the dead.
9. A ____________ is a large piece of plastic or cotton material used to enclose a body after death.
10. ____________ occurs when the individual perceives no solutions to a problem.
11. An individual who conducts rituals of mourning (e.g., funeral) is said to be in which of the following of Engel's stages of grieving?
    a. Shock and disbelief
    b. Developing awareness
    c. Restitution
    d. Resolving the loss
12. More than ____________ nurses in the United States are nationally certified in hospice and palliative care.
    a. 9,000
    b. 14,000
    c. 18,000
    d. 24,000

13. A(An) ____________ is a large piece of plastic or cotton material used to enclose a body after death.
    a. Undertaker
    b. Hospice
    c. Mortician
    d. Shroud
14. Which of the following age groups has the following beliefs/attitudes about the concept of death?
    - Understands death as the inevitable end of life.
    - Begins to understand own mortality, expressed as interest in afterlife or as fear of death.

    a. Infancy to 5 years
    b. 5 to 9 years
    c. 9 to 12 years
    d. 12 to 18 years
15. An individual who is displaying the behavioral response of separation anxiety would be in which of Sander's phases of bereavement?
    a. Shock
    b. Awareness of loss
    c. Conservation/withdrawal
    d. Healing: the turning point

FOCUSED STUDY TIPS

1. Discuss the dying person's bill of rights.
2. Describe the types and sources of losses.
3. Discuss selected frameworks for identifying stages of grieving.
4. Identify clinical symptoms of grief.
5. Discuss factors affecting a grief response.
6. Identify measures that facilitate the grieving process.
7. List clinical signs of impending and actual death.
8. Describe helping clients die with dignity.
9. Describe nursing measures for care of the body after death.
10. Describe the role of the nurse in working with families or caregivers of dying clients.
11. Define grief, bereavement, and mourning.
12. List the factors influencing the loss and grief responses.
13. Discuss various responses to dying and death.

14. Explain the steps in postmortem care.

15. Discuss the physiological needs of the dying client.

16. Discuss the psychosocial needs of the dying client.

CASE STUDY

1. You are visiting with a 22-year-old male client. During the assessment phase, you discover his father passed away last week from a terminal illness. The client tells you he was very close to his father.
   a. Which type of loss is the client experiencing?
   b. Explain grief, bereavement, and mourning.
   c. List four appropriate questions to ask during the assessment.

REVIEW QUESTIONS

1. Bereavement is:
   1. The total response to the emotional experience related to loss.
   2. The subjective response experienced by the surviving loved ones after the death of a person with whom they have shared a significant relationship.
   3. The behavioral process through which grief is eventually resolved or altered; it is often influenced by culture, spiritual beliefs, and custom.
   4. An actual or potential situation in which something that is valued is changed or no longer available.
2. A nurse's client just passed away. The nurse understands that rigor mortis is the stiffening of the body that occurs about ____________ hours after death.
   1. 2 to 4
   2. 5 to 7
   3. 8 to 10
   4. 11 to 13
3. A nurse is taking care of a client who just lost her husband to a terminal illness. The client is refusing to believe that loss is happening. Which of Kübler-Ross's stages of grieving is the client experiencing?
   1. Denial
   2. Anger
   3. Bargaining
   4. Depression
4. A nurse is caring for a client who just lost her brother to suicide. The client accepts the situation intellectually, but denies it emotionally. Which of Engel's stages of grieving is the client experiencing?
   1. Shock and disbelief
   2. Developing awareness
   3. Restitution
   4. Resolving the loss

5. Which of the following is a correct description of Sander's conservation/withdrawal phase of bereavement?
   1. The bereaved move from distress about living without their loved one to learning to live more independently.
   2. The survivors feel a need to be alone to conserve and replenish both physical and emotional energy.
   3. Friends and family resume normal activities. The bereaved experience the full significance of their loss.
   4. The survivors are left with feelings of confusion, unreality, and disbelief that the loss has occurred.
6. A nurse is evaluating a nursing student who is caring for a dying client's physiological needs. Which of the following actions demonstrates a need for further teaching?
   1. For an unconscious client with an airway clearance problem, the nursing student places him in Fowler's position.
   2. The client is diaphoretic; the nursing student gives the client frequent baths and changes the linen.
   3. The nursing student regularly changes client's position.
   4. The nursing student provides the client with skin care in response to incontinence of urine or feces.
7. A nurse is planning a seminar on the dying person's bill of rights. Which of the following statements is NOT part of the dying person's bill of rights?
   1. I have the right to express my feelings and emotions about my approaching death in my own way.
   2. I have the right to expect continuing medical and nursing attention even though cure goals must be changed to comfort goals.
   3. I have the right to be free from pain.
   4. I have the right to die alone.
8. The nurse is providing care to an unconscious client who is dying. Which of the following is NOT a clinical manifestation of impending clinical death?
   1. Difficulty swallowing and gradual loss of the gag reflex
   2. Mottling and cyanosis of the extremities
   3. Rapid, shallow, irregular, or abnormally slow respirations
   4. Faster and weaker pulse
9. At what age does a client typically believe his or her own death can be reversible?
   1. Infancy to 5 years
   2. 5 to 9 years
   3. 9 to 12 years
   4. 12 to 18 years
10. Which of the following actions is NOT appropriate for the nurse providing postmortem care?
    1. One pillow is placed under the head and shoulders to prevent blood from discoloring the face by settling in it.
    2. The eyelids are closed and held in place for a few seconds so they remain closed.
    3. Dentures are always removed and placed with the client's personal belongings.
    4. All jewelry is removed, except a wedding band in some instances, which is taped to the finger.

CHAPTER 44

ACTIVITY AND EXERCISE

KEY TERM REVIEW

Match each term with its appropriate definition.

1. _______ Active ROM exercises
2. _______ Aerobic exercise
3. _______ Anabolism
4. _______ Anaerobic exercise
5. _______ Basal metabolic rate
6. _______ Catabolism
7. _______ Foot drop
8. _______ Functional strength
9. _______ Isokinetic (resistive) exercise
10. _______ Isometric (static or setting) exercise
11. _______ Isotonic (dynamic) exercise
12. _______ Lateral position
13. _______ Metabolism
14. _______ Orthopneic position
15. _______ Orthostatic hypotension
16. _______ Passive ROM exercises
17. _______ Prone position
18. _______ Range of motion (ROM)
19. _______ Relaxation response (RR)
20. _______ Spastic
21. _______ Supine position
22. _______ Tripod (triangle) position
23. _______ Valsalva maneuver

a. Occurs when a stronger muscle dominates the opposite muscle

b. Another person moves each of the client's joints through its complete range of movement

c. Protein breakdown

d. Isotonic exercises in which the client moves each joint in the body through its complete range of movement

e. The ability of the body to perform work

f. Involves activity in which the muscles cannot draw out enough oxygen from the bloodstream; used for endurance training

g. Protein synthesis

h. Muscle contraction or tension against resistance

i. The minimal energy expended for maintenance of physical and chemical processes of the body

j. Muscle contraction without moving the joint

k. Crutch positioned in front of feet about 40 cm (15 in.), out laterally about 15 cm (6 in.)

l. Activity during which the amount of oxygen taken in the body is greater than that used to perform the activity

m. Client sits either in bed or on the side of the bed with an overbed table across the lap

n. Side-lying position

o. Sum of all the physical and chemical processes by which living substance is formed and maintained, and by which energy is made available for use by the body

p. Decreased blood pressure as a result of changing from a sitting or lying position to a standing position

q. Exercise can counteract some of the harmful effects of stress on the body

r. With too much muscle tone

s. The maximum movement that is possible for that joint

t. Refers to holding the breath and straining against a closed glottis

u. Those in which the muscle shortens to produce muscle contraction and active movement

v. Client positioned on the abdomen with the head turned to one side

w. Lying on back; dorsal recumbent

KEY TOPIC REVIEW

1. An activity-exercise pattern refers to an individual's routine of exercise, activity, leisure, and recreation.

   a. True

   b. False

2. An individual maintains balance as long as the line of gravity (an imaginary horizontal line drawn through the body's center of gravity) passes through the center of gravity.

   a. True

   b. False

3. The base of support is the foundation on which the body rests.

   a. True

   b. False

4. The range of motion (ROM) of a joint is the maximum movement that is possible for that joint.

   a. True

   b. False

5. Proprioception is the term used to describe awareness of posture, movement, and changes in equilibrium and the knowledge of position, weight, and resistance of objects in relation to the body.

   a. True

   b. False

6. ___________ is commonly seen in the arm muscles of a tennis player, the leg muscles of a skater, and the arm and hand muscles of a carpenter.

7. ___________ is a condition in which the bones become brittle and fragile due to calcium depletion.

8. Unused muscles ___________, losing most of their strength and normal function.

9. When the muscle fibers are not able to shorten and lengthen, eventually a ___________ forms, limiting joint mobility.

10. Without movement, the collagen tissues at the joint become ___________.

11. Match the following terms with the correct definition.

a. Physical activity	______	The ability to move freely, easily, rhythmically, and purposefully in the environment; is an essential part of living
b. Exercise	______	Bodily movement produced by skeletal muscle contraction that increases energy expenditure
c. Isotonic (dynamic) exercises	______	A type of physical activity defined as a planned, structured, and repetitive bodily movement performed to improve or maintain one or more components of physical fitness
d. Aerobic exercise	______	Exercise in which the muscle shortens to produce muscle contraction and active movement
e. Mobility	______	Exercise in which there is muscle contraction without moving the joint (muscle length does not change)
f. Anaerobic exercise	______	Involve muscle contraction or tension against resistance; thus, they can be either isotonic or isometric
g. Isokinetic (resistive) exercises	______	Activity during which the amount of oxygen taken in by the body is greater than that used to perform the activity
h. Osteoporosis	______	Involves activity in which the muscles cannot draw out enough oxygen from the bloodstream, and anaerobic pathways are used to provide additional energy for a short time
i. Ventilation	______	Air circulating into and out of the lungs
j. Isometric (static or setting) exercises	______	A condition in which the bones become brittle and fragile due to calcium depletion

12. Which of the following is defined as having too much muscle tone?
    a. Meningitis
    b. Paresis
    c. Flaccid
    d. Spastic

13. ____________ refers to holding the breath and straining against a closed glottis.
    a. Valsalva maneuver
    b. Orthostatic hypotension
    c. Stasis
    d. Venous vasodilation

14. Which of the following is NOT one of the three factors that collectively predispose a client to the formation of a thrombophlebitis?
    a. Increased oil in the diet
    b. Impaired venous return to the heart
    c. Hypercoagulability of the blood
    d. Injury to a vessel wall

15. ____________ refers to the sum of all the physical and chemical processes by which living substance is formed and maintained and by which energy is made available for use by the body.

a. Metabolism

b. Catabolism

c. Anabolism

d. Anorexia

FOCUSED STUDY TIPS

1. Discuss how the U.S. Department of Health and Human Services defines exercise and physical activity.
2. Describe the effects of exercise on cognitive function.
3. List some of the factors that affect an individual's body alignment, mobility, and daily activity level.
4. Define and discuss the term *body mechanics*.
5. Describe the three different ways the intensity of exercise can be measured.
6. Discuss the importance of the musculoskeletal system.
7. Describe how to use safe practices when positioning, moving, lifting, and ambulating clients.
8. Describe a variety of movement interventions and therapies to improve physical health, mobility, strength, balance, mood, and cognition.
9. Develop nursing diagnoses and outcomes related to activity, exercise, and mobility problems.
10. Discuss the activity-exercise pattern, alignment, mobility capabilities and limitations, activity tolerance, and potential problems related to immobility.
11. Identify factors influencing a person's body alignment and activity.
12. Compare the effects of exercise and immobility on body systems.
13. Differentiate isotonic, isometric, isokinetic, aerobic, and anaerobic exercise.
14. Describe four basic elements of normal movement.
15. List some of the factors that increase the potential for lower back injuries.
16. Describe how increased venous pressure leads to edema.
17. Describe the factors that predispose a client to the development of thrombophlebitis.

CASE STUDY

1. A 43-year-old client is recovering from a back injury and is receiving care from a home health nurse. A major aspect of discharge planning involves instru ctional needs of the client and the client's family. *Provide the client and the client's family education about the following topics:*
   - Maintaining musculoskeletal function
   - Preventing injury
   - Managing energy to prevent fatigue
   - Preventing back injuries

REVIEW QUESTIONS

1. A nurse is planning a seminar on preventing back injuries. Which of the following statements is correct?
   1. When sitting for a period of time, periodically move legs and hips, flex one hip and knee, and rest your foot on an object if possible.
   2. When sitting, keep your knees slightly lower than your hips.
   3. Use a hard mattress and firm pillow that provide good body support at natural body curvatures.
   4. Exercise regularly to maintain overall physical condition and regulate weight; include exercises that strengthen the pelvic, abdominal, and spinal muscles.
2. During discharge planning, the nurse is evaluating the client's understanding of wheelchair safety. Which of the following statements indicates a need for further teaching?
   1. Always lock the brakes on both wheels of the wheelchair when the client transfers in or out of it.
   2. Lower the footplates before transferring the client into the wheelchair.
   3. Lower the footplates after the transfer, and place the client's feet on them.
   4. Ensure the client is positioned well back in the seat of the wheelchair.
3. A nurse is evaluating a nursing student's understanding of stretcher safety. Which of the following statements demonstrates a need for further teaching?
   1. Never leave a client unattended on a stretcher unless the wheels are locked and the side rails are raised on both sides and/or the safety straps are securely fastened across the client.
   2. Always push a stretcher from the end where the client's head is positioned. This position protects the client's head in the event of a collision.
   3. Maneuver the stretcher when entering the elevator so that the client's feet go in first.
   4. Fasten safety straps across the client on a stretcher, and raise the side rails.
4. Which of the following actions is appropriate for the nurse performing active ROM exercises?
   1. Perform each ROM exercise as taught to the point of slight resistance, but not beyond, and never to the point of discomfort.
   2. Perform the movements systematically, using a different sequence during each session.
   3. Perform each exercise five times.
   4. Perform each series of exercises three times daily.

5. During discharge planning, the nurse is teaching the client how to control postural hypotension. Which of the following statements is correct?
    1. Bend down all the way to the floor and stand up quickly after stooping.
    2. Wear elastic stockings day and night to inhibit venous pooling in the legs.
    3. Use a rocking chair to improve circulation in the lower extremities.
    4. Get out of a hot bath very quickly, because high temperatures can lead to venous pooling.
6. Isotonic (dynamic) exercises:
    1. Are those in which there is muscle contraction without moving the joint (muscle length does not change).
    2. Involve muscle contraction or tension against resistance; thus, they can be either isotonic or isometric.
    3. Are activities during which the amount of oxygen taken in by the body is greater than that used to perform the activity.
    4. Are those in which the muscle shortens to produce muscle contraction and active movement.
7. A nurse is evaluating a nursing student's understanding of positioning clients. Which of the following statements indicates a need for further teaching?
    1. Positioning a client in good body alignment and changing the position regularly (every 3 hours) and systematically are essential aspects of nursing practice.
    2. Any position, correct or incorrect, can be detrimental if maintained for a prolonged period.
    3. For all clients, it is important to assess the skin and provide skin care before and after a position change.
    4. Frequent change of position helps to prevent muscle discomfort, undue pressure resulting in pressure ulcers, damage to superficial nerves and blood vessels, and contractures.
8. Fowler's position is a bed position:
    1. In which the head and trunk are raised 45° to 60°.
    2. In which the client's head and shoulders are slightly elevated on a small pillow.
    3. In which the client lies on the abdomen with the head turned to one side.
    4. In which the person lies on one side of the body. Flexing the top hip and knee and placing this leg in front of the body creates a wider, triangular base of support and achieves greater stability.
9. General guidelines for transfer techniques include all of the following EXCEPT:
    1. Obtain essential equipment before starting (e.g., transfer belt, wheelchair), and check its function.
    2. Always support or hold equipment rather than the client to ensure safety and dignity.
    3. Remove obstacles from the area used for the transfer.
    4. Explain the transfer to the nursing personnel who are helping; specify who will give directions (one person needs to be in charge).
10. Which of the following actions is appropriate for the nurse assisting a client with crutches?
    1. The client lies in a prone position and the nurse measures from the anterior fold of the axilla to the heel of the foot and adds 2.5 cm (1 in.).
    2. The client stands erect and positions the crutch. The nurse makes sure the shoulder rest of the crutch is at least three fingerwidths, that is, 2.5 to 5 cm (1 to 2 in.), below the axilla.
    3. The client stands upright and supports the body weight by the axilla.
    4. The nurse measures the angle of elbow flexion. It should be about 10°.

CHAPTER 45

SLEEP

KEY TERM REVIEW

Match each term with its appropriate definition.

1. _______ Biological rhythms
2. _______ Electroencephalogram (EEG)
3. _______ Electromyogram (EMG)
4. _______ Electro-oculogram (EOG)
5. _______ Hypersomnia
6. _______ Insomnia
7. _______ Narcolepsy
8. _______ Nocturnal emissions
9. _______ NREM sleep
10. _______ Parasomnia
11. _______ Polysomnography
12. _______ REM sleep
13. _______ Sleep
14. _______ Sleep apnea
15. _______ Sleep architecture
16. _______ Sleep hygiene

a. Orgasm and release of semen during sleep
b. Naturally occurring altered state of consciousness in which perceptions and reactions are decreased
c. Basic organization of normal sleep
d. Individual obtains sufficient sleep at night but has difficulty staying awake during the day
e. Excessive daytime sleepiness caused by lack of chemical in area of the CNS that regulates sleep
f. Use of several monitoring and recording devices used to measure sleep objectively
g. Occurs about every 90 minutes; essential for psychosocial and mental equilibrium
h. Controlled within the body and synchronized with environmental factors
i. Characterized by frequent, short breathing pauses during sleep
j. Inability to fall asleep or remain asleep
k. Records brain waves
l. Four stages; essential for physiological well-being
m. Interventions used to promote and enhance the quality of client's sleep
n. Records muscle activity
o. Behavior that may interfere with sleep, and may occur during sleep
p. Records eye movement

KEY TOPIC REVIEW

1. Somnology is the study of sleep.
   a. True
   b. False
2. Stage 1 is the deepest stage of sleep.
   a. True
   b. False
3. Most dreams take place during REM sleep, but usually will not be remembered unless the individual arouses briefly at the end of the REM period.
   a. True
   b. False
4. Sleep apnea is characterized by frequent short breathing pauses during sleep.
   a. True
   b. False
5. Sleep hypnotics is a term referring to interventions used to promote sleep.
   a. True
   b. False
6. ___________ has come to be considered an altered state of consciousness in which the individual's perception of and reaction to the environment are decreased.
7. Biological ___________ exist in plants, animals, and humans.
8. REM sleep usually recurs about every ___________ minutes and lasts 5 to 30 minutes.
9. ___________ is described as the inability to fall asleep, remain asleep, or awaken feeling rested.
10. ___________ is a disorder of excessive daytime sleepiness caused by lack of the chemical hypocretin in the area of the central nervous system that regulates sleep.
11. Match the following terms with the correct definition.

a. Sundown syndrome	_____	The study of sleep
b. Insomnia	_____	The basic organization of normal sleep
c. Cognitive therapy	_____	A pattern of symptoms (e.g., agitation, anxious, aggressive, and sometimes delusional) that occur in the late afternoon
d. Sleep quality	_____	A subjective characteristic, often determined by whether or not a person wakes up feeling energetic or not
e. Narcolepsy	_____	The total time the individual sleeps
f. Hypersomnia	_____	The most common sleep complaint in America
g. Quantity of sleep	_____	Learning to develop positive thoughts and beliefs about sleep
h. Stimulus control	_____	Creating a sleep environment that promotes sleep
i. Sleep architecture	_____	Conditions where the affected individual obtains sufficient sleep at night but still cannot stay awake during the day
j. Somnology	_____	A disorder of excessive daytime sleepiness caused by the lack of the chemical hypocretin in the area of the central nervous system that regulates sleep

12. Newborns sleep ___________ hours a day, on an irregular schedule with periods of 1 to 3 hours spent awake.

    a. 10 to 12

    b. 12 to 14

    c. 14 to 16

    d. 12 to 18

13. Most healthy adults need ___________ hours of sleep a night.

    a. 7 to 9

    b. 9 to 11

    c. 11 to 13

    d. 13 to 15

14. Stress is considered by most sleep experts to be the number ___________ cause of short-term sleeping difficulties.

    a. one

    b. two

    c. three

    d. four

15. By the end of the first year, how many hours of sleep should an infant receive during the day?

    a. 7 to 8

    b. 9 to 12

    c. 12 to 13

    d. 14 to 15

16. Approximately ___________ million Americans have a chronic disorder of sleep and wakefulness that hinders daily functioning and adversely affects health.

    a. 10 to 30

    b. 30 to 50

    c. 50 to 70

    d. 70 to 90

FOCUSED STUDY TIPS

1. Identify factors that affect normal sleep.
2. Describe variations in sleep patterns throughout the life span.
3. Identify the characteristics of the sleep states of NREM and REM sleep.
4. Explain the functions and the physiology of sleep.
5. Discuss the following three types of sleep apnea: obstructive apnea, central apnea, and mixed apnea.
6. Identify items included in and the purpose of a sleep diary.

7. Summarize the major goal for clients with sleep disturbances.
8. Discuss the importance of bedtime rituals.
9. List several of the factors that can affect sleep.
10. Discuss several techniques for reducing environmental distractions in hospitals.
11. Discuss three nursing responsibilities to help clients sleep.
12. List seven drugs that may disrupt REM sleep, delay onset of sleep, or decrease sleep time.
13. Describe common sleep disorders.
14. Identify the components of a sleep pattern assessment.
15. Describe interventions that promote normal sleep.
16. Describe the reticular activating system (RAS) and its involvement in the sleep/wake cycle.

CASE STUDY

1. A 21-year-old client presented to the clinic today complaining of difficulty sleeping. The client is a part-time college student and also works 40 to 50 hours per week at an automotive body shop. The client is not taking any prescription medications and has an occasional alcoholic beverage at special events.
   a. Explain the two types of sleep.
   b. Describe factors that affect sleep.
   c. Explain the information that should be included in a sleep diary.

REVIEW QUESTIONS

1. During discharge planning, the nurse is teaching the client how to maintain a sleep diary. Which of the following statements is correct?
   1. Document the activities you perform 5 to 6 hours before going to bed.
   2. Document the consumption of caffeinated beverages and alcohol and amounts of those beverages.
   3. Do not list the bedtime rituals before bed.
   4. List only the prescribed medications taken during the day.
2. A nurse is evaluating a client's understanding of comfort measures that are essential to help fall asleep and stay asleep. Which of the following client statements indicates a need for further teaching?
   1. "I should wear loose-fitting nightwear."
   2. "I will void before bedtime."
   3. "I will perform hygienic routines prior to bedtime."
   4. "When I'm in pain, I will take the prescribed analgesics 1 hour before I go to sleep."

3. A nurse is evaluating a nursing student's understanding of medications. Which of the following statements by the nursing student indicates a need for further teaching?
   1. "Antianxiety medications decrease levels of arousal by facilitating the action of neurons in the CNS that suppress responsiveness to stimulation."
   2. "Sleep medications vary in their onset and duration of action and will impair waking function as long as they are chemically active."
   3. "Sleep medications affect NREM sleep more than REM sleep."
   4. "Initial doses of medications should be low and increases added gradually, depending on the client's response."
4. Hypersomnia is:
   1. A condition in which the affected individual obtains sufficient sleep at night but still cannot stay awake during the day.
   2. A disorder of excessive daytime sleepiness caused by the lack of the chemical hypocretin in the area of the central nervous system that regulates sleep.
   3. A condition characterized by frequent short breathing pauses during sleep.
   4. A behavior that may interfere with sleep and/or occurs during sleep.
5. Which stage of NREM (slow-wave) sleep lasts only about 10 to 15 minutes, during which the eyes are generally still, the heart and respiratory rates decrease slightly, and body temperature falls?
   1. Stage 1
   2. Stage 2
   3. Stage 3
   4. Stage 4
6. A nurse is evaluating a nursing student who is discussing physiological changes during NREM sleep. Which of the following statements by the nursing student demonstrates a need for further teaching?
   1. Arterial blood pressure falls.
   2. Pulse rate decreases.
   3. Peripheral blood vessels constrict.
   4. Cardiac output decreases.
7. When planning interventions to reduce environmental distractions in hospitals, which of the following would NOT be included in the client's plan of care?
   1. Lower the ring tone of nearby telephones.
   2. Discontinue use of the paging system after a certain hour or reduce its volume.
   3. Keep required staff conversations at low levels; conduct nursing reports or other discussions in a separate area away from client rooms.
   4. Perform noisy activities only during the day, never during sleeping hours.

8. A nurse is planning a seminar on promoting sleep. Which of the following is correct information?
    1. Establish a regular bedtime and wake-up time for all days of the week to enhance biologic rhythm.
    2. Complete office work or discuss family problems before bedtime.
    3. Get adequate exercise during the day to reduce stress, but avoid excessive physical exertion 1 hour before bedtime.
    4. Establish a regular, relaxing bedtime routine before sleep such as exercising or taking a cool shower.
9. When planning interventions to promote sleep, which of the following would be included in the client's plan of care?
    1. Create a sleep-conducive environment that is dark, quiet, comfortable, and cool.
    2. Give analgesics 3 hours before bedtime to relieve aches and pains.
    3. If a bedtime snack is necessary, give only high-carbohydrate snacks or a milk drink.
    4. Avoid giving the client heavy meals 4 to 5 hours before bedtime.
10. A nurse is evaluating a client's understanding of her child's night terrors. Which of the following statements indicates a need for further teaching?
    1. Night terrors are usually seen in children 3 to 6 years of age.
    2. Children usually cannot be wakened during night terrors, but should be protected from injury, helped back to bed, and soothed back to sleep.
    3. Children do not remember the night terror the next day, and there is no indication of a neurologic or emotional problem.
    4. Night terrors are partial awakenings from non-REM stage 1 or 2 sleep.

CHAPTER 46

PAIN MANAGEMENT

KEY TERM REVIEW

Match each term with its appropriate definition.

1. _______ Acute pain
2. _______ Agonist analgesic
3. _______ Agonist–antagonist analgesic
4. _______ Allodynia
3. _______ Chronic pain
4. _______ Coanalgesic
5. _______ Dysesthesia
6. _______ Effleurage
7. _______ Equianalgesia
8. _______ Hyperalgesia
9. _______ Hyperpathia
10. _______ Nerve block
11. _______ Neuropathic pain
12. _______ Nociceptive pain
13. _______ Nonsteroidal anti-inflammatory drugs (NSAIDs)
14. _______ Pain threshold
15. _______ Pain tolerance
16. _______ Patient-controlled analgesia (PCA)
17. _______ Peripheral neuropathic pain
18. _______ Pseudoaddiction
19. _______ Referred pain
20. _______ Somatic pain
21. _______ Sympathetically maintained pain
22. _______ Transcutaneous electrical nerve stimulation (TENS)
23. _______ Visceral pain

a. Type of massage consisting of long, slow, gliding strokes

b. Experienced when an intact, properly functioning nervous system sends signals that tissues are damaged

c. Chemical interruption of a nerve pathway, effected by injecting a local anesthetic into the nerve

d. Prolonged, usually recurring or lasting more than 3 months; interferes with functioning

e. A nonopioid pain medication that has anti-inflammatory, analgesic, and antipyretic effects

f. Heightened responses to a painful stimulus

g. Sudden or slow onset, regardless of its intensity

h. Appear to arise in different areas to other parts of the body

i. Associated with damaged or malfunctioning nerves due to illness, injury, or undetermined reasons

j. Hyperalgesia

k. Interactive method of pain management that permits clients to treat their pain by self-administering doses of analgesics

l. Refers to relative potency of various opioid analgesics compared to a standard dose of parenteral morphine

m. Originates in skin, muscles, bone, or connective tissue

n. Can act like opioids and relieve pain when given to a client who has not taken any pure opioids

o. Condition that results from the undertreatment of pain where the client may become hyperfocused on obtaining medication

p. May occur with abnormal connections between pain fibers and the sympathetic nervous system

q. Phantom limb pain

r. Pure opioid drugs that provide maximum pain inhibition

s. Not classified as a pain medication but may reduce pain alone or in combination with other analgesics; may potentiate the effects of pain medications

t. Least amount of stimuli necessary for a person to label a sensation as pain

u. Nonpainful stimulus that produces pain

v. Method of applying electrical stimulation directly over identified pain areas; stimulation through to block transmission of nociceptive impulse

w. Unpleasant, abnormal sensation that can be either spontaneous or evoked

x. The most pain an individual is willing or able to bear before taking evasive actions

y. Pain arising from organs

KEY TOPIC REVIEW

1. Central neuropathic pain occurs occasionally when abnormal connections between pain fibers and the sympathetic nervous system perpetuate problems with both the pain and sympathetically controlled functions.

   a. True

   b. False

2. Pain tolerance is the least amount of stimulus that is needed for a person to feel a sensation he or she labels as pain.

   a. True

   b. False

3. Pain management is the alleviation of pain or a reduction in pain to a level of comfort that is acceptable to the client.

   a. True

   b. False

4. Preemptive analgesia is the administration of analgesics prior to an invasive or operative procedure in order to treat pain before it occurs.

   a. True

   b. False

5. Pain threshold is the maximum amount of painful stimuli that a person is willing to withstand without seeking avoidance of the pain or relief.

   a. True

   b. False

6. A full agonist ___________ includes morphine (e.g., Kadian, MS Contin), oxycodone (e.g. Percocet, OxyContin), and hydromorphone (e.g., Dilaudid, Palladone).

7. Partial agonists have a ___________ effect in contrast to a full agonist.

8. ___________ refers to the relative potency of various opioid analgesics compared to a standard dose of parenteral morphine.

9. ___________ is "any medication or procedure, including surgery, that produces an effect in a client because of its implicit or explicit intent and not because of its specific physical or chemical properties."

10. ___________ drug therapy is advantageous in that it delivers a relatively stable plasma drug level and is noninvasive.

11. Match the following terms with the correct definition.

a. Chronic pain	______	Appear to arise in different areas
b. Mild pain	______	Pain arising from organs or hollow viscera
c. Physiological pain	______	When pain lasts only through the expected recovery period
d. Peripheral neuropathic pain	______	Prolonged, usually recurring or persisting over 6 months or longer, and interferes with functioning
e. Neuropathic pain	______	Pain in the 1–3 range of a 0-10 scale
f. Referred pain	______	Experienced when an intact, properly functioning nervous system sends signals that tissues are damaged, requiring attention and proper care
g. Somatic pain	______	Originates in the skin, muscles, bone, or connective tissue
h. Visceral pain	______	Experienced by people who have damaged or malfunctioning nerves
i. Moderate pain	______	Follow damage and/or sensitization of peripheral nerves
j. Acute pain	______	Pain in the 4–6 range of a 0-10 scale

12. A (An) ___________ block is a chemical interruption of a nerve pathway, effected by injection of a local anesthetic into the nerve.

    a. Nerve

    b. Anesthetic

    c. Chemical

    d. Pathway

13. Which of the following is NOT a type of pain stimuli?
    a. Mechanical
    b. Thermal
    c. Electrical
    d. Chemical
14. Which of the following terms is described as a painful sensation felt from a part of the body that has been amputated?
    a. Nociceptive pain
    b. Phantom pain
    c. Neuropathic pain
    d. Sensitization
15. All of the following are reasons clients may be reluctant to report pain EXCEPT:
    a. Unwillingness to trouble staff who are perceived as busy.
    b. Do not want to be labeled as "complainers" or "bad" patients.
    c. Concern that use of drugs now will render the drug inefficient later in life.
    d. Belief that others will think they are strong if they express pain.

FOCUSED STUDY TIPS

1. List the four physiological processes that are involved in nociception.
2. What is the "fifth vital sign"?
3. Describe the World Health Organization's step ladder approach developed for cancer pain control.
4. Describe pharmacologic interventions for pain.
5. Compare and contrast barriers to effective pain management.
6. Identify examples of nursing diagnoses for clients with pain.
7. Identify subjective and objective data to collect and analyze when assessing pain.
8. Describe the gate control theory and its application to nursing care.
9. Describe how the contribution of physical, mental, spiritual, and social aspects of pain contribute to concepts such as pain tolerance, suffering, and pain behavior.
10. Describe the four processes involved in nociception and how pain interventions can work during each process.
11. Discriminate between physiological and neuropathic pain categories.
12. Give an example of rational polypharmacy as described by the American Pain Society.
13. Differentiate between tolerance, dependence, and addiction.
14. Identify risks and benefits of various analgesic delivery routes and analgesic delivery technologies.

15. Describe nonpharmacologic pain control interventions.

16. List two interventions for reducing client's misconceptions about pain.

17. List three methods that nurses may use to acknowledge and accept a client's pain.

CASE STUDY

1. A 43-year-old client is complaining of abdominal pain. The client locates his pain in the epigastric region. On a 0–10 scale, he rates his pain as an 8. He describes the pain as "constant throbbing."
   a. As the fifth vital sign, pain should be screened for every time vital signs are evaluated. Define pain.
   b. Identify the two major components of a pain assessment.
   c. Explain the pain intensity scale.

REVIEW QUESTIONS

1. Which of the following statements about pain is true?
   1. Pain is a sign, not a symptom.
   2. Pain presents only physiological dangers to health and recovery.
   3. Severe pain is viewed as an emergency situation.
   4. Pain is a low-priority problem.
2. When pain lasts only through the expected recovery period, it is described as:
   1. Chronic pain.
   2. Acute pain.
   3. Referred pain.
   4. Visceral pain.
3. Pain tolerance is:
   1. The least amount of stimuli that is needed for an individual to feel a sensation labeled as pain.
   2. The maximum amount of painful stimuli that an individual is willing to withstand without seeking avoidance of the pain or relief.
   3. An unpleasant, abnormal sensation.
   4. A situation in which nonpainful stimuli (e.g., contact with linen, water, or wind) produce pain.
4. A client who describes her pain as 3 on a scale of 0–10 is having:
   1. Mild pain.
   2. Moderate pain.
   3. Severe pain.
   4. Intense pain.

5. The nurse is evaluating a client's understanding of acute pain and chronic pain. The nurse recognizes that further teaching is necessary when which of the following statements is made by the client?
   1. Acute pain increases a client's pulse rate.
   2. With chronic pain the client appears depressed and withdrawn.
   3. With chronic pain the client exhibits behavior indicative of pain: crying, rubbing area, and holding area.
   4. Acute pain increases a client's respiratory rate.
6. Which of the following would be a misconception of pain?
   1. The individual who experiences the pain is the only authority about its existence and nature.
   2. Pain is a subjective experience, and the intensity and duration of pain vary considerably among individuals.
   3. Even with severe pain, periods of physiological and behavioral adaptation can occur.
   4. The amount of tissue damage is directly related to the amount of pain.
7. Which of the following statements about nonopioids is true?
   1. Nonopioids alone are often sufficient to relieve severe pain, but they are an important part in the total analgesic plan.
   2. A nonopioid should not be given at the same time as an opioid.
   3. Side effects from long-term use of NSAIDs are considerably less severe and life threatening than the side effects from daily doses of oral morphine or other opioids.
   4. Giving a dose of nonopioid at the same time as a dose of opioid poses no more danger than giving the doses at different times.
8. A nurse is planning a seminar on COLDERR, which is a mnemonic for pain assessment. Which of the following statements is NOT correct?
   1. *Character* describes the sensation of the pain (e.g., sharp, aching, burning).
   2. *Location* is where the pain hurts (all locations).
   3. *Onset* is when the pain started and how it has changed.
   4. *Relief* means a pattern of shooting/spreading/location of pain away from its origin.
9. A nurse is evaluating a nursing student's understanding of transcultural differences in responses to pain. Which of the following actions demonstrates a need for further teaching?
   1. The African American culture believes pain and suffering is a part of life and is to be endured.
   2. The Mexican American culture believes that enduring pain is a sign of strength.
   3. The Asian American culture tends to be loud and outspoken in expressions of pain.
   4. Native Americans are quiet, less expressive verbally and nonverbally, and may tolerate a high level of pain.
10. The nurse evaluating a practice guideline for a client with pain at a seminar, recognizes that further teaching is necessary when which of the following statements is made by a participant?
    1. A trusting relationship promotes expression of the client's thoughts and feelings and enhances effectiveness of planned pain therapies.
    2. Consider the client's ability and willingness to participate actively in pain relief measures.
    3. Provide measures to relieve pain before it becomes severe.
    4. Maintain a biased attitude about what may relieve the pain.

CHAPTER 47

NUTRITION

KEY TERM REVIEW

Match each term with its appropriate definition.

1. _______ Anabolism
2. _______ Basal metabolic rate (BMR)
3. _______ Body mass index (BMI)
4. _______ Calorie
5. _______ Catabolism
6. _______ Complete proteins
7. _______ Disaccharides
8. _______ Enzymes
9. _______ Essential amino acids
10. _______ Fatty acids
11. _______ Glycogen
12. _______ Ideal body weight (IBW)
13. _______ Incomplete proteins
14. _______ Kilocalorie (Kcal)
15. _______ Kilojoule (kJ)
16. _______ Lipoproteins
17. _______ Malnutrition
18. _______ Metabolism
19. _______ Monosaccharides
20. _______ Monounsaturated fatty acids
21. _______ Nitrogen balance
22. _______ Nonessential amino acids
23. _______ Polyunsaturated fatty acids
24. _______ Saturated fatty acids
25. _______ Unsaturated fatty acid

a. Building tissue

b. Breaking down tissue

c. Contain all of the essential amino acids plus many of the nonessential ones

d. Those that cannot be manufactured in the human body

e. Rate at which the body metabolizes food to maintain the energy requirements of a person awake and at rest

f. Basic structural units of most lipids

g. Lack of necessary or appropriate food substances

h. Soluble end product of lipid digestion

i. A large compound molecule of glucose stored in the body

j. Biologic catalysts that speed up chemical reactions

k. All biochemical and physiological processes by which the body grows and maintains itself

l. Single molecule sugars such as glucose

m. Unit of heat energy

n. Fatty acid with one double carbon bond

o. One that could accommodate more hydrogen atoms

p. Weight recommended for optimal health

q. One in which all carbon atoms are filled to capacity with hydrogen; butter

r. Indicator of changes in body fat stores

s. Measure of degree of protein anabolism and catabolism

t. Double molecule sugars

u. Those that the body can manufacture

v. Amount of work energy required when a force of 1 newton moves 1 kilogram of weight 1 meter distance

w. Fatty acids with more than one double bond; vegetable oil

x. Lack one or more essential amino acids; usually plant based

y. Large calorie

KEY TOPIC REVIEW

1. Foods differ greatly in their nutritive value (the nutrient content of a specified amount of food), and no single food provides all essential nutrients.

   a. True

   b. False

2. The body's most basic nutrient need is water.

   a. True

   b. False

3. Micronutrients—vitamins and minerals—are those required in small amounts (e.g., milligrams or micrograms) to metabolize the energy-providing nutrients.

   a. True

   b. False

4. Sugars, the most complex of all carbohydrates, are fat soluble and are produced naturally by both plants and animals.

   a. True

   b. False

5. Of the three monosaccharides (glucose, fructose, and galactose), fructose is by far the most abundant simple sugar.

   a. True

   b. False

6. ____________ is the sum of all the interactions between an organism and the food it consumes. In other words, nutrition is what a person eats and how the body uses it.

7. ____________ are organic and inorganic substances found in foods that are required for body functioning.

8. ____________ are the insoluble, nonsweet forms of carbohydrate.

9. ____________, a complex carbohydrate derived from plants, supplies roughage, or bulk, to the diet.

10. ____________ are biologic catalysts that speed up chemical reactions.

11. Match the following terms with the correct definition.

a. Complete proteins	______	Organic molecules made up primarily of carbon, hydrogen, oxygen, and nitrogen, which combine to form proteins
b. Incomplete proteins	______	Those that cannot be manufactured in the body and must be supplied as part of the protein ingested in the diet
c. Amino acids	______	Those that the body can manufacture
d. Oils	______	Contain all of the essential amino acids plus many nonessential ones
e. Monounsaturated fatty acids	______	Lack one or more essential amino acids (most commonly lysine, methionine, or tryptophan) and are usually derived from vegetables
f. Nonessential amino acids	______	Organic substances that are greasy and insoluble in water but soluble in alcohol or ether
g. Fats	______	Lipids that are solid at room temperature
h. Fatty acids	______	Lipids that are liquid at room temperature
i. Lipids	______	Made up of carbon chains and hydrogen; are the basic structural units of most lipids
j. Essential amino acids	______	Fatty acids with one double bond

12. Which of the following is NOT one of the three major functions of nutrients?
    a. Provide energy for body processes and movement.
    b. Provide structural material for body tissues.
    c. Regulate body processes.
    d. Replace the natural nutrients found in food with supplemental nutrients.

13. All of the following are considered macronutrients EXCEPT:
    a. Vitamins.
    b. Carbohydrates.
    c. Fats.
    d. Protein.

14. Every cell in the body contains some protein, and about ____________ of body solids are proteins.
    a. One eighth
    b. One fourth
    c. Two thirds
    d. Three quarters

15. ___________ have (has) three fatty acids and account for more than 90% of the lipids in food and in the body.
    a. Triglycerides
    b. Cholesterol
    c. Glycerides
    d. Minerals
16. Carbohydrates are composed of all of the following elements EXCEPT:
    a. Nitrogen.
    b. Carbon.
    c. Hydrogen.
    d. Oxygen.

FOCUSED STUDY TIPS

1. Discuss energy balance in terms of energy intake and energy output.
2. List several of the factors affecting nutrition.
3. Discuss some of the psychological factors that can affect nutrition.
4. Describe how to correctly assist with special diets (e.g., clear liquid, full liquid, soft, diet as tolerated, and modification for disease).
5. Describe the term *body mass index* (BMI) and give an example of how it is calculated.
6. Discuss nursing interventions when caring for clients with nutritional problems.
7. Describe nursing interventions that promote optimal nutrition.
8. Identify risk factors for and clinical signs of malnutrition.
9. Discuss essential components and purposes of nutritional screening and nutritional assessment.
10. Identify developmental nutritional considerations.
11. Identify factors influencing nutrition.
12. Discuss body weight and body mass standards.
13. Explain essential aspects of energy balance.
14. Describe normal digestion, absorption, and metabolism of carbohydrates, proteins, and lipids.
15. Identify essential nutrients and their dietary sources.
16. Describe symptoms of iron deficiency anemia.
17. List the steps involved in inserting a nasogastric tube.

CASE STUDIES

1. A 37-year-old African American client is experiencing loss of appetite.
   a. Explain the combinations of plant proteins that provide complete proteins.
   b. Identify ways this client can improve his or her appetite.
   c. Describe possible variations in nutritional practices and preferences among this client's culture.

REVIEW QUESTIONS

1. Which of the following is considered a micronutrient?
   1. Carbohydrates
   2. Fats
   3. Proteins
   4. Vitamins
2. A nurse is evaluating a nursing student's understanding of nutrition. Which of the following statements demonstrates a need for further teaching?
   1. Starches are the insoluble, nonsweet forms of carbohydrate.
   2. Most sugars are produced naturally by plants, especially fruits, sugar cane, and sugar beets.
   3. Fiber, a complex carbohydrate derived from plants, supplies roughage, or bulk, to the diet.
   4. Fiber is present in the inner layer of grains, bran, and in the skin, seeds, and pulp of many vegetables and fruits.
3. The student nurse is learning about nutrition. Which of the following statements indicates a need for further teaching?
   1. Essential amino acids are those that cannot be manufactured in the body and must be supplied as part of the protein ingested in the diet.
   2. The essential amino acids are alanine, aspartic acid, cystine, glutamic acid, glycine, hydroxyproline, proline, serine, and tyrosine.
   3. Nonessential amino acids are those that the body can manufacture.
   4. Most animal proteins, including meats, poultry, fish, dairy products, and eggs, are complete proteins.
4. During discharge planning, the nurse is teaching the client about lipids. Which of the following statements is correct?
   1. Lipids are inorganic substances that are greasy and soluble in water but soluble in alcohol or ether.
   2. In common use, the terms *fats* and *lipids* are used interchangeably.
   3. Fats are lipids that are liquid at room temperature.
   4. Oils are lipids that are solid at room temperature.
5. The nurse is calculating a client's BMI. The client's height is 1.5 m and his weight is 70 kg. Which of the following calculations is the correct BMI?
   1. 31.11
   2. 46.67
   3. 30.02
   4. 36.16

6. Which of the following suggestions will NOT help parents meet the child's nutritional needs and promote effective parent–child interactions?
   1. Make mealtime a pleasant time by avoiding tensions at the table and discussions of bad behavior.
   2. Routinely use sweet desserts after dinners.
   3. Schedule meals, sleep, and snack times that will allow for optimum appetite and behavior.
   4. Offer a variety of simple, attractive foods in small portions.
7. A food diary is a:
   1. Recall of all the food and beverages the client consumes during a typical 24-hour period when at home.
   2. Detailed record of measured amounts (portion sizes) of all food and fluids a client consumes during a specified period, usually 3 to 7 days.
   3. Comprehensive, time-consuming assessment of a client's food intake that involves an extensive interview by a nutritionist or dietitian.
   4. Checklist that indicates how often general food groups or specific foods are eaten.
8. A nurse is evaluating a nursing student's understanding of special diets. Which of the following statements demonstrates a need for further teaching?
   1. A clear liquid diet is limited to water, tea, coffee, clear broths, ginger ale, or other carbonated beverages, strained and clear juices, and plain gelatin.
   2. A full liquid diet contains only liquids or foods that turn to liquid at body temperature, such as ice cream.
   3. A soft diet is easily chewed and digested.
   4. Note that the word "clear" in clear diet means "colorless."
9. Enteral feedings can be given intermittently or continuously. Intermittent feedings are the administration of ____________ mL of enteral formula several times per day.
   1. 50 to 100
   2. 100 to 200
   3. 300 to 500
   4. 600 to 700
10. When planning interventions to improve a client's appetite, which of the following would be included in the client's plan of care?
    1. Unpleasant or uncomfortable treatments can be performed before or after a meal.
    2. Provide unfamiliar food to try.
    3. Encourage or provide oral hygiene after mealtime.
    4. Provide a tidy, clean environment that is free of unpleasant sights and odors.

CHAPTER 48

URINARY ELIMINATION

KEY TERM REVIEW

Match each term with its appropriate definition.

1. _______ Anuria
2. _______ Bladder training
3. _______ Blood urea nitrogen (BUN)
4. _______ Creatinine clearance
5. _______ Detrusor muscle
6. _______ Dialysis
7. _______ Diuresis
8. _______ Diuretics
9. _______ Dysuria
10. _______ Enuresis
11. _______ Glomerulus
12. _______ Ileal conduit
13. _______ Nephrostomy
14. _______ Neurogenic bladder
15. _______ Oliguria
16. _______ Polydipsia
17. _______ Polyuria
18. _______ Suprapubic catheter
19. _______ Ureterostomy
20. _______ Urgency
21. _______ Urinary frequency
22. _______ Urinary hesitancy
23. _______ Urinary incontinence (UI)
24. _______ Urinary retention
25. _______ Urination

a. Painful urination

b. One or both ureters are brought to side of abdomen to form small stoma

c. Lack of urine production

d. Also known as diuresis

e. Excessive thirst

f. Measurement of end product of protein metabolism

g. Voiding at frequent intervals

h. Tuft of capillaries in the nephron

i. Occurs with impaired bladder emptying; may result in distended bladder

j. Urine output of less than 500 mL/day for an adult

k. The smooth muscle layer of the bladder wall

l. Filtering of the blood done in the presence of inadequate kidney function

m. Uses urine and serum levels to determine glomerular filtration rate

n. Common urinary diversion that creates a pouch and stoma

o. Impaired neurologic function that results in inability of the client to feel bladder fullness

p. Involuntary leakage of urine

q. Increase urine formation by preventing reabsorption of water and electrolytes

r. Surgically inserted through abdominal wall above symphysis pubis into urinary bladder

s. Sudden strong desire to void

t. Requires client to postpone voiding; voiding according to a timetable, in order to stabilize bladder, diminish urgency

u. Process of emptying the urinary bladder

v. Involuntary urination in children beyond the normal age of bladder control

w. Delay and difficulty in initiating voiding

x. Diverts urine from the kidney to a stoma

y. Increased production of urine

KEY TOPIC REVIEW

1. The most common urinary diversion is the ileal conduit or ileal loop.

   a. True

   b. False

2. Urinary tract infections (UTIs) are the most common infection in children.

   a. True

   b. False

3. The paired kidneys are situated on either side of the spinal column, behind the peritoneal cavity.

   a. True

   b. False

4. The urinary bladder (vesicle) is a hollow, muscular organ that serves as a reservoir for urine and as the organ of excretion.

   a. True

   b. False

5. The female urethra serves only as a passageway for the elimination of urine.

   a. True

   b. False

6. ____________ increase urine formation by preventing the reabsorption of water and electrolytes from the tubules of the kidney into the bloodstream.
7. Clients who have a ____________ bladder may use manual pressure on the bladder to promote bladder emptying.
8. ____________ is a flushing or washing out with a specified solution.
9. A ____________ diverts urine from the kidney to a stoma.
10. A ____________ may be formed when the bladder is left intact but voiding through the urethra is not possible (e.g., due to an obstruction or a neurogenic bladder).
11. Match the following terms with the correct definition.

a. Anuria	______	Bed-wetting
b. Polyuria (diuresis)	______	The production of abnormally large amounts of urine by the kidneys, often several liters more than the client's usual daily output
c. Nocturnal enuresis	______	Low urine output
d. Residual urine	______	Refers to a lack of urine production
e. Bladder training	______	Voiding two or more times at night
f. Creatinine clearance	______	Voiding that is either painful or difficult
g. Dysuria	______	Urine remaining in the bladder following the voiding
h. Habit training	______	A test that uses 24-hour urine and serum creatinine levels to determine the glomerular filtration rate, a sensitive indicator of renal function
i. Oliguria	______	Requires that the client postpone voiding, resist or inhibit the sensation of urgency, and void according to a timetable rather than according to the urge to void
j. Nocturia	______	Referred to as timed voiding or scheduled toileting, attempts to keep clients dry by having them void at regular intervals

12. Normal bladder capacity is between ____________ mL of urine.
    a. 300 and 600
    b. 600 and 900
    c. 900 and 1,200
    d. 1,200 and 1,500
13. An infant may urinate as often as ____________ times a day.
    a. 5
    b. 10
    c. 15
    d. 20
14. About ____________% of all 6-year-olds experience difficulty controlling the bladder.
    a. 10
    b. 20
    c. 30
    d. 40

15. Although patterns of urination are highly individual, most individuals void about ____________ times a day.
    a. 3 to 4
    b. 5 to 6
    c. 7 to 8
    d. 9 to 10
16. Which statement is true regarding urinary elimination and the aging process?
    a. Kidney function significantly decreases.
    b. The number of functioning nephrons remains the same.
    c. Excretion time is decreased
    d. Excretion time is increased

FOCUSED STUDY TIPS

1. Discuss several practice guidelines to prevent catheter-associated urinary infections.
2. What are the accuracy and clinical benefits of using a bladder scanner?
3. List and discuss several factors that influence urinary elimination.
4. Problems of urinary elimination also may become the etiology for other problems experienced by the client. Discuss several of these other problems.
5. Describe and list several of the different types of urinary catheters.
6. List several medications that may cause urinary retention.
7. Explain the care of clients with retention catheters or urinary diversions.
8. Discuss ways to prevent urinary infection.
9. Develop nursing diagnoses, desired outcomes, and interventions related to urinary elimination.
10. Identify normal and abnormal characteristics and constituents of urine.
11. Describe nursing assessment of urinary function including subjective and objective data.
12. Identify common causes of selected urinary problems.
13. Identify factors that influence urinary elimination.
14. Describe the process of urination, from urine formation through micturition.
15. List the various organs and elements that form the pelvic floor.

CASE STUDY

1 A 68-year-old client has been experiencing urinary elimination problems. He has given you a urine specimen and asks how to maintain normal urinary elimination.

a. List the steps a nurse must follow to measure fluid output.

b. Identify various goals for clients with urinary elimination problems.

c. Explain how this client can maintain normal urinary elimination.

REVIEW QUESTIONS

1. What is oliguria?
   1. Low urine output
   2. Increased urine output
   3. Excessive fluid intake
   4. A lack of urine production
2. What is urinary frequency?
   1. Voiding two or more times at night
   2. Voiding at frequent intervals
   3. The sudden and strong desire to void
   4. Voiding that is either painful or difficult
3. During discharge planning, the nurse is teaching the client ways to prevent a recurrence of a UTI. Which of the following actions is correct?
   1. Drink six 6-ounce glasses of water per day to flush bacteria out of the urinary system.
   2. Wear nylon rather than cotton underclothes.
   3. Girls and women should always wipe the perineal area from back to front following urination or defecation in order to prevent introduction of gastrointestinal bacteria into the urethra.
   4. Avoid tight-fitting pants or other clothing that can irritate the urethra and prevents ventilation of the perineal area.
4. A nurse is evaluating a client's understanding of intermittent self-catheterization. Which of the following statements indicates a need for further teaching? Intermittent self-catheterization:
   1. Reduces the incidence of urinary tract infection.
   2. Enables the client to retain independence and gain control of the bladder.
   3. Allows normal sexual relations without incontinence.
   4. Protects the lower urinary tract from reflux.
5. Which of the following is an abnormal color or clarity of urine?
   1. Straw
   2. Amber
   3. Dark amber
   4. Transparent

6. A nurse is testing urine for specific gravity. Which of the following would be considered a normal range for the test result?
   1. 0.100 to 0.999
   2. 1.000 to 1.050
   3. 1.010 to 1.025
   4. 1.050 to 1.100
7. The nurse is performing urethral urinary catheterization on a male client. Which of the following actions by the nurse is correct?
   1. Lubricates the catheter 1 to 2 inches.
   2. Picks up a cleansing ball with the forceps in the nondominant hand and wipes from the top of the meatus in a circular motion around the glans.
   3. Grasps the catheter firmly 2 to 3 inches from the tip; asks the client to take a slow deep breath and inserts the catheter as the client exhales.
   4. Puts on examination gloves.
8. A nurse evaluating a class on facilitating and promoting urinary elimination recognizes that further teaching is necessary when which of the following statements is made by a participant?
   1. Advise the client and family to install grab bars and elevated toilet seats as needed.
   2. Teach the client to empty the bladder completely at each voiding.
   3. Emphasize the importance of drinking five to six 8-ounce glasses of water daily.
   4. Suggest clothing that is easily removed for toileting, such as elastic-waist pants or pants with Velcro closures.
9. During discharge planning, the nurse is teaching the client how to perform pelvic muscle exercises (Kegels). Which of the following actions is correct?
   1. Initially perform each contraction 10 times, five times daily. Gradually increase the count to a full 10 seconds for both contraction and relaxation.
   2. To control episodes of stress incontinence, perform a pelvic muscle contraction only after activities that increase intra-abdominal pressure, such as coughing, laughing, sneezing, or lifting.
   3. Develop a schedule that will help remind you to do these exercises, for example, before getting out of bed in the morning.
   4. Contract your pelvic muscles whereby you pull your rectum, urethra, and vagina up inside, and hold for a count of 1 to 2 seconds. Then relax the same muscles for a count of 1 to 2 seconds.
10. A nurse is evaluating a client's understanding of preventing catheter-associated urinary infections. Which of the following statements indicates a need for further teaching?
    1. Maintain a sterile closed-drainage system.
    2. Always disconnect the catheter and drainage tubing.
    3. Provide routine perineal hygiene, including cleansing with soap and water after defecation.
    4. Prevent contamination of the catheter with feces.

CHAPTER 49

FECAL ELIMINATION

KEY TERM REVIEW

Match each term with its appropriate definition.

1. _______ Bowel incontinence
2. _______ Carminatives
3. _______ Cathartics
4. _______ Chyme
5. _______ Colostomy
6. _______ Commode
7. _______ Constipation
8. _______ Defecation
9. _______ Diarrhea
10. _______ Enema
11. _______ Fecal impaction
12. _______ Fecal incontinence
13. _______ Flatus
14. _______ Gastrocolic reflex
15. _______ Gastrostomy
16. _______ Haustra
17. _______ Haustral churn ing
18. _______ Hemorrhoids
19. _______ Ileostomy
20. _______ Jejunostomy
21. _______ Mass peristalsis
22. _______ Meconium
23. _______ Ostomy
24. _______ Peristalsis
25. _______ Stoma

a. Opening through the abdominal wall into the ileum

b. Mass or collection of hardened feces in the folds of the rectum

c. Portable chair with a toilet seat

d. Expulsion of feces from the anus and rectum

e. An opening for the gastrointestinal, urinary, or respiratory tract onto the skin

f. Herbal oils known to help expel gas from the stomach and intestines

g. Air and by-products of carbohydrate digestion

h. Distended veins in the rectum

i. A wave of powerful muscular contraction that moves over large areas of the colon

j. An opening through the abdominal wall into the stomach

k. Increased peristalsis of colon after food has entered the stomach

l. Fewer than three bowel movements per week

m. Pouches that form due to the enlarging and lengthening of the large intestine

n. Waste products that leave the stomach and small intestine

o. An opening through the abdomen into the jejunum

p. Loss of voluntary ability to control fecal and gaseous discharges through the anal sphincter

q. Bowel incontinence

r. Wavelike movement produced by the circular and longitudinal muscle fibers in the intestine walls

s. Drugs that induce defecation

t. The opening created in the abdominal wall by an ostomy

u. Passage of liquid feces and increased frequency of defecation

v. First fecal material passed by a newborn

w. An opening through the abdominal wall into the colon

x. A solution introduced into the rectum and large intestine

y. Moving back and forth of the chyme within the intestinal pouches

KEY TOPIC REVIEW

1. Elimination of the waste products of digestion from the body is essential to health.

   a. True

   b. False

2. The small intestine extends from the ileocecal (ileocolic) valve, which lies between the large and small intestines, to the anus.

   a. True

   b. False

3. Normal feces are made of about 25% water and 75% solid materials.

   a. True

   b. False

4. Constipation is the most common bowel-management problem in older populations.

   a. True

   b. False

5. The colon (large intestine) in the adult is generally about 125 to 150 cm (50 to 60 in.) long.

   a. True

   b. False

6. ____________ is the presence of excessive flatus in the intestines and leads to stretching and inflation of the intestines.

7. A(An) ____________ is an opening for the gastrointestinal, urinary, or respiratory tract onto the skin.

8. Clients restricted to bed may need to use a ____________, a receptacle for urine and feces.

9. A(An) ____________ is a solution introduced into the rectum and large intestine.

10. ____________ are drugs that induce defecation.

11. Match the following terms with the correct definition.

a. Hemorrhoids	______	The act of eating food
b. Laxatives	______	Waste products leaving the stomach through the small intestine and then passing through the ileocecal valve
c. Bowel/fecal incontinence	______	A condition that can occur when the veins become distended, as can occur with repeated pressure
d. Constipation	______	The expulsion of feces from the anus and rectum
e. Diarrhea	______	Increased peristalsis of the colon after food has entered the stomach
f. Defecation	______	Medications that stimulate bowel activity and so assist fecal elimination
g. Fecal impaction	______	Fewer than three bowel movements per week
h. Ingestion	______	A mass or collection of hardened feces in the folds of the rectum
i. Gastrocolic reflex	______	The passage of liquid feces and an increased frequency of defecation
j. Chyme	______	The loss of voluntary ability to control fecal and gaseous discharges through the anal sphincter

12. The contents of the colon normally represent foods ingested over the previous ____________ days.
    a. 2
    b. 3
    c. 4
    d. 5

13. All of the following may be causes and factors that contribute to constipation EXCEPT:
    a. A lack of privacy.
    b. Daily routines.
    c. Insufficient fiber intake.
    d. Insufficient fluid intake.

14. All of the following are thought to contribute to constipation EXCEPT:
    a. Overuse of laxatives.
    b. Bland diets.
    c. Irregular defecation habits.
    d. Exercise.

15. Which of the following feces consistencies would be considered abnormal?
    a. Soft
    b. Moist
    c. Semisolid
    d. Dry

FOCUSED STUDY TIPS

1. Distinguish normal from abnormal characteristics and constituents of feces.
2. List the seven parts of the colon (large intestine).
3. Identify factors that influence fecal elimination and patterns of defecation.
4. Discuss the physiology of defecation.
5. Discuss regular exercise and how it helps clients develop a regular defecation pattern.
6. Discuss some of the ways to reduce or expel flatus.
7. Describe methods used to assess the intestinal tract.
8. Identify examples of nursing diagnoses, outcomes, and interventions for clients with elimination problems.
9. List and describe the three types of movements that occur in the large intestine.
10. Identify measures that maintain normal fecal elimination patterns.
11. Describe the purpose and action of commonly used enema solutions.
12. List four common problems that are related to fecal elimination.
13. Describe essentials of fecal stoma care for clients with an ostomy.
14. List and discuss the three primary sources of flatus.
15. Describe how to administer an enema.
16. Discuss ways in which the nurse can provide holistic care to a client who may be uncomfortable with procedures associated with bowel elimination.
17. Describe the appropriate documentation after administering an enema to a client.

CASE STUDY

1. A 37-year-old client has been experiencing diarrhea for the past 12 hours.
    a. Identify ways for the client to manage diarrhea.
    b. Provide the client with information about healthy defecation.
    c. Identify three major causes of diarrhea.

REVIEW QUESTIONS

1. What is a gastrostomy?
   1. An opening through the abdominal wall into the stomach
   2. An opening through the abdominal wall into the jejunum
   3. An opening into the colon.
   4. An opening into the ileum
2. Which type of enema is given primarily to expel flatus?
   1. Retention
   2. Carminative
   3. Return-flow
   4. Cleansing
3. Which of the following actions is NOT appropriate for the nurse removing a fecal impaction?
   1. Place a bed pad under the client's buttocks and a bedpan nearby to receive stool.
   2. Ask the client to assume a right side-lying position, with the knees flexed and the back toward the nurse.
   3. Drape the client for comfort and to avoid unnecessary exposure of the body.
   4. Gently insert the index finger into the rectum and move the finger along the length of the rectum.
4. A nurse is evaluating a client's understanding of healthy defecation. Which of the following statements indicates a need for further teaching?
   1. "I will include high-fiber foods, such as vegetables, fruits, and whole grains, in my diet."
   2. "I will maintain a fluid intake of 4,000 to 5,000 mL each day."
   3. "I will allow time to defecate, preferably at the same time each day."
   4. "I will avoid over-the-counter medications to treat constipation and diarrhea."
5. During discharge planning, the nurse is teaching the client how to manage diarrhea. Which of the following actions is NOT correct?
   1. Drink at least eight glasses of water per day to prevent dehydration.
   2. Eat foods with sodium and potassium.
   3. Increase foods containing insoluble fiber, such as high-fiber whole-wheat bread..
   4. Limit fatty foods.
6. A nurse is evaluating a client's understanding of ostomy care. Which of the following client statements indicates a need for further teaching?
   1. "The ostomy pouch is emptied when it is one-third to one-half full."
   2. "The ostomy pouch can be applied for up to 10 days."
   3. "Most ostomy pouches contain odor barrier material."
   4. "If the ostomy pouch overfills, it can cause stool to come in contact with the skin."

7. A nurse is evaluating a nursing student's understanding of colostomies. Which of the following statements demonstrates a need for further teaching?

   1. "The single stoma is created when one end of bowel is brought out through an opening onto the anterior abdominal wall."
   2. "With a loop colostomy, a loop of bowel is brought out onto the abdominal wall and supported by a plastic bridge, or a piece of rubber tubing."
   3. "The divided colostomy consists of two edges of bowel brought out onto the abdomen but separated from each other."
   4. "The loop colostomy is often used in situations where spillage of feces into the distal end of the bowel needs to be avoided."

8. The nurse is promoting regular defecation for a client whom she is taking care of. Which of the following actions by the nurse is NOT correct?

   1. A client should be encouraged to defecate when the urge is recognized.
   2. Regular exercise helps clients develop a regular defecation pattern.
   3. Although the squatting position best facilitates defecation, the best position for most clients seems to be leaning backward while on a toilet seat.
   4. For clients who have difficulty sitting down and getting up from the toilet, an elevated toilet seat can be attached to a regular toilet.

9. A primary care provider orders examination of stool for signs of intestinal infection. What color of stool would the nurse expect to see?

   1. Red
   2. Green
   3. Black
   4. White

10. A nurse is evaluating a nursing student's understanding of the actions of enema solutions. Which of the following statements demonstrates a need for further teaching?

    1. Hypertonic solutions draw water into the colon.
    2. Hypotonic solutions distend the colon, stimulate peristalsis, and soften feces.
    3. Isotonic solutions lubricate the feces and the colonic mucosa.
    4. Soapsuds solutions irritate the mucosa and distend the colon.

CHAPTER 50

OXYGENATION

KEY TERM REVIEW

Match each term with its appropriate definition.

1. _______ Apnea
2. _______ Atelectasis
3. _______ Biot's (cluster) respiration
4. _______ Bradypnea
5. _______ Cheyne-Stokes respirations
6. _______ Cyanosis
7. _______ Dyspnea
8. _______ Emphysema
9. _______ Eupnea
10. _______ Hemothorax
11. _______ Hypercapnia
12. _______ Hyperinflation
13. _______ Hypoxemia
14. _______ Hypoxia
15. _______ Intrapleural pressure
16. _______ Intrapulmonary pressure
17. _______ Kussmaul's breathing
18. _______ Noninvasive ventilation
19. _______ Orthopnea
20. _______ Pleural effusion
21. _______ Pneumothorax
22. _______ Stridor
23. _______ Surfactant
24. _______ Tachypnea
25. _______ Tidal volume

a. Collapsed alveoli

b. Harsh, high-pitched sound during inspiration

c. Shallow breaths interrupted by apnea

d. Air collected in the pleural space

e. Abnormally slow breathing

f. Marked rhythmic waxing and waning of respirations, from very shallow to very deep, with short periods of apnea

g. Normal respirations

h. Excessive fluid in the pleural space

i. Accumulation of blood in the pleural space

j. Difficult or labored breathing

k. The body's attempts to compensate for increased metabolic acidosis by blowing of acid in the form of CO_2

l. Absence of any breathing

m. Insufficient oxygen anywhere in the body

n. The amount of air inspired and expired with each breath

o. Oxygen concentrations play a major role in regulating respiration; decreased oxygen concentrations are the main stimuli for receptors because the increased carbon dioxide levels desensitize the central chemoreceptors

p. Faster than normal breathing

q. Pressure within the lungs

r. Bluish discoloration of the skin, nail beds, and mucous membranes

s. Lipoprotein that reduces surface tension in lungs without which lung expansion is exceedingly difficult

t. Inability to breathe easily unless sitting upright

u. Increased levels of CO_2

v. Low levels of oxygen in the blood

w. Pressure in the pleural cavity surrounding the lungs

x. Delivery of air or oxygen under pressure without the need for an invasive tube

y. Involves giving client breaths of greater volume than set on ventilator or via manual resuscitation bag

KEY TOPIC REVIEW

1. Postural drainage is the drainage by gravity of secretions from various lung segments.

   a. True

   b. False

2. Suctioning is aspirating secretions through a catheter connected to a suction machine or wall suction outlet.

   a. True

   b. False

3. Hyperoxygenation involves giving the client breaths that are 1 to 1.5 times the tidal volume set on the ventilator through the ventilator circuit or via a manual resuscitation bag.

   a. True

   b. False

4. When air collects in the pleural space, it is known as a hemothorax.

   a. True

   b. False

5. Hyperinflation can be done with a manual resuscitation bag or through the ventilator and is performed by increasing the oxygen flow (usually to 100%) before suctioning and between suction attempts.

   a. True

   b. False

6. ____________ is a clear, odorless gas that constitutes approximately 21% of the air we breathe, and is necessary for proper functioning of all living cells.

7. ____________ pressure (pressure within the lungs) always equalizes with atmospheric pressure.

8. ____________ is a collapse of a portion of the lung.

9. ____________ is the movement of gases or other particles from an area of greater pressure or concentration to an area of lower pressure or concentration.

10. ____________ is the cessation of breathing.

11. Match the following terms with the correct definition.

a. Surfactant	______	A lipoprotein produced by specialized alveolar cells; acts like a detergent, reducing the surface tension of alveolar fluid
b. Sputum	______	Oxygen-carrying red pigment
c. Cyanosis	______	Red blood cells (RBCs)
d. Expectorate	______	A condition of insufficient oxygen anywhere in the body, from the inspired gas to the tissues
e. Hemoglobin	______	Bluish discoloration of the skin, nail beds, and mucous membranes, due to reduced hemoglobin-oxygen saturation
f. Bradypnea	______	An abnormally slow respiratory rate
g. Humidifiers	______	The inability to breathe except in an upright or standing position
h. Hypoxia	______	Coughed-up material
i. Orthopnea	______	Spit out
j. Erythrocytes	______	Devices that add water vapor to inspired air

12. ____________ is a series of vigorous quiverings produced by the hands that are placed flat against the client's chest wall in an effort to mobilize retained secretions.

    a. Hemoglobin

    b. Hematocrit

    c. Oxyhemoglobin

    d. Vibration

13. ____________ is the continual tendency of the lungs to collapse away from the chest wall.

    a. Atelectasis

    b. Lung recoil

    c. Diffusion

    d. Lung compliance

14. ____________ is a condition of insufficient oxygen anywhere in the body, from the inspired gas to the tissues.

a. Hypoxia

b. Emphysema

c. Hypercarbia

d. Hypercapnia

15. ____________ refers to reduced oxygen in the blood and is characterized by a low partial pressure of oxygen in arterial blood or a low hemoglobin saturation.

a. Cyanosis

b. Tachypnea

c. Hypoxemia

d. Bradypnea

16. Normal respiration (____________) is quiet.

a. Orthopnea

b. Apnea

c. Dyspnea

d. Eupnea

FOCUSED STUDY TIPS

1. Discuss what an obstructed airway is and how to assess and maintain a patent airway.
2. List and explain some of the types of medications that can be used for clients with oxygenation problems.
3. Explain how chest tubes are inserted.
4. Discuss the overall outcomes/goals for a client with oxygenation problems.
5. List and explain the nursing responsibilities regarding drainage systems.
6. Discuss some of the NANDA diagnostic labels for clients with oxygenation problems.
7. State outcome criteria for evaluating client responses to measures that promote adequate oxygenation.
8. Explain the use of therapeutic measures such as medications, inhalation therapy, oxygen therapy, artificial airways, airway suctioning, and chest tubes to promote respiratory function.
9. Describe nursing measures to promote respiratory function and oxygenation.
10. Identify common manifestations of impaired respiratory function.
11. Identify factors influencing respiratory function.
12. Explain the role and function of the respiratory system in transporting oxygen and carbon dioxide to and from body tissues.
13. Describe the processes of breathing (ventilation) and gas exchange (respiration).
14. Outline the structure and function of the respiratory system.

15. Discuss the procedure for obtaining an arterial blood gas (ABG) sample. List the precautions required when performing this procedure.

16. Describe a pulmonary function test (PFT) and interventions that may be used for a client undergoing this procedure.

CASE STUDY

1. You are a nursing student's preceptor today. This is the nursing student's first semester in nursing school. When the student first arrives on the unit, she asks you several questions:

   a. Which factors does adequate ventilation depend on?

   b. Which factors affect the rate of oxygen transport from the lungs to the tissues?

   c. Which factors that influence oxygenation affect the cardiovascular system as well as the respiratory system?

   d. What are oxygen therapy safety precautions?

REVIEW QUESTIONS

1. Which of the following is NOT a factor that determines adequate ventilation?
   1. Clear airways
   2. Adequate pulmonary compliance and recoil
   3. An intact endocrine system
   4. An intact thoracic cavity capable of expanding and contracting

2. Eupnea is best defined as:
   1. A normal respiration.
   2. A rapid rate.
   3. An abnormally slow respiratory rate.
   4. The cessation of breathing.

3. Which of the following is marked rhythmic waxing and waning of respirations from very deep to very shallow breathing and temporary apnea?
   1. Biot's (cluster) respirations
   2. Orthopnea
   3. Cheyne-Stokes respirations
   4. Dyspnea

4. The nonrebreather mask delivers the highest oxygen concentration possible (95% to 100%) by means other than intubation or mechanical ventilation, at liter flows of ___________ L per minute.
   1. 2 to 6
   2. 5 to 8
   3. 6 to 10
   4. 10 to 15

5. Which type of mask delivers oxygen concentrations varying from 24% to 40% or 50% at liter flows of 4 to 10 L per minute?
   1. Nonrebreather
   2. Venturi
   3. Simple face
   4. Partial rebreather
6. A nurse is evaluating a nursing student's understanding of endotracheal tubes. Which of the following statements indicates a need for further teaching?
   1. Endotracheal tubes are most commonly inserted for clients who have had general anesthetics or for those in emergency situations where mechanical ventilation is required.
   2. An endotracheal tube is inserted by the primary care provider, nurse, or respiratory therapist with specialized education.
   3. An endotracheal tube is inserted through the mouth or the nose and into the trachea with the guide of a laryngoscope.
   4. The client is able to speak while an endotracheal tube is in place but is unable to swallow.
7. Which of the following is the amount of air remaining in the lungs after maximal exhalation?
   1. TLC
   2. RV
   3. VC
   4. ERV
8. The spouse of a client is explaining to the nurse what she learned about a cough reflex. Which of the following indicates a need for further teaching? The spouse states:
   1. The epiglottis and glottis (vocal cords) close.
   2. A large inspiration of approximately 3.5 L occurs.
   3. Nerve impulses are sent through the vagus nerve to the medulla.
   4. A strong contraction of abdominal and internal intercostal muscles dramatically raises the pressure in the lungs.
9. A nurse is evaluating a nursing student's understanding of oxygen therapy precautions. Which of the following statements indicates a need for further teaching?
   1. Place cautionary signs reading "No Smoking: Oxygen in Use" on the client's door, at the foot or head of the bed, and on the oxygen equipment.
   2. Be sure that electric monitoring equipment, suction machines, and portable diagnostic machines are all electrically grounded.
   3. Make known the location of fire extinguishers, and make sure personnel are trained in their use.
   4. The use of volatile, flammable materials, such as oils, greases, alcohol, ether, and acetone (e.g., nail polish remover) near clients receiving oxygen is acceptable with a primary care provider's order.
10. Which of the following actions is NOT appropriate for the nurse providing tracheostomy care?
    1. Clean the lumen and entire inner cannula thoroughly using a brush or pipe cleaners moistened with sterile normal saline.
    2. Rinse the inner cannula thoroughly in the sterile normal saline.
    3. After rinsing, gently tap the cannula against the inside edge of the sterile saline container.
    4. Put on sterile gloves. Keep your nondominant hand sterile during the procedure.

CHAPTER 51

CIRCULATION

KEY TERM REVIEW

Match each term with its appropriate definition.

1. _______ Afterload
2. _______ Atherosclerosis
3. _______ Atria
4. _______ Atrioventricular (AV) node
5. _______ Atrioventricular (AV) valves
6. _______ Automaticity
7. _______ Bundle of His
8. _______ Cardiac output (CO)
9. _______ Coronary arteries
10. _______ C-reactive protein (CRP)
11. _______ Creatine kinase (CK)
12. _______ Diastole
13. _______ Heart failure
14. _______ Homocysteine
15. _______ Ischemia
16. _______ Myocardial infarction (MI)
17. _______ Peripheral vascular resistance (PVR)
18. _______ Preload
19. _______ Purkinje fibers
20. _______ Semilunar valves
21. _______ Sinoatrial (SA or sinus) node
22. _______ Stroke volume (SV)
23. _______ Systole
24. _______ Troponin
25. _______ Ventricles

a. Amino acid that may indicate an increased risk for circulatory events when elevated

b. Valves between the ventricles and the great vessels

c. Valves between the atria and the ventricles

d. Amount of blood ejected with each contraction

e. Relaxation of heart muscle; characterized by ventricular filling

f. Area of the heart where electrical impulses from SA node converge prior to initiating ventricular contraction

g. Degree to which muscle fibers in the ventricle are stretched at the end of diastole

h. Two upper chambers within the heart

i. Enzyme released as result of cell membrane damage during an MI; measured with CK

j. Enzyme that is released into the blood as a result of cell membrane damage to cardiac muscle

k. Screening test for inflammatory process in cardiovascular disease

l. Primary pacemaker of the heart

m. Two lower chambers within the heart

n. The buildup of fatty plaques within the arteries

o. Contraction of heart muscle and ejection of blood

p. Ability of cardiac muscle to generate electrical impulses and contractions independently of the nervous system

q. Network of vessels that supply heart muscle with oxygen and nourishment

r. Condition in which cardiac tissue becomes necrotic and dies

s. Impedes blood flow to the tissues

t. One of three ventricular conduction pathways

u. Inability of the heart to keep up with the body's need for oxygen and nutrients to the tissues

v. Lack of blood supply due to obstructed circulation

w. The resistance that the ventricle must overcome during systole to eject blood into the circulation

x. Terminate in ventricular muscle, stimulating contraction

y. Amount of blood pumped by the ventricles in 1 minute

KEY TOPIC REVIEW

1. Cardiac muscle contraction is a mechanical event that occurs in response to electrical stimulation.
   a. True
   b. False
2. Heart rates are highest and most variable in adults.
   a. True
   b. False
3. Congenital heart disease affects less than 1% of all live births, but is the leading cause of early death from all congenital anomalies.
   a. True
   b. False
4. The American Heart Association (AHA) recommends at least 100 minutes per week of moderate exercise for adults.
   a. True
   b. False

5. Recent studies suggest that moderate alcohol use (1 to 2 oz of alcohol per day) may actually reduce the risk of heart disease.

   a. True

   b. False

6. ____________ is a lack of blood supply due to obstructed circulation.

7. The ____________ is a hollow, cone-shaped organ about the size of a fist.

8. Cardiac output is calculated by multiplying the ____________ ____________ (the amount of blood ejected with each contraction) by the heart rate (HR).

9. ____________ is the degree to which muscle fibers in the ventricle are stretched at the end of the relaxation period (diastole) and largely depends on the amount of blood returning to the heart from the venous circulation.

10. ____________ is the resistance against which the heart must pump to eject the blood into circulation.

11. Match the following terms with the correct definition.

a. Blood pressure (BP)	______	A major component of red blood cells (erythrocytes), the predominant type of cell present in blood
b. Hemoglobin	______	The buildup of fatty plaque within the arteries; is the major contributor to cardiovascular disease, the leading cause of death in North America
c. Blood	______	Serves as the transport medium within the cardiovascular system, bringing oxygen and nutrients from the environment (via the lungs and gastrointestinal system) to the cells
d. Atherosclerosis	______	A ______ arrest (pulmonary arrest) is the cessation of breathing.
e. Systemic	______	The study of the forces or pressures involved in blood circulation
f. Cardiovascular	______	A lack of blood supply due to obstructed circulation
g. Hemodynamics	______	The molecule that oxygen attaches to; it gives an indication of the oxygen-carrying capacity of the blood
h. Hemoglobin	______	The heart and the blood vessels make up the ______ system that, together with blood, is the major system for transporting oxygen and nutrients to the tissues, and waste products away from the tissues for elimination.
i. Ischemia	______	A type of blood vessel that carries blood to the tissues through a system of arteries, arterioles, and capillaries and returns it to the heart through the venules, veins, and the venae cavae
j. Respiratory	______	The force exerted on arterial walls by the blood flowing within the vessel

12. Electrocardiography most commonly uses ___________ "leads" or different views of the heart.

   a. 6

   b. 8

   c. 10

   d. 12

13. Each health care facility has policies and procedures for announcing cardiac/respiratory arrest and initiating interventions. In many institutions this emergency is called a Code ____________, and the announcement is referred to as "calling a code."

    a. Blue

    b. Red

    c. Green

    d. Yellow

14. Cardiac output (CO) is the amount of blood pumped by the ventricles in ____________ minute.

    a. 1

    b. 2

    c. 3

    d. 4

15. With each contraction, a certain amount of blood, known as the stroke volume, is ejected from the ventricles into circulation. In adults, the average stroke volume is about ____________ mL per beat.

    a. 40

    b. 50

    c. 60

    d. 70

16. Nearly ____________ of the adult population of the United States is overweight or obese.

    a. 1/4

    b. 1/3

    c. 1/2

    d. 2/3

FOCUSED STUDY TIPS

1. Explain what a modifiable risk factor is and list several examples.

2. List the signs of anemia.

3. Explain arterial circulation.

4. Discuss the steps in cardiopulmonary resuscitation (CPR).

5. Describe the cardiac cycle.

6. Discuss the importance of homocysteine levels.

7. Summarize venous return.

8. What is cardiac monitoring and what is it used for?

9. List the signs of impaired peripheral arterial circulation.

10. Discuss physical assessment as it relates to the cardiovascular system.

11. Discuss life span considerations in relation to the cardiovascular system.

12. Discuss serum lipid levels and coronary artery disease.

13. Explain what a nonmodifiable risk factor is and give some examples.

14. Define hypertension.

15. List the three cardinal signs of a cardiac arrest.

16. List the five risk factors for metabolic syndrome.

17. List the three cardiovascular risk factors that are considered nontraditional.

CASE STUDY

1. A 43-year-old female client has just been diagnosed with hypertension and also has elevated serum lipid levels. The client asks you the following questions:
   a. Why is the health care provider concerned about my lipid levels being elevated?
   b. What is hypertension?
   c. What are the risk factors for coronary heart disease?

REVIEW QUESTIONS

1. The spouse of a client is recalling the modifiable risk factors for coronary heart disease. Which statement by the client's spouse indicates a need for further teaching?
   1. "My wife's age is a modifiable risk factor."
   2. "Diabetes is a modifiable risk factor for my wife."
   3. "Obesity is a modifiable risk factor for my wife."
   4. "My wife's sedentary lifestyle is a modifiable risk factor."
2. The nurse is teaching a client about methods to decrease the client's homocysteine level. Which statement by the client indicates a need for further teaching?
   1. "Homocysteine is an amino acid that may increase my risk for developing heart disease."
   2. "Homocysteine levels may be decreased by taking a multivitamin with folate."
   3. "Homocysteine is an enzyme that increases my cholesterol level, which increases my risk for developing heart disease."
   4. "Homocysteine levels may be decreased by taking a multivitamin with B_6 and B_{12}."
3. Normal changes of aging may contribute to problems of circulation in older adults, even when there is no actual pathology. Which of the following is NOT a correct statement regarding the aging process and the cardiovascular system?
   1. A decrease of muscle tone in the heart results in a decrease in cardiac output.
   2. Blood vessels become less elastic and have an increase in calcification.
   3. Impaired valve function in the heart is often the result of increased stiffness and calcification and results in a decrease in cardiac output.
   4. An increase in baroreceptor response to blood pressure changes makes the heart and blood vessels more responsive to exercise and stress.

4. A nurse is planning a seminar on promoting a healthy heart. Which of the following statements is incorrect?
    1. Reduce stress and manage anger.
    2. Exercise at least 20 minutes, three times a week.
    3. Do not smoke.
    4. Eat a diet low in total fat, saturated fats, and cholesterol.
5. A nurse is evaluating a nursing student's understanding of the heart. Which of the following statements demonstrates a need for further teaching?
    1. There are four hollow chambers within the heart: two upper atria and two lower ventricles.
    2. The heart is a hollow, cone-shaped organ about the size of a fist.
    3. The heart is located in the mediastinum, between the lungs and underlying the sternum.
    4. Deoxygenated blood from the veins enters the left side of the heart through the superior and inferior venae cavae.
6. Which of the following statements by the nurse is NOT correct?
    1. Systole is when the heart ejects (propels) the blood into the pulmonary and systemic circulations.
    2. At the end of the systolic phase, the atria contract, adding an additional volume to the ventricles.
    3. The diastolic phase of the cardiac cycle is twice as long as the systolic phase.
    4. Diastole is largely a passive process.
7. The primary pacemaker of the heart is the:
    1. SA node.
    2. Bundle of His.
    3. AV node.
    4. Purkinje fibers.
8. PVR is determined by all of the following EXCEPT:
    1. Blood vessel length.
    2. Blood vessel diameter.
    3. The viscosity of the blood.
    4. The fineness of the blood.
9. Which of the following would be a sign of heart failure?
    1. Pulmonary congestion; adventitious lung sounds
    2. Decreased respiratory rate
    3. Warm, red extremities
    4. Decreased heart rate

CHAPTER 52

FLUID, ELECTROLYTE, AND ACID–BASE BALANCE

KEY TERM REVIEW

Match each term with its appropriate definition.

1. _______ Acid
2. _______ Acidosis
3. _______ Alkalosis
4. _______ Anions
5. _______ Arterial blood gases (ABGs)
6. _______ Cations
7. _______ Colloid osmotic pressure
8. _______ Colloids
9. _______ Crystalloids
10. _______ Dehydration
11. _______ Extracellular fluid (ECF)
12. _______ Fluid volume deficit (FVD)
13. _______ Fluid volume excess (FVE)
14. _______ Hydrostatic pressure
15. _______ Hypertonic
16. _______ Hypervolemia
17. _______ Hypotonic
18. _______ Hypovolemia
19. _______ Isotonic
20. _______ Metabolic acidosis
21. _______ Metabolic alkalosis
22. _______ Osmolality
23. _______ pH
24. _______ Respiratory acidosis
25. _______ Respiratory alkalosis

a. Condition that occurs when carbonic acid levels fall, more carbon dioxide than normal is exhaled, and pH rises to greater than 7.45

b. Same osmolality as ECF

c. Substance that releases hydrogen ions in solution

d. Occurs when body loses both water and electrolytes from the ECF in similar proportions

e. Negatively charged ions

f. Happens when the ratio of bicarbonate to carbonic acid is upset with the depletion of bicarbonate

g. Provide an accurate reflection of the gas exchange in the pulmonary system

h. Substances that do not readily dissolve in true solutions

i. Concentration of solutes in body fluids

j. Hyperosmolar fluid imbalance; water lost from body leaving client with excess sodium

k. Occurs when the amount of bicarbonate in the body exceeds the normal 20–1 ratio

l. Pressure exerted by plasma proteins whichpull water from the interstitial space into the vascular compartment when necessary

m. Ions that carry a positive charge

n. Found outside the cells

o. Occurs when the body retains both water and sodium in similar proportions to normal ECF

p. May be caused by decreased fluid intake, bleeding

q. Rise in pH that can be due to depletion of carbonic acid

r. Pressure exerted by a fluid within a closed system against the walls of the container in which it is contained

s. Higher osmolality than ECF

t. Increased blood volume; FVE

u. Salts that dissolve readily into true solutions

v. Lower osmolality than ECF

w. The relative acidity or alkalinity of a solution

x. Occurs when bicarbonate levels are low in relation to the amount of carbonic acid in the body

y. Any condition that causes carbonic acids to increase, carbon dioxide to be retained, and pH to fall below 7.35

KEY TOPIC REVIEW

1. Approximately 90% of the average healthy adult's weight is water, the primary body fluid.
   a. True
   b. False
2. The body fluid compartments are separated from one another by cell membranes and the capillary membrane.
   a. True
   b. False
3. Osmosis is the movement of water across cell membranes, from the less concentrated solution to the more concentrated solution.
   a. True
   b. False
4. Diffusion is the power of a solution to draw water across a semipermeable membrane.
   a. True
   b. False
5. The kidneys are the primary regulator of body fluids and electrolyte balance.
   a. True
   b. False

6. The most common electrolyte imbalances are deficits or excesses in sodium, potassium, and ______.

7. Fluid volume excess (FVE) is also referred to as ____________.

8. Human ____________ is commonly classified into four main groups: A, B, AB, and O.

9. The number of drops delivered per milliliter of an intravenous solution varies with different brands and types of infusion sets. This rate is called the ____________ factor.

10. ____________, or wing-tipped, needles with plastic flaps attached to the shaft are sometimes used for IV catheters.

11. Match the following terms with the correct definition.

a. Extracellular fluid (ECF)	______	The chemical combining power of the ion, or the capacity of cations to combine with anions to form molecules
b. Cations	______	The continual intermingling of molecules in liquids, gases, or solids brought about by the random movement of the molecules
c. Milliequivalent	______	Found outside the cells and accounts for about one third of total body fluid
d. Filtration	______	Have a low hydrogen ion concentration and can accept hydrogen ions in solution
e. Acid	______	Also known as hyperosmolar imbalance, this occurs when water is lost from the body, leaving the client with excess sodium
f. Buffers	______	Prevent excessive changes in pH by removing or releasing hydrogen ions
g. Hyponatremia	______	A sodium deficit, or serum sodium level of less than 135 mEq/L
h. Dehydration	______	A substance that releases hydrogen ions (H^+) in solution
i. Bases or alkalis	______	A process whereby fluid and solutes move together across a membrane from one compartment to another
j. Diffusion	______	Ions that carry a positive charge

12. ____________ is a potassium deficit or a serum potassium level of less than 3.5 mEq/L.

a. Hypokalemia

b. Hypocalcemia

c. Hyperkalemia

d. Hypercalcemia

13. Hypoventilation and carbon dioxide retention cause carbonic acid levels to increase and the pH to fall below 7.35, a condition known as:

a. Compensation.

b. Respiratory acidosis.

c. Hyperphosphatemia.

d. Respiratory alkalosis.

14. ____________ is an indicator of urine concentration that can be performed quickly and easily by nursing personnel.

a. Arterial blood gases

b. Hematocrit

c. Specific gravity

d. Volume expander

15. The ____________ is inserted in the basilic or cephalic vein just above or below the antecubital space of the arm. The tip of the catheter rests in the superior vena cava.

a. Central dripping catheter

b. Centrally elongated catheter

c. Central venous catheter

d. Peripherally inserted central venous catheter (PICC)

16. ____________ is the movement of molecules through a semipermeable membrane from an area of higher concentration to an area of lower concentration.

a. Osmosis

b. Diffusion

c. Filtration

d. Oncotic pressure

FOCUSED STUDY TIPS

1. Discuss the selection and screening of blood donors.
2. List several examples of cations.
3. Discuss the pathophysiology of dehydration.
4. Discuss gender and body size and its effects on total body water.
5. Compare and contrast diffusion, filtration, and osmosis..
6. Identify three factors that generally result in fluid volume deficit.
7. List three of the six measurements that are commonly used to interpret arterial blood gas tests.
8. What is a volume expander? Give one example.
9. List and discuss the three main mechanisms that can cause edema.
10. List several of the items usually included in intravenous solution infusion sets.
11. Discuss lifestyle and its effect on fluid, electrolyte, and acid–base balance.
12. Describe acid–base balance and its regulation.
13. List three of the four routes of fluid output.

14. List symptoms of hypokalemia.

15. List symptoms of hypercalcemia.

CASE STUDY

1. A 77-year-old male client has just been admitted to the unit. His fluid intake has been about 500 mL per day. He then tells you he sometimes forgets to drink water throughout the day.

   a. Why is water vital to health and normal cellular function?

   b. Explain the thirst mechanism.

   c. List the four routes of fluid output.

REVIEW QUESTIONS

1. A nurse is evaluating a nursing student's understanding of body water. Which of the following statements indicates a need for further teaching?

   1. Approximately 60% of the average healthy adult's weight is water, the primary body fluid.
   2. Infants have the highest proportion of water, accounting for 70% to 80% of their body weight.
   3. Men have a lower percentage of body water than women.
   4. Water makes up a greater percentage of a lean individual's body weight than an obese individual's.

2. Which of the following information about osmosis is NOT correct?

   1. Osmosis is the continual intermingling of molecules in liquids, gases, or solids brought about by the random movement of the molecules.
   2. Osmosis is an important mechanism for maintaining homeostasis and fluid balance.
   3. Osmosis occurs when the concentration of solutes on one side of a selectively permeable membrane, such as the capillary membrane, is higher than on the other side.
   4. Osmolality is determined by the total solute concentration within a fluid compartment and is measured as parts of solute per kilogram of water.

3. Which of the following is a sodium deficit, or serum sodium level of less than 135 mEq/L?

   1. Hypernatremia
   2. Hypokalemia
   3. Hyponatremia
   4. Hyperkalemia

4. Which of the following events occurs when an individual hyperventilates?

   1. Less carbon dioxide than normal is exhaled.
   2. Carbonic acid levels increase.
   3. pH rises to greater than 7.45.
   4. More oxygen than normal is exhaled.

5. The following are normal values of arterial blood gases EXCEPT:
   1. PaO_2 = 50–70 mm Hg.
   2. pH = 7.35–7.45.
   3. $PaCO_2$ = 35–45 mm Hg.
   4. HCO_3^- = 22–26 mEq/L.
6. Which of the following actions is NOT appropriate for the nurse who is starting an intravenous (IV) infusion? The nurse:
   1. Adjusts the IV pole so that the solution container is suspended about 1 m (3 ft) above the client's head.
   2. Completely fills the drip chamber with solution.
   3. Uses the client's nondominant arm, unless contraindicated.
   4. Cleans the skin at the site of entry with a topical antiseptic swab.
7. A nurse is planning a seminar on wellness care and promoting fluid and electrolyte balance. Which of the following statements is correct? (Select all that apply.)
   1. Consume 9 to 10 glasses of water daily.
   2. Limit alcohol intake because it has a diuretic effect.
   3. Avoid excess amounts of foods or fluids high in salt, sugar, and caffeine.
   4. Increase fluid intake before, during, and after strenuous exercise.
   5. Limit fluid intake before bedtime.
8. The nurse who is starting an intravenous infusion should avoid using all of the following EXCEPT a vein that is:
   1. Damaged by previous use, phlebitis, infiltration, or sclerosis.
   2. In an area of flexion.
   3. Not as visible, because it will tend to roll away from the needle.
   4. Continually distended with blood, or knotted or tortuous.
9. A nurse is evaluating a nursing student's understanding of blood transfusions. Which of the following statements demonstrates a need for further teaching?
   1. A blood transfusion is the introduction of whole blood or blood components into the venous circulation.
   2. To avoid transfusing incompatible red blood cells, both blood donor and recipient are typed and their blood is crossmatched.
   3. Stop the transfusion immediately if signs of a reaction develop.
   4. Human blood is commonly classified into four main groups: A, AB, O, and AO.
10. Which of the following actions is NOT appropriate for the nurse administering blood to a client?
    1. Blood is usually administered through a #18- to #20-gauge intravenous needle or catheter.
    2. Saline is used to prime the set and flush the needle before administering blood.
    3. A transfusion should be completed within 4 hours of initiation.
    4. An S-type blood transfusion set with an in-line or add-on filter is used when administering blood.

ANSWER KEY

CHAPTER 1

Key Term Review

1. h 2. j 3. g 4. i 5. l 6. m

7. n 8. c 9. o 10. p 11. q 12. v

13. a 14. t 15. e 16. k 17. f 18. r

19. u 20. d 21. y 22. s 23. b 24. w

25. x

Key Topic Review Answers

1. To promote wellness, prevent illness, restore health, care for the dying
2. a, d
3. b
4. b
5. f, a, h, j, d, g, b, i, e, c
6. Consumer, patient, client
7. a, d
8. professionalization
9. b
10. a
11. diagnosisrelated groups
12. c
13. the right to accept or refuse care; the ability to use advanced directives
14. Continuing education (CE)

Case Study Answers

1. *What role is the nurse acting in by representing the client's needs and wishes and assisting the client in behavior modification plans?* The nurse is acting as a change agent in this role. Nurses are continually dealing with change in the health care system.
2. *The nurse is in the process of helping the client recognize and cope with both the asthma condition and the tobacco cessation program. The nurse is acting as a change agent, and what other role is the nurse representing?* The nurse is acting as a client advocate to protect the client. The nurse may represent the client's needs to other health care providers. The nurse may suggest some medications to assist the client in his smoking cessation program, such as Zyban.
3. *According to Benner's stages of nursing expertise, in what stage is the nurse functioning?* The nurse has been practicing for 4 years. The nurse is thus at Stage IV, Proficient. (Refer to <LINK>Box 1–3</LINK> in the textbook.)

Review Question Answers

1. ***Answer:*** 1 (Objective: 2) ***Rationale:*** The traditional nursing role has always entailed humanistic caring, nurturing, comforting, and supporting. Religion has also played a significant role in the development of nursing. The Christian value of "love thy neighbor as thyself" and Christ's parable of the Good Samaritan both had a significant impact on the development of Western nursing. Wars accentuate the need for nurses. Greater financial support provided through public and private health insurance programs has increased the demand for nursing care. ***Nursing Process:*** Assessment ***Client Need:*** Safe, Effective Care Environment
2. ***Answer:*** 3 (Objective: 6) ***Rationale:*** A nurse who has an advanced education and is a graduate of a nurse practitioner program is considered a nurse practitioner. Nurse practitioners usually deal with nonemergency acute or chronic illness and provide primary ambulatory care. ***Nursing Process:*** Assessment ***Client Need:*** Safe, Effective Care Environment

3. *Answer:* 2 (Objective: 8) ***Rationale:*** Stage III, Competent, is able to coordinate multiple complex care demands and focuses on the important aspects of care. ***Nursing Process:*** Assessment ***Client Need:*** Safe, Effective Care Environment

4. *Answer:* 3 (Objective: 1) ***Rationale:*** Workplace issues include inadequate staffing, heavy workloads, increased use of overtime, and difficulty recruiting and retaining nurses. ***Nursing Process:*** Assessment ***Client Need:*** Safe, Effective Care Environment

5. *Answer:* 4 (Objective: 1) ***Rationale:*** The ANA is actively working to improve the image of nursing. The radio commercial will most likely include information to help shape the listener's image of contemporary nursing. ***Nursing Process:*** Assessment ***Client Need:*** Safe, Effective Care Environment

6. *Answer:* 2 (Objective: 2) ***Rationale:*** The goal of illness prevention programs is to maintain optimal health by preventing disease. Nursing activities that prevent illness include immunizations, prenatal and infant care, and prevention of sexually transmitted infections. ***Nursing Process:*** Planning ***Client Need:*** Health Promotion and Maintenance

7. *Answer:* 1 (Objective: 4) ***Rationale:*** Although nurse practice acts differ in various jurisdictions, they all have a common purpose: to protect the public. ***Nursing Process:*** Assessment ***Client Need:*** Safe, Effective Care Environment

8. *Answer:* 3 (Objective: 3) ***Rationale:*** The caregiver role has traditionally included those activities that assist the client physically and psychologically while preserving the client's dignity. ***Nursing Process:*** Assessment ***Client Need:*** Safe, Effective Care Environment

9. *Answer:* 2 (Objective: 9) ***Rationale:*** Professionalization is the process of becoming professional, that is, of acquiring characteristics considered to be professional. ***Nursing Process:*** Implementation ***Client Need:*** Safe, Effective Care Environment

10. *Answer:* 4 (Objective: 7) ***Rationale:*** Demography is the study of population, including statistics about distribution by age and place of residence, mortality (death), and morbidity (incidence of disease). From demographic data, population needs for nursing services can be assessed. ***Nursing Processes:*** Assessment ***Client Need:*** Safe, Effective Care Environment

CHAPTER 2

Key Term Review

1. i 2. m 3. a 4. n 5. l 6. f

7. g 8. o 9. p 10. q 11. r 12. k

13. w 14. s 15. b 16. t 17. u 18. h

19. v 20. d 21. e 22. j 23. c

Key Topic Review Answers

1. Evidence-based practice

2. "Right not to be harmed" either physically, emotionally, legally, financially, or socially; "right to full disclosure" without deception about what participating in a study would involve; "right to self-determination" without feeling pressured to participate in studies and without constraints, coercion, or any undue influence to participate in a study; "right to privacy and confidentiality," such as ensuring anonymity of the participant

3. confidentiality

4. research is the application of the scientific approach to generate empirical knowledge.

5. Research

6. a. 2; b. 2; c. 1; d. 2; e. 1

7. a, b, d, e

8. i, c, a, f, j, h, d, g, e, b

9. e, c, a, b, d

10. Quantitative research is the systematic collection, statistical analysis, and interpretation of numerical data; qualitative research: systematic collection and thematic analysis of narrative data

11. b

12. a

13. b

14. Feasibility

15. pilot study

Case Study Answers

1. No; one research study alone does not provide adequate evidence for changing practice.

2. The nurse should first analyze the study framework for validity and then conduct a literature search to determine if further support for the findings in the original study exists.

3. This is a quantitative study because it involves scientific research and empirical data.

Review Question Answers

1. ***Answer:*** 1 (Objective 7) ***Rationale:*** Hidden inducements, such as suggestions that by taking part in a study they might become famous or make an important contribution to science, must be strictly avoided. Sharing client information with the pharmaceutical company may be a violation of the client's right to privacy. Providing basic care to the client is a basic nursing function. Giving the client information about the study is part of full disclosure that is a basic client right. ***Nursing Process:*** Implementation ***Client Need:*** Safe, Effective Care Environment

2. ***Answer:*** 3 (Objective: 5) ***Rationale:*** A qualitative study is not linear like quantitative research. The intent of qualitative research is to describe and then explain a phenomenon. The technique most often used to collect data for this type of research is interviews. Quantitative research progresses through systematic, logical steps according to a specific plan to collect numerical information, often under conditions of considerable control that is analyzed using statistical procedures. Ethnographic inquiry is related to selective topics specific to a group with the same beliefs or lifestyles. Pilot studies are often a tentative probe to see if further research study is needed on a topic. ***Nursing Process:*** Assessment ***Client Need:*** Safe, Effective Care Environment

3. ***Answer:*** 1, 2, 4 (Objective: 4) ***Rationale:*** Answers 1, 2, and 4 are examples of the professional nurse's activities in nursing research. One of the nurse's responsibilities with research is in safeguarding the rights of the client, which includes informed consent. ***Nursing Process:*** Implementation ***Client Need:*** Safe, Effective Care Environment

4. ***Answer:*** 4 (Objective: 1) ***Rationale:*** The nursing student should not document any identifiers on paperwork that would be made public or could cause potential embarrassment to the client. The use of identifiers would violate the right of privacy and confidentiality for the client. ***Nursing Process:*** Implementation ***Client Need:*** Safe, Effective Care Environment

5. ***Answer:*** 2 (Objective 5) ***Rationale:*** A strategy for identifying key terms when locating research literature is PICO. *P* stands for patient, population, or problem of interest. *I* stands for intervention or therapy to consider for the subject of interest. *C* stands for comparison of interventions, such as no treatment. *O* stands for outcome of the intervention. ***Nursing Processes:*** Assessment, Implementation ***Client Need:*** Safe, Effective Care Environment

6. ***Answer:*** 2 (Objective 5) ***Rationale:*** Formulating a research problem is facilitated by performing a literature review. ***Nursing Processes:*** Implementation ***Client Need:*** Safe, Effective Care Environment

7. ***Answer:*** 1, 2 (Objective: 3) ***Rationale:*** New scientific knowledge acquired with new discoveries regarding health and cultural changes that are continuously changing as time progresses are two reasons for continually revising nursing education curricula. Disease and treatments evolve as time passes so nurses must keep up to date on all medical breakthroughs. ***Nursing Process:*** Assessment ***Client Need:*** Health Promotion and Maintenance

8. ***Answer:*** 1 (Objective: 6) ***Rationale:*** Scientific and technologic advances are key factors in keeping abreast of the changing health care environment. ***Nursing Process:*** Assessment ***Client Need:*** Health Promotion and Maintenance

9. ***Answer:*** 1, 3, 4, 5 (Objective: 7) ***Rationale:*** The research process involves identifying the problem or question, collecting data using various means such as computer searches and/or questionnaires, analyzing the data and writing up the results , and publishing or presenting the research findings to expand the body of nursing knowledge. ***Nursing Process:*** Assessment ***Client Need:*** Health Promotion and Maintenance

10. ***Answer:*** 2 (Objective: 6) ***Rationale:*** All nurses involved in research have a role in safeguarding the client's rights. ***Nursing Process:*** Implementation ***Client Need:*** Safe, Effective Care Environment

11. ***Answer:*** 1 (Objective: 5) ***Rationale:*** The dependent variable is a behavior, characteristic, or outcome that the researcher wishes to explain or predict. ***Nursing Process:*** Implementation ***Client Need:*** Safe, Effective Care Environment

CHAPTER 3

Key Term Review

1. f 2. i 3. h 4. j 5. e 6. a

7. k 8. c 9. b 10. l 11. d 12. m

13. g

Key Topic Review Answers

1. *Theory* has been defined as a supposition or system of ideas that is proposed to explain a given phenomenon. Characteristics of a theory include: (Student will choose two.)
   a. It is an articulated idea about something important.
   b. It is used to describe, predict, and control phenomena.

c. It offers ways of looking at or conceptualizing the central interests of a discipline.

2. In a practice discipline, the main function of theory (and research) is to provide new possibilities for understanding the discipline's practice (music, art, management, and nursing).

3. a

4. soft; hard

5. concepts

6. conceptual framework; grand; conceptual model

7. paradigm

8. a. Person or client; the recipient of nursing care (includes individuals, families, groups, and communities).

   b. Environment; the internal and external surroundings that affect the client. This includes people in the physical environment, such as families, friends, and significant others.

   c. Health; the degree of wellness or well-being experienced by the client.

   d. Nursing; the attributes, characteristics, and actions of the nurse providing care on behalf of or in conjunction with the client.

9. Nightingale's theories, interactive theories, systems theories, and developmental theories

10. Orem (b), Nightingale (a), Peplau (c), Parse (c), Henderson (a), Roy (b), Neuman (c), Rogers (b), Leininger (c), Watson (a), King (b)

11. Florence Nightingale

12. philosophy

13. a

14. a. Client (person): recipient of nursing care (individuals, families, groups)

    b. Environment: internal/external surroundings that affect the client (includes people in the physical environment—families, friends, significant others)

    c. Health: degree of wellness and well-being experienced by the client

    d. Nursing: attributes, characteristics, and actions of the nurse providing care on behalf of or in conjunction with the client

15. Nursing is considered to be a practice discipline because the central focus is performance of a professional role (nursing, teaching, management, music).

Case Study Answers

1. *Choose the best nursing theory on which to base the revised philosophy of nursing for this particular facility.* Imogene King's theory of goal attainment would work well in the long-term facility and the assisted living facility. King developed a transactional model that describes the nature of and standard for nurse–client interactions that lead to goal attainment—that nurses purposefully interact and mutually set, explore, and agree to means to achieve goals.

2. *Explain your rationale for using the theory that you have chosen.* The rationale for the theory should be based on the main ideals supported by the concepts. The answer will depend on which theory the student chooses.

Review Question Answers

1. ***Answer:*** 2 (Objective: 1) ***Rationale:*** *Theory* is defined as a supposition or system of ideas that is proposed to explain a given phenomenon. Concepts are called the "building blocks" of theories and are difficult to explain or define. *Paradigm* refers to a pattern of shared understandings and assumptions about reality and the world. *Conceptual models* or *frameworks* are defined as a group of related ideas, statements, or concepts. They articulate a broad range of the significant relationships among the concepts of a discipline. ***Nursing Process:*** Assessment ***Client Need:*** Safe, Effective Care Environment

2. ***Answer:*** 2 (Objective: 3) ***Rationale:*** Concepts are labels given to ideas, objects, and/or events—a summary of thoughts or a way to categorize thoughts or ideas. Intelligence, motivation, learned helplessness, and/or obesity are examples of a construct, which is a group of concepts. A theory is the organization of concepts or constructs that shows the relationship of the ideas with the intent of describing, explaining, or predicting. An example of a theory includes self-care, adaptation, caring, behavioral system, unitary man, hierarchy of needs, interpersonal relationships, humanistic, and/or nurse–client transactions. ***Nursing Process:*** Assessment ***Client Need:*** Safe, Effective Care Environment

3. ***Answer:*** 4 (Objective: 2) ***Rationale:*** Jean Watson's theory is based on a humanistic and caring concept of nursing. The holistic outlook addresses the impact and importance of altruism, sensitivity, trust, and interpersonal skills. Imogene King's theory is based on systems theory and the behavioral sciences. A transactional model of interaction between the nurse and client was developed. Creation, spirituality, the client, and the environment are the basis of Roy's model of nursing. Orem's theory of nursing is based on self-care and restoring the client to the highest level of functioning. ***Nursing Process***: Planning ***Client Need:*** Psychosocial Integrity

4. ***Answer:*** 1 (Objective: 3) ***Rationale:*** Peplau's psychodynamic nursing model is an example of a middle-range theory. Watson's, Orem's, and King's theories are considered grand theories. ***Nursing Process:*** Assessment ***Client Need:*** Safe, Effective Care Environment

5. ***Answer:*** 4 (Objective: 3) ***Rationale:*** Virginia Henderson's theory explains the 14 essential functions toward independence that a client must meet to achieve the highest level of health. Myra Estrin Levine's theory was based on four conservation principles of inpatient client resources. Dorothea Orem uses nursing interventions to meet clients' self-care needs. Madeline Leininger's theory uses transcultural nursing and caring nursing, in which the concepts are aimed toward caring and the components of a culture care theory. ***Nursing Process:*** Assessment ***Client Need:*** Safe, Effective Care Environment

6. ***Answer:*** 1 (Objective: 4) ***Rationale:*** Maintenance of system equilibrium is one of the goals of Betty Neuman's nursing theory. Orem's model is based on assisting the client to achieve the highest level of self-care. Internal and external stimuli are based on Roy's adaptation model. The last choice in this grouping of answers is not a factor in any of the nursing theories. ***Nursing Process:*** Planning ***Client Need:*** Psychosocial Integrity

7. ***Answer:*** 2 (Objective: 4) ***Rationale:*** It was an early effort to define nursing phenomena that serves as the basis for later theoretical formulations. ***Nursing Process:*** Assessment ***Client Need:*** Safe, Effective Care Environment

8. ***Answer:*** 3 (Objective: 5) ***Rationale:*** Disciplines without a strong theory and research base historically were referred to as "soft," a negative comparison with the "hard" natural sciences. Many of the soft disciplines attempted to emulate the sciences, so theory and scientific research became a more important part of academic life, both in the practice disciplines and in the humanities. ***Nursing Process:*** Assessment ***Client Need:*** Safe, Effective Care Environment

9. ***Answer:*** 1 (Objective: 1) ***Rationale:*** A conceptual framework is a group of related ideas, statements, or concepts. A paradigm refers to a pattern of shared understandings and assumptions about reality and the world. A philosophy is a belief system, often an early effort to define nursing phenomena, and serves as the basis for later theoretical formulations. Critical theory is the way to elucidate how social structures affect a wide variety of human experiences, from art to social practices. ***Nursing Process:*** Assessment ***Client Need:*** Safe, Effective Care Environment

10. ***Answer:*** 1, 2, 3, and 5 (Objective: 4) ***Rationale:*** The four major concepts are considered to be person or client, the recipient of nursing care (includes individuals, families, groups, and communities); the environment, the internal and external surroundings that affect the client—the environment includes people in the physical environment, such as families, friends, and significant others; health, the degree of wellness or well-being that the client experiences; and nursing, the attributes, characteristics, and actions of the nurse providing care on behalf of or in conjunction with the client. ***Nursing Process:*** Planning ***Client Need:*** Psychosocial Integrity

11. ***Answer:*** ______c____ A nurse performing non-contact therapeutic touch.

______a____ A nurse measuring the client's intake and output

______b____ A nurse demonstrating therapeutic communication with a client who has been diagnosed with depression.

______d___ A nurse who plans care with the client to establish mutual goals and outcomes.

Rationale: Martha Rogers' Science of Unitary Human Beings states the idea of non-contact therapeutic touch. This is the idea that humans are dynamic energy fields in continuous exchange with environmental fields, both of which are infinite. Florence Nightingale's Environmental Theory linked health with five environmental factors: (1) pure or fresh air, (2) pure water, (3) efficient drainage, (4) cleanliness, and (5) light, especially direct sunlight. Deficiencies in these five factors produced lack of health or illness. In addition to those factors, Nightingale also stressed the importance of keeping the client warm, maintaining a noise-free environment, and attending to the client's diet in terms of assessing intake, timeliness of the food, and its effect on the person. Peplau's Interpersonal Relations Model introduces the existence of a therapeutic relationship between the nurse and the client. Imogene King's Goal Attainment Theory describes the nature of and standard for nurse–client interactions that lead to goal attainment—that nurses purposefully interact and mutually set, explore, and agree to means to achieve goals. Goal attainment represents outcomes. ***Nursing Process:*** Implementation. ***Client Need:*** Safe and Effective Care Environment

CHAPTER 4

Key Term Review Answers

1. l	2. c	3. k	4. j	5. n	6. b
7. m	8. a	9. i	10. d	11. e	12. y
13. o	14. w	15. p	16. x	17. r	18. g
19. s	20. h	21. u	22. v	23. q	24. f
25. t					

Key Topic Review Answers

1. It is important because nurses are accountable for their professional judgments and actions.

2. Accountability is the ability and willingness to assume responsibility for one's actions and to accept the consequences of one's behavior.

   a. To ensure that the nurse's decisions and actions are consistent with current legal principles.

   b. To protect the nurse from liability.

3. Functions of laws in nursing are: (Student will choose two.)

   a. They provide a framework for establishing the nursing actions while caring for clients.

   b. They differentiate the nurse's responsibility from those of other members of the health care team.

   c. They help to establish the boundaries of independent nursing action.

   d. They help to maintain a standard of nursing practice by making nurses accountable under the law.

4. a

5. a

6. Types of law include: (Student will choose two.)

   a. Public law refers to the body of law that deals with relationships between individuals and the government and/or governmental agencies.

   b. Criminal law refers to the body of law that deals with disputes between an individual and the society as a whole.

   c. Private law refers to the body of law that deals with relationships among private individuals.

   d. Contract law refers to the body of law that involves enforcement of agreements among individuals.

   e. Tort law defines and enforces duties and rights among individuals that are not based on contract law.

7. b, d, e

8. litigation

9. a, e, d, b, c

10. a, b, c, d

11. a

12. mutual recognition; interstate

13. Certification

14. Standards of care are the skills and learning commonly possessed by members of a profession. The purpose is to protect the consumer. Two standards of care include:

    a. Internal standards

    b. External standards

15. Four examples of external standards of care are:

    a. Nurse practice acts

    b. Professional organizations

    c. Nursing specialty-practice organizations

    d. Federal organizations and federal guidelines

16. a

17. A contract is considered to be expressed when the two parties discuss and agree, either orally or in writing, to terms and conditions during the creation of the contract. One example of an expressed contract is when a travel nurse works at a hospital for a stated length of time and under stated conditions. An implied contract is one that has not been explicitly agreed to by the parties, but that the law nevertheless considers as existing. An example of an implied contract is when the hospital is expected to provide the necessary supplies and equipment needed to provide competent nursing care.

18. A right is a privilege or fundamental power to which an individual is entitled unless it is revoked by law or given up voluntarily. A responsibility is the obligation associated with a right. See Table 4–2 in Chapter 4 of the text for examples of the responsibilities and rights associated with each role.

19. strike

20. The two types of consent include:

    a. Expressed consent may take the form of either an oral or written agreement. Usually, the more invasive a procedure or the greater the potential for risk to the client, the greater the need for written permission.

    b. Implied consent is when the client's behavior indicates agreement or when a medical emergency occurs and the client cannot express consent.

21. b; it is the responsibility of the health care provider who is performing the procedure.

22. The nurse's signature confirms three things:

    a. The client has no further questions about the procedure and is ready to give consent.

b. The individual signing the consent is the appropriate individual (either the client or the individual with legal responsibility for the client, such as a parent).

c. The nurse is not aware of any factor that could cause the client to be considered incompetent (such as administration of narcotics, court order declaring the client incompetent, etc.).

23. The nurse must verify that the client is aware of the pros and cons of refusal and is making an informed decision. Documentation is essential and must include notification of the health care provider, the concerns of the client, the understanding of refusal of the client, and any witnesses to the refusal.

24. The nurse needs to know the state Nurse Practice Act because it will assist the nurse in delegation of duties among the various personnel, and also in the recognition of what is involved in the scope of nursing practice. Nurses are accountable and will be held responsible for following the Nurse Practice act in his or her practicing state.

25. a

26. The Americans with Disabilities Act prohibits discrimination on the basis of disability in employment, public services, and public accommodations. The nurse assists individuals with disabilities to comprehend the opportunities provided by law. Also, the nurse needs to be familiar with this law because nurses with disabilities may be refused employment opportunities inappropriately, and the nurse manager must know the laws in order to avoid discrimination of others.

27. b; federal laws regulate controlled substances

28. Stress

29. The definitions of the following terms and certain responsibilities of nurses are:

a. Advance directives: Allow individuals to specify aspects of care that he or she wishes to receive should that individual become unable to make or communicate his or her own preferences. Nurses need to assess whether clients and families have an accurate understanding of advance directives and give instructions as necessary. Also, nurses must know the laws in his or her practicing state regarding patient self-determination.

b. Autopsies: Are also called postmortem examinations. An autopsy is an examination of the body after death and is only performed in certain cases. It examines the organs and tissues to establish the exact cause of death. The nurse must understand the process to answer family's questions and to obtain a signed consent when the autopsy is performed voluntarily.

c. Certification of death: The formal determination of death or pronouncement that must be performed by a physician, a coroner, or a nurse. The granting of the authority of nurses to pronounce death is regulated by the state or province. It is necessary by law to complete this form.

d. Do-not-resuscitate orders (DNRs): These are generally written by the provider when the client or proxy has expressed the wish for no resuscitation in the event of respiratory or cardiac arrest. It is written to indicate that the goal of treatment is a comfortable, dignified death and that further life-sustaining measures are not indicated. The nurse can request a change in assignment if a DNR is contrary to the nurse's personal beliefs. The responsibility of the nurse is to make sure that the health care team is aware of any DNR orders.

e. Euthanasia: The act of painlessly putting to death persons suffering from incurable or chronically painful disease. It is illegal in both Canada and the majority of the United States to perform any type of euthanasia. Some states have laws that allow clients to end their lives through the voluntary self-administration of lethal medications, expressly prescribed by a physician for that purpose. Some states have right-to-die statutes and honor living wills. These states legally recognize the right-to-die statutes as the client's right to refuse treatment. Nurses must know their state's policies and Nurse Practice Act in order to make any decisions regarding this matter.

f. Inquests: Legal inquiries into the cause or manner of a death. An inquest is usually performed when the death is a result of an accident to determine any blame. Agency policy dictates who is responsible for reporting deaths to the coroner or medical examiner.

g. Organ donation: The donation of organs that an individual 18 years or older and of sound mind can endorse. Individuals can make a gift of any organs or his or her body for the following purposes: medical or dental education and research, the advancement of medical or dental science, therapy, and/or transplantation. Nurses may serve as witnesses for individuals consenting to donate organs.

30. Tort

31. c, d

32. HIPAA is the first nationwide legislation to protect the privacy of health information. The four specific areas of HIPAA include:

a. The electronic transfer of information among organizations

b. Standardized numbers for identifying providers, employers, and health plans

c. Security rules providing for a uniform level of protection of all health care information

d. Privacy rules that set standards defining appropriate disclosure to protect health information

33. Nurses should question any order a client questions; any order if the client's condition has changed; any verbal orders to avoid miscommunications; and any orders that are illegible, unclear, or incomplete.

Case Study Answers

1. *Did the surgeon adhere to the signed consent form that the client signed before the surgery?* No, the surgeon did not adhere to the signed consent form because the appendix was not listed in the original signed consent.

2. *Under the circumstances, what type of tort is the surgeon liable for?* Battery is the type of tort because the surgeon has intentionally and wrongfully performed an act without the client's permission.

3. *What was the operating nurse's role in this incident?* The operating nurse should have questioned the removal of the appendix since it is assumed that she reviewed the informed consent and is considered the patient's advocate.

Review Question Answers

1. ***Answer:*** 4 (Objective: 2) ***Rationale:*** The nurse with a master's degree and a certificate in maternal–infant nursing is deemed an expert in that field because of the advanced preparation. The other choices do not address the needed expertise. ***Nursing Process:*** Assessment ***Client Needs:*** Safe, Effective Care Environment

2. ***Answer:*** 2, 5 (Objective: 4) ***Rationale:*** Of these options, the parents of the 14-year-old child and the competent older client would be the best persons to make health care decisions. The other responses are incorrect due to the altered mental state and age of consent limitations. If the child with the laceration was hemorrhaging, implied consent would be adequate enough in order to save the child's life. ***Nursing Process:*** Assessment ***Client Need:*** Safe, Effective Care Environment

3. ***Answer:*** 1 (Objective: 1) ***Rationale:*** Failing to provide discharge instructions is a form of malpractice. The nurse should document in the client's chart that discharge instructions were given verbally, the client expressed understanding of the discharge instructions, and/or a copy of the discharge instructions were given to the client or caregiver. Negligence is misconduct or practice that is below the standard expected of an ordinary, reasonable, and prudent person. Assault can be described as an attempt or threat to touch another person unjustifiably. Assault precedes battery; it is the act that causes the person to believe a battery is about to occur. ***Battery is the willful touching of a person (or the person's clothes or even something the person is carrying) that may or may not cause harm. Nursing Process:*** Implementation ***Client Need:*** Safe, Effective Care Environment

4. ***Answer:*** *3* (Objective: 4) ***Rationale:*** In order for consent to be considered informed, the physician must describe the procedure, explain risks of the procedure, and alternative treatment options; the client must verbalize understanding of the explanation; and the informed consent form must be signed and witnessed. The client cannot sign the consent before the procedure is explained by the surgeon, cannot have the son give express consent for surgery if the client is competent to give consent for himself, and consent would need to be obtained if the client has been declared incompetent. ***Nursing Process:*** Assessment ***Client Needs:*** Safe, Effective Care Environment

5. ***Answer:*** 1 (Objective: 7) ***Rationale:*** A living will provides specific instructions about what medical treatment the client chooses to omit or refuse in the event that the client is unable to make those decisions. A durable power of attorney for health care is a notarized or witnessed statement that appoints someone to make health care decisions when the client is unable to do so. designates who should make medical decisions if the client is incapable of making independent decisions. Neither a living will nor a durable power of attorney describes determining real estate or health care provider's actions when the client is unable to make his or her own health care decisions. ***Nursing Process:*** Assessment ***Client Need:*** Safe, Effective Care Environment

6. ***Answer:*** 4 (Objective: 11) ***Rationale:*** Assault is the attempt or threat to touch another person unjustifiably. It often precedes battery. Battery is the willful touching of a person that may or may not cause harm. ***Nursing Process:*** Assessment ***Client Needs:*** Planning; Management of Care; Safety

7. ***Answer:*** 1, 3 (Objective 1) ***Rationale:*** The nurse defamed the health care provider's reputation by use of the word *incompetent* in the documentation. The nurse also committed libel because the defamation was by means of print, writing, or pictures. The nurse did not commit slander, defamation by spoken word. Unprofessional conduct includes incompetence or gross negligence, conviction for practicing without a license, falsification of client records, illegally obtaining, using, or possessing controlled substances. ***Nursing Process:*** Implementation ***Client Need:*** Management of Care

8. ***Answer:*** 3 (Objective: 1) ***Rationale:*** Unprofessional conduct is defined by the *Code of Ethics for Nurses*. Unethical conduct may also be addressed in nurse practice acts. It includes violation of professional ethical codes, breach of confidentiality, fraud, or refusing to care for clients of specific socioeconomic or cultural origins. ***Nursing Process:*** Assessment ***Client Needs:*** Safety; Safe, Effective Care Environment

9. ***Answer:*** 2 (Objective: 15) ***Rationale:*** The conscience clauses give hospitals the right to deny admission to abortion clients and give health care personnel, including nurses, the right to refuse to

participate in abortions. When these rights are exercised, the statutes also protect the agency and employee from discrimination or retaliation. ***Nursing Process:*** Implementation ***Client Need:*** Management of Care

10. ***Answer:*** 4 (Objective: 2) ***Rationale:*** Hospital policies are not included in the laws of nursing. The other three items are functions of nursing laws. ***Nursing Process:*** Assessment ***Client Need:*** Management of Care

CHAPTER 5

Key Term Review

1. d	2. g	3. f	4. m	5. a	6. s
7. o	8. n	9. p	10. j	11. k	12. b
13. q	14. t	15. r	16. e	17. h	18. i
19. l	20. c				

Key Topic Review Answers

1. Values are enduring beliefs or attitudes about the worth of a person, object, idea, or action. Values are important because they influence decisions and actions, including nurses' ethical decision making.

2. Beliefs (or opinions) are interpretations that people accept as true. Beliefs do not always involve values. Values give direction to life and form the basis of behavior.

3. Attitudes

4. a. altruism b. autonomy c. human dignity d. integrity e. social justice

5. Whenever clients hold detrimental or conflicting values regarding their health, the nurse could use values clarification as a nursing intervention.

6. Bioethics or nursing ethics

7. Morality

8. a

9. b, a, c, b, a, a and b, c, b

10. A statement on compassion has been added and the duty to protect patients has been broadened to include all patient rights.

11. To reach a mutual peaceful agreement that is in the best interests of the client.

12. Inform, support, and mediate

13. Beneficence

14. Justice

15. Veracity

16. Accountability; responsibility

Case Study Answers

1a. *What considerations should you take into account in assisting the client to make those decisions?* You should consider the client and family's outlook and past experiences, the client's fears about and abilities to cope with this disorder, and the client's religious beliefs. As the nurse, you could use the seven questions to facilitate values clarification for the client. The process is listed in the text.

1b. *In what way could you assist the client in reaching decisions about further health care?* You need to let the client and family make their own choices, help guide the client and family in working through their emotions, maintain professional relationships with both the client and the family, and be aware of your own thoughts and feelings regarding this issue. You should be sure not to impose your own feelings on the client or family members.

1c. *Would an ethics committee be involved in this matter?* An ethics committee would be helpful in the decision-making process and would give recommendations. The committee is a multidisciplinary team and assists with ethical issues, client values, and professional obligations.

1d. *What principles of autonomy are applied to this situation?* Autonomy is defined as having independence or freedom from control by external forces. The final decision regarding the extent of life-promoting activities is in the hands of the client. The nurse could inform the client about advance directives and other methods that may be helpful in this matter.

2a. *What are his rights as a client?* According to the Patient's Bill of Rights and HIPAA regulations, he should have a right to privacy and anonymity as a client in the hospital.

2b. *Could he take legal actions?* He would have the right to sue the hospital for privacy invasion. It would have to be proven in a court of law.

Review Question Answers

1. ***Answers:*** 1, 2 (Objective: 1) ***Rationale:*** The feelings of shame and guilt, along with use of feeling words such as *should*, *ought to*, *right*, *wrong*, *good*, and *bad*, both indicate the morality involved in a specific situation. Legislative regulations, infringing on individual human rights such as the right to life or privacy, and fear of imprisonment indicate a legal situation. ***Nursing Process:*** Assessment ***Client Need:*** Safe and Effective Care Environment

2. ***Answer:*** 4 (Objective: 3) ***Rationale:*** Altruism is a concern for the welfare and well-being of others. In professional practice, altruism is reflected by the nurse's concern for the welfare of patients, other nurses, and other health care providers. Turning the patient every 4 hours is an example of standards of practice more than altruism because failure to do so would result in malpractice and negligence. ***Nursing Process:*** Assessment ***Client Need:*** Physiological Integrity

3. ***Answer:*** 3 (Objective: 2) ***Rationale:*** When clients hold unclear or conflicting values that are detrimental to their health, the nurse should use values clarification as an intervention. The client who has multiple admissions to the chemical dependency program is demonstrating unclear self-values, while the other answer choices display individuals who are clear regarding self-values. ***Nursing Process:*** Planning ***Client Needs:*** Safe, Effective Care Environment; Education and Health Promotion

4. ***Answer:*** 1 (Objective: 4) ***Rationale:*** Ethics committees include nurses and can be asked to provide guidance to a competent client, an incompetent client's family, or health care providers. These committees ensure that relevant facts of a case are brought out, provide a forum in which diverse views can be expressed, provide support for caregivers, and can reduce the institution's legal risks. These committees do not decide when a law has been violated; rather, these committees are formed to provide ethical guidance. ***Nursing Process:*** Assessment ***Client Need:*** Safe, Effective Care Environment

5. ***Answer:*** 1 (Objective: 7) ***Rationale:*** The relationships-based (caring) theories stress courage, generosity, commitment, and the need to nurture and maintain relationships. ***Nursing Process:*** Implementation ***Client Need:*** Safe, Effective Care Environment

6. ***Answer:*** 2 (Objective: 6) ***Rationale:*** Unintentional harm occurs when the risk could not have been anticipated. The other examples are examples of intentional harm. Harm can be intentionally causing harm, placing someone at risk of harm, and unintentionally causing harm. A client may be at risk of harm as a known consequence of a nursing intervention that is intended to be helpful. ***Nursing Process:*** Implementation ***Client Need:*** Safe, Effective Care Environment

7. ***Answer:*** 1, 3, 4 (Objective: 5) ***Rationale:*** Invasion of privacy is an intentional tort and nurses and nursing staff can be held liable if convicted. HIPAA, the American Health Insurance Portability and Accountability Act of 1996, requires that health information about clients be secured in such a way that only those with the right and need to acquire the information are able to do so. The clinical faculty would already know the client they had assigned to the student. The nurse should not randomly discard any items of a client's without express permission. If the cousin is not listed on a signed release from the client and hospital, then the cousin should not be allowed to review the client's record. ***Nursing Process:*** Implementation ***Client Need:*** Safe, Effective Care Environment

8. ***Answer:*** 3 (Objective: 6) ***Rationale:*** The nurse should inform the health care provider about the lack of education and/or experience and refuse to do the procedure or task. All of the other answers would make the nurse and health care provider negligent. However, if the nurse does not inform the health care provider, only the nurse would be liable. ***Nursing Process:*** Implementation ***Client Need:*** Safe, Effective Care Environment

9. ***Answer:*** 1 (Objective: 2) ***Rationale:*** All facts and information regarding a person's condition, treatment, care, progress, refusal or consent of treatment, and response to illness and treatment should be documented in the chart. ***Nursing Process:*** Assessment ***Client Need:*** Safe, Effective Care Environment

10. ***Answer:*** 2, 3 (Objective: 2) ***Rationale:*** The National Organ Transplant Act prohibits the selling of organs and/or marketing of body parts. The other examples are acceptable. ***Nursing Process:*** Assessment ***Client Need:*** Safe, Effective Care Environment

CHAPTER 6

Key Term Review

1. k	2. h	3. l	4. i	5. p	6. o
7. m	8. a	9. d	10. b	11. e	12. g
13. f	14. c	15. q	16. j	17. n	

Key Topic Review Answers

1. a. Primary prevention
   b. Secondary prevention
   c. Tertiary prevention

2. a

3. c

4. b

5. a. Increase quality and years of healthy life.
   b. Achieve health equity and eliminate health disparities.
   c. Create healthy environments for everyone.
   d. Promote health and quality life across the life span.

6. a

7. Public Health Service (PHS) of the U.S. Department of Health and Human Services

8. Occupational health clinics are an important setting for employee health care. They are responsible for worker safety, health education, annual employee health screening for tuberculosis, and maintenance of immunization information. Other screenings for health concerns can be conducted at the discretion of the nurse or companies.

9. Factors affecting health care delivery include the following: (Student will choose four.)
   a. Increasing number of older adults
   b. Advances in technology
   c. Economics
   d. Women's health
   e. Uneven distribution of services
   f. Access to health insurance

10. fastest; 76.5; 90

11. One of the major alterations in how health care is practiced in this country may be attributed to HIPAA. The new regulations were instituted to protect the privacy of individuals by safeguarding individually identifiable health care records, including electronic media. Violations of HIPAA regulations by health care providers or agencies can result in heavy fines for this breach of trust.

12. A critical pathway is an interdisciplinary plan or tool that specifies interdisciplinary assessments, interventions, treatments, and outcomes for health-related conditions across a time line. Case management may be used as a cost-containment strategy in managed care. Both of the systems often use critical pathways to track a client's progress.

13. a. These centers permit the client to live at home while obtaining necessary health care.

    b. These centers free up costly hospital beds for seriously ill clients.

Case Study Answers

1a *What type of health care coverage is the client almost guaranteed of carrying?* Everyone in the United States over age 65 is eligible for Medicare. The client may also carry other insurance plans, however Medicare is guaranteed if she is a citizen of the United States.

1b. *If the client's income is below the poverty level, what type of coverage could also be included in the health care coverage plan?* Medicaid is offered to individuals with low income and can be carried in addition to Medicare to reduce copayments.

2a. *What roles do the physical therapist and dietitian fulfill?* The physical therapy could be performed by the physical therapist. Physical therapists treat movement dysfunctions by means of heat, water, exercise, massage, and electric current. They also assess client mobility and strength, provide therapeutic measures, and teach new skills. A dietitian has special knowledge about the diets required to maintain health and treat disease.

2b. *Where could the client receive the services, and what type of coverage could possibly pay for these services?* Services may be found in acute care outpatient facilities, long-term care facilities that offer rehabilitation services, or in free-standing facilities in the community. Medicare Part B, in addition to Medicaid and/or private insurance, will cover the cost of these services.

3a. *What is the true regarding clients with chronic conditions or disabilities and access to care? There is a high prevalence of impaired access to care among those with chronic conditions or disabilities.*

3b. *What are the nursing implications when caring for clients with chronic conditions or disabilities? Nurses are* often the health care providers who have the most contact with clients who have disabilities and chronic health conditions. Nurses are in an ideal position to assist clients in obtaining the care they need at the most appropriate facilities and cost, often bridging the gap for the client who has decreased access to appropriate care.

Review Question Answers

1. ***Answer:*** 1, 4 (Objective: 5) ***Rationale:*** Managed care and team nursing are used as frameworks for care in today's health care system, which supports continuity of care and cost effectiveness. ***Nursing Process:*** Assessment ***Client Need:*** Safe, Effective Care Environment

2. ***Answer:*** 3 (Objective: 5) ***Rationale:*** The Medicare plan is divided into two parts, Part A and Part B. Part A is available to people with disabilities and people ages 65 years and older. It provides insurance toward hospitalization, home care, and hospice care. Part B is voluntary and provides partial coverage of outpatient and physician services to people eligible for Part A. Part D is the voluntary prescription drug plan begun in January 2006. Medicaid is a federal public assistance program paid out of general

taxes to people who require financial assistance, such as people with low incomes. ***Nursing Process:*** Assessment ***Client Need:*** Psychosocial Integrity

3. ***Answer:*** 2 (Objective: 5) ***Rationale:*** The Medicare plan is divided into two parts, Part A and Part B. Part A is available to people with disabilities and people ages 65 years and older. It provides insurance toward hospitalization, home care, and hospice care. Part B is voluntary and provides partial coverage of outpatient and physician services to people eligible for Part A. Part D is the voluntary prescription drug plan begun in January 2006. Medicaid is a federal public assistance program paid out of general taxes to people who require financial assistance, such as people with low incomes. ***Nursing Process:*** Assessment ***Client Need:*** Safe and Effective Care Environment

4. ***Answer:*** 1 (Objective: 5) ***Rationale:*** The Medicare plan is divided into two parts, Part A and Part B. Part A is available to people with disabilities and people ages 65 years and older. It provides insurance toward hospitalization, home care, and hospice care. Part B is voluntary and provides partial coverage of outpatient and physician services to people eligible for Part A. Part D is the voluntary prescription drug plan begun in January 2006. Medicaid is a federal public assistance program paid out of general taxes to people who require financial assistance, such as people with low incomes. ***Nursing Process:*** Assessment ***Client Need:*** Safe and Effective Care Environment

5. ***Answer:*** 4 (Objective: 5) ***Rationale:*** The Medicare plan is divided into two parts, Part A and Part B. Part A is available to people with disabilities and people ages 65 years and older. It provides insurance toward hospitalization, home care, and hospice care. Part B is voluntary and provides partial coverage of outpatient and physician services to people eligible for Part A. Part D is the voluntary prescription drug plan begun in January 2006. Medicaid is a federal public assistance program paid out of general taxes to people who require financial assistance, such as people with low incomes. ***Nursing Process:*** Assessment ***Client Need:*** Safe and Effective Care Environment

6. ***Answer:*** 1, 2, 5 (Objective: 5) ***Rationale:*** Supplemental Security Income (SSI) is for individuals with disabilities, individuals who are blind, or those who may not be eligible for Social Security. The benefits are not restricted to health care costs. Clients often use this money to purchase medicines or to cover the costs of extended health care. ***Nursing Process:*** Assessment ***Client Need:*** Health Promotion and Maintenance

7. ***Answer:*** 4 (Objective: 5) ***Rationale:*** Diagnosis-related groups (DRGs) are a prospective payment system limiting the amount paid to hospitals that are reimbursed by Medicare. The system has categories that establish pretreatment diagnosis billing categories. ***Nursing Process:*** Assessment ***Client Need:*** Safe and Effective Care Environment

8. ***Answer:*** 1 (Objective: 4) ***Rationale:*** Private health insurance pays either the entire bill or a percentage of the costs of health care services. ***Nursing Process:*** Assessment ***Client Need:*** Psychosocial

9. ***Answer:*** 3 (Objective: 2) ***Rationale:*** Prepaid group plans include HMOs, PPOs, PPAs, IPAs, and PHOs. Medicare and Medicaid are government programs, and Blue Cross and Blue Shield are private-pay insurance plans. Social Security and Supplemental Security Income are government programs. ***Nursing Process:*** Assessment ***Client Need:*** Safe and Effective Care Environment

10. ***Answer:*** 1 (Objective: 1) ***Rationale:*** Immunization is an illness prevention strategy that is primary prevention, not secondary. Caring for a dying client is palliative care and tertiary care. Assisting a stroke victim is rehabilitative care—also tertiary care. Secondary prevention is the diagnosis and treatment of disease, illness, or injury. ***Nursing Process:*** Assessment ***Client Need:*** Health Promotion and Maintenance

CHAPTER 7

Key Term Review

1. g 2. i 3. a 4. e 5. f 6. b

7. k 8. j 9. l 10. c 11. d 12. h

Key Topic Review Answers

1. a, c, d, f

2. (Student will choose four.)
   a. Community participation is provider directed.
   b. Professional's role is expert, provider, authority, and team leader.
   c. Collaboration occurs among members of the health care team.
   d. The individual or the family is the focus.
   e. Access is limited.
   f. Health care is available within given health care institutions.
   g. Empowerment is a provider-assisted process.

3. (Student will choose four.)
   a. Community participation is client directed.
   b. The professional's role is facilitator, consultant, and resource person.
   c. Collaboration goes beyond the health care sector.
   d. The community or some aggregate is the focus.
   e. Access is universal.
   f. Health care is available where people live and work.

g. Empowerment is a collaborative, enabling process.

4. community

5. population

6. (Student will choose four.)

   a. Type: integrated health care system

   Definition: System that makes all levels of care available in an integrated form—primary care, secondary care, and tertiary care. The goals are to facilitate care across settings, recovery, positive health outcomes, and the long-term benefits of modifying harmful lifestyles through health promotion and disease prevention.

   b. Type: community initiatives

   Definition: These initiatives, called healthy cities and healthier communities, involve members of the community to establish health priorities, set measurable goals, and determine actions to reach these goals. If a community agency is initiating this project, the associated hospital generally contributes human resources to assist in the endeavor.

   c. Type: community coalitions

   Definition: Alliances that bring together individuals and groups for the shared purpose of improving the community's health. Nurses are major participants and contributors in these coalitions and often assume leadership positions.

   d. Type: managed care

   Definition: A common model in health care restructuring. Health care providers (hospitals, physicians, nurse practitioners, insurance carriers, and so on) join to meet health needs across the care continuum. The managed care organization serves as a "go-between" or "gatekeeper" with the client, provider, and payer. Providers are organized into groups and the client must select one from the group to which they belong. Managed care aims in this way to enhance the quality and cost effectiveness of health care.

   e. Type: case management

   Definition: An integrative health care model that tracks client needs and services through a variety of care settings to ensure continuity. The case manager is familiar with clients' health needs and resources available through their insurance coverage so they can receive cost-effective care. Another important aspect of case management is assisting the client and family to understand and navigate their way through the health care system.

   f. Type: outreach programs

   Definition: Methods of linking underserved or high-risk populations with the formal health care system. These programs can minimize or reduce barriers to health care, increase access to services, and thus improve the health status of the community. Outreach programs involve partnerships between nurses and members of the community.

7. a.

8. a, c, d

9. a.

10. a

Case Study Answers

1. *What are some types of community nursing that could be considered?* Occupational health nursing, school nursing, parish nursing, telehealth, public health nursing, correctional nursing, camp nurse, home health, or community nursing centers are all possible options.

2. *What skills would be needed for community nursing that might not be used in the pediatric unit?* The nurse would need to utilize roles of the nurse such as collaborator, educator, advocate, manager, and clinician. With the experience from the pediatric ward, the nurse should consider the school nurse position role.

Review Question Answers

1. ***Answer:*** 2 (Objective: 6) ***Rationale:*** The key elements necessary for collaboration among health care providers include communication skills, mutual respect, and shared decision making. Negotiation and conflict management are important skills for the nurse to acquire and use; however, these are not the key elements necessary for collaboration. ***Nursing Process:*** Planning ***Client Needs:*** Safety, Safe and Efficient Care Environment

2. ***Answer:*** 1, 2, 3, 4 (Objective: 6) ***Rationale:*** The nurse collaborator shares personal expertise with other nurses and elicits the expertise of others to ensure quality client care, seeks opportunities to collaborate with and within professional organizations, offers expert opinions on legislative initiatives related to health care, and collaborates with other health care providers and consumers on health care legislation to best serve the needs of the public. ***Nursing Process:*** Implementation ***Client Need:*** Safe and Efficient Care Environment

3. ***Answer:*** 2 (Objective: 7) ***Rationale:*** Discharge planning is initiated for all clients on admission to any health care setting. Effective discharge planning involves ongoing assessment to obtain comprehensive information about the client's ongoing needs and nursing care plans to ensure those needs are met. ***Nursing Process:*** Planning ***Client Need:*** Safe and Efficient Care Environment

4. *Answer:* 1 (Objective: 4) ***Rationale:*** The older adult client without caregivers would need a referral to meet his or her health care needs. In this case, the patient should be referred to a long-term care facility, a community-based health care facility. ***Nursing Process:*** Assessment ***Client Need:*** Safe, Effective Care Environment

5. *Answer:* 2 (Objective: 2) ***Rationale:*** The major focus of integrated health care systems is health promotion and maintenance and disease prevention. ***Nursing Processes:*** Planning ***Client Need:*** Safe, Effective Care Environment

6. *Answer:* 2, 3, 4 (Objective: 4) ***Rationale:*** There are five main functions of community. These include production, distribution, and consumption of goods and services; socialization; social control and social interparticipation; and mutual support. ***Nursing Process:*** Assessment ***Client Need:*** Health Promotion and Maintenance

7. *Answer:* 1, 2, 3, 4 (Objective: 3) ***Rationale:*** The role of the parish nurse includes that of personal health counselor, health educator, referral source, and integrator of faith and health. ***Nursing Process:*** Implementation ***Client Need:*** Health Promotion and Maintenance

8. *Answer:* 1, 3 (Objective: 4) ***Rationale:*** The larger numbers of advanced practice nurses in recent years have resulted in the provision of primary care to many consumers who had previously been neglected—those living in rural areas, people with low incomes, undocumented immigrants, older adults, and women and infants. The incarcerated adult and homeless individual are the most likely consumers cared for by the advanced practice nurse. ***Nursing Process:*** Assessment ***Client Need:*** Safe, Effective Care Environment

CHAPTER 8

Key Term Review

1. e 2. d 3. a 4. b 5. c 6. f

7. g

Key Topic Review Answers

1. A number of factors have contributed to the growth in home health care. Some of these factors include rising health care costs, an aging population, and a growing emphasis on managing chronic illness and stress, preventing illness, and enhancing the quality of life.

2. Home care today involves a wide range of health care professionals providing services in the home setting to individuals recovering from an acute illness/injury, individuals with disabilities, or individuals with chronic conditions.

3. Hospice

4. :

   a. Intimacy and familiarity of the home setting.

   b. Sharing between the client, nurse, and family members.

   c. The ability of the nurse to function independently.

5. a. Resources may not be available in the event of a crisis.

   b. The burden of caregiving and family dynamic roles are often more apparent to the home health nurse.

   c. Home health nurses enter homes where the living conditions are less than desirable (e.g., homes with no running water or electricity).

6. (Student will choose four.)

   a. Performs physical assessments.

   b. Changes wound dressings.

   c. Inserts and maintains intravenous access for various therapies.

   d. Establishes and monitors indwelling urinary catheters.

   e. Monitors exercise or nutritional therapies.

7. a

8. _____c____ Institutions that rely on private pay sources or "third-party" reimbursement

   _____b____ United Way

   _____d____ Hospital home health agencies

   _____a____ State health department

9. a. Hand hygiene

   b. Use of gloves

   c. Handling of linens

   d. Disposal of wastes and soiled dressings

Case Study Answers

1. *What interventions will the home health nurse likely perform when caring for Mrs. Campos?* Providing client education is an essential skill of the home health nurse. The home health nurse will provide client education on diabetic care, including information on the proper use of new equipment or supplies. In addition, the nurse will provide education on medication management, especially if the client is nonadherent to the medication regimen. Additional teaching may include safety precautions and chronic disease management of the client's comorbidities. Most agencies have a packet that includes forms for consent to treatment; physical, psychosocial, and spiritual assessment; medications; pain assessment; family data; financial assessment including insurance verification; client's bill of rights; care plan; and daily visit notes.

2. *What unique cultural considerations will the nurse take when caring for Mrs. Campos?* Mrs. Campos does not speak English well and it is the home health nurse's obligation to ensure that the information provided to the client is well understood. The nurse should make sure that handouts, pamphlets, and forms are written in the client's first language.

3. *What age-related considerations will the nurse plan?* All clients should be assessed for safety; however, older adult clients have an increased risk for falls and the nurse must consider this age-related factor. In addition, adult clients tend to take multiple medications for various chronic diseases and conditions. This factor may lead to medication reactions or adverse effects, and client teaching on prevention of falls and multiple-medication reactions is essential.

Review Question Answers

1. ***Answer:*** 3 (Objective: 3) ***Rationale:*** A durable medical equipment (DME) company supplies health care equipment for the client at home. ***Nursing Process:*** Assessment ***Client Need:*** Safe, Effective Care Environment

2. ***Answer:*** 3 (Objective: 4) ***Rationale:*** The major roles of the home health nurse are those of advocate, caregiver, educator, and case manager. The nurse who is instructing the client on the diabetic diet is in the role of an educator. An example of the caregiver role is changing the Foley catheter, documenting the care is an example of case management, and a nurse in the advocate role would refer the client for a social work consultation. ***Nursing Process:*** Implementation ***Client Need:*** Health Promotion and Maintenance

3. ***Answer:*** 2 (Objective: 4) ***Rationale:*** The major roles of the home health nurse are those of advocate, caregiver, educator, and case manager. An example of the advocate role is referring the client for a social work consultation. The nurse who is instructing the client on the diabetic diet is in the role of an educator. An example of the caregiver role is changing the Foley catheter and documenting the care is an example of case management. ***Nursing Process:*** Implementation ***Client Need:*** Health Promotion and Maintenance

4. ***Answer:*** 1 (Objective: 4) ***Rationale:*** The major roles of the home health nurse are those of advocate, caregiver, educator, and case manager. An example of the caregiver role is changing the Foley catheter. The nurse who is instructing the client on the diabetic diet is in the role of an educator, documenting the care is an example of case management, and a nurse in the advocate role would refer the client for a social work consultation. ***Process:*** Implementation ***Client Need:*** Safe, Effective Care Environment

5. ***Answer:*** 4 (Objective: 5) ***Rationale:*** Education is ongoing and can be considered the core concept of home care practice; its goal is to help clients learn to manage as independently as possible. ***Nursing Process:*** Assessment ***Client Need:*** Health Promotion and Maintenance

6. ***Answer:*** 1, 2, 4 (Objective: 7) ***Rationale:*** Clinical manifestations of caregiver role strain include decreased energy, anxiety, and difficulty performing routine tasks. Difficulty concentrating is not a manifestation of caregiver role strain. ***Nursing Process:*** Assessment ***Client Need:*** Psychosocial Integrity

7. ***Answer:*** 3 (Objective: 1) ***Rationale:*** Daily wound care is a skilled nursing task. The other tasks are not dependent on nursing care. ***Nursing Process:*** Assessment ***Client Need:*** Safe, Effective Care Environment

8. ***Answer:*** 3 (Objective: 3) ***Rationale:*** Hospice nursing is the support and care of an individual who is terminally ill and his or her family. Hospice services are frequently delivered to terminally ill clients in their residence. ***Nursing Process:*** Assessment ***Client Need:*** Psychosocial Integrity

9. ***Answer:*** 3 (Objective: 8) ***Rationale:*** The referral process to home care services often occurs prior to discharge from the hospital. ***Nursing Process:*** Assessment ***Client Need:*** Health Promotion and Maintenance

CHAPTER 9

Key Term Review

1. d 2. f 3. j 4. i 5. k 6. g

7. e 8. h 9. b 10. a 11. c

Key Topic Review Answers

1. a. Design plans to enhance the nurse's ability to use EHRs to improve health care delivery.
   b. Have more nurses engaged in the design of national health care information systems infrastructure.
   c. Speed adoption of technology that can enhance health care safety and effectiveness.
2. privacy; confidentiality
3. a. management information systems (MIS)
   b. hospital information systems (HIS)
4. a. Admissions
   b. Medical records
   c. Clinical laboratory
   d. Pharmacy
   e. Order entry
   f. Finance
5. a. Record client assessments
   b. Medication administration
   c. Progress notes
   d. Care plan updating
   e. Client acuity
   f. Accrued changes
6. online; network
7. (Student will choose one,)
   a. Word processing programs: programs that provide the ability to save and manipulate words; probably the most used computer applications. They can be used in any facility in the health care setting.
   b. Databases: programs that manage detailed information. One example of a database is that of a pharmacy that lists the mediation it has in stock and the strength, quantity, locations, price, and manufacturer for each of the medications.
   c. Spreadsheets: programs that manipulate words and numbers. The data is arranged into columns and rows. It can be used to manage budgets for a health care facility.
   d. Communications software: software that connects computers and remote communication devices for the purpose of sending and receiving data. An important type of communications software is electronic mail (e-mail). E-mail has become a standard method of communication worldwide.
   e. Presentation graphics programs: software programs used to create charts, graphs, tables, pictures, videos, audio, and other nontext files. They have become increasingly popular. Users can create so-called "slide shows" for use in teaching or research presentations.
8. Health Insurance Portability and Accountability Act (HIPAA) of 1996
9. a. Access to literature
   b. Computer-assisted instruction
   c. Classroom technologies
   d. Strategies for learning at a distance
10. a. Communicate
    b. Manage knowledge
    c. Mitigate error
    d. Support decision making

Case Study Answers

1. *If the client's results are entered into computer-based patient records (CPRs), who would be able to legally access her medical information?* Any member of the client's health care team can access the CPRs with the necessary passwords.
2. *The chest x-ray is abnormal and the physician wishes to consult a respiratory specialist. If he sends the x-ray film electronically to the consulting physician, that is an example of what type of medicine?* Telemedicine.
3. *What are the advantages of this type of consultation?* By using telemedicine, the client does not physically have to be seen by the specialist unless it is deemed necessary. It could possibly save time and resources, and enable quicker health care.
4. *Does the client have to sign any consent forms with regard to her electronic medical records?* The client has a right to confidentiality and privacy. The hospital should have a consent form that should be signed prior to the entering of any data into the system.

Review Question Answers

1. ***Answer:*** 1 (Objective: 4) ***Rationale:*** Paper records have already been tested by the legal community and are already understood. Paper medical records are not standardized, the records take up a large amount of storage space, and protection of client health information is not ensured. ***Nursing Process:*** Assessment ***Client Need:*** Safe, Effective Care Environment

2. *Answer:* 2 (Objective: 1) ***Rationale:*** The World Wide Web (WWW) refers to the complex links among web pages or websites, accessed through "addresses" called universal resource locators (URLs). URLs begin with the designation http://, often followed by www. URLs end with a designation that denotes the type of site. ***Nursing Process:*** Assessment ***Client Need:*** Safe and Effective Care Environment Integrity

3. *Answer:* 3 (Objective: 1) ***Rationale:*** Universal resource locators (URLs) are also called "addresses." URLs begin with the designation http://, often followed by www. URLs end with a designation that denotes the type of site. ***Nursing Process:*** Assessment ***Client Need:*** Psychosocial Integrity

4. *Answer:* 3 (Objective: 3) ***Rationale:*** Telemedicine uses technology to transmit electronic data about clients to people at distant locations. Despite its advantages, however, there are legal and ethical concerns over the use of telemedicine. ***Nursing Process:*** Assessment ***Client Need:*** Safe, Effective Care Environment

5. *Answer:* 2 (Objective: 4) ***Rationale:*** URLs end with a designation that denotes the type of site. For example, .com is used for commercial sites, .org for organizations, .edu for educational institutions, and .gov for government facilities. ***Nursing Process:*** Assessment ***Client Need:*** Psychosocial Integrity

6. *Answer:* 2 (Objective: 3) ***Rationale:*** Distance learning may be categorized as asynchronous when the individuals involved are not interacting at the same "real" time or as synchronous when teachers and students are communicating simultaneously. In this case, the teachers and students are interacting at the same time so they are using synchronous distance learning. ***Nursing Process:*** Assessment ***Client Need:*** Safe, Effective Care Environment

7. *Answer:* 2 (Objective: 6) ***Rationale:*** A nurse administrator may use a computer system to manage personnel, budgets, human resources, staffing, and other measures. The other tasks may be performed by a nurse administrator; however these tasks do not fit within that role for the nurse. ***Nursing Process:*** Assessment ***Client Need:*** Safe, Effective Care Environment

8. *Answer:* 1 (Objective: 3) ***Rationale:*** Software programs enhance the education of nurses, make it easier to adjust to the use of software programs, and assist nurses in meeting educational needs for credentialing. ***Nursing Process:*** Assessment ***Client Need:*** Safe, Effective Care Environment

9. *Answer:* 4 (Objective: 4) ***Rationale:*** Confidentiality and privacy are major concerns in any health care–related field. Nurses should participate in the ongoing debate about and development of federal laws designed to ensure patient privacy and confidentiality. HIPAA plays a major role in establishing privacy for health care clients. ***Nursing Process:*** Implementation ***Client Need:*** Safe, Effective Care Environment

10. *Answer:* 4 (Objective: 7) ***Rationale:*** Maintaining the privacy and security of health care data is a significant issue. The Health Insurance Portability and Accountability Act (HIPAA) of 1996 established legal requirements for the protection, security, and appropriate sharing of client personal health information. The various hospitals, state governments, and a patient bill of rights currently do not set these legal requirements. ***Nursing Process:*** Implementation ***Client Need:*** Safe, Effective Care Environment

CHAPTER 10

Key Term Review

1. j 2. m 3. n 4. k 5. h 6. i

7. g 8. c 9. b 10. d 11. o 12. l

13. a 14. e 15. f

Key Topic Review Answers

1. problem solving; decision making

2. a. Trial and error: a number of approaches are tried until a solution is found. Trial and error can be dangerous because the client might suffer harm if an approach is inappropriate.

   b. Intuition: the understanding or learning of things without the conscious use of reasoning; also known as the "sixth sense." Its use is not recommended for novices or students.

   c. Nursing process: a systemic, rational method of planning and providing individualized nursing care. The phases of the nursing process are assessing, diagnosing, planning, implementing, and evaluating.

   d. Scientific method: most useful when the researcher is working in a controlled situation. Refer to Table 10–4 of the text for further information.

   e. Modified scientific method: a formalized, logical, systematic approach to solving problems that is often used by health care professionals. Refer to Table 10–4 in the text for further information.

3. Critical thinking

4. Inductive reasoning moves from specific examples (premises) to a generalized conclusion. Deductive reasoning is reasoning that moves from general premises to a specific conclusion.

5. Socratic questioning

6. (Student will choose five.)

   a. Independence

   b. Fair-mindedness

   c. Insight

   d. Intellectual humility

   e. Intellectual courage to challenge the status quo and rituals

   f. Integrity

   g. Perseverance

   h. Confidence

   i. Curiosity

7. Reflection

8. a. Identify the purpose.

   b. Set the criteria.

   c. Weigh the criteria.

   d. Seek alternatives.

   e. Examine alternatives.

   f. Project.

   g. Implement.

   h. Evaluate the outcome.

9. Decision making is a critical thinking process for choosing the best actions to meet a desired goal. For example, the individual who wishes to become a nurse in the United States has several possible courses of action: a diploma program, an associate degree program, or a baccalaureate program. Prospective students must choose between the options. Therefore, they must evaluate the different types of programs, as well as personal circumstances, to make a decision appropriate to their situations.

10. a

11. a. Hierarchical maps: the arrangement of a concept and attributes in a hierarchical pattern; typically constructed in a descending order of importance. Relationships are identified between a concept and its attributes.

   b. Spider maps. depictions of the interrelatedness of the concept and its attributes.

   c. Flowchart maps: linear diagrams that demonstrate sequence or cause-and-effect relationships

   d. Systems maps: inputs and outputs illustrate relationships between a concept and its attributes.

Case Study Answers

1. a. *Questions about the decision or problem:* This problem about lack of financial planning is correctly identified, important, and clear.

   b. *Questions about assumptions:* Your friend seems to be assuming that she is always overdrawn at the bank. Is that so?

   c. *Questions about point of view:* Can this be seen in any other way? There are two possible ways that this could be viewed. One, your friend is spending more money than she puts into her checking account. Two, your friend may not be listing all the checks and/or service fees correctly in her checkbook.

   d. *Questions about evidence and reasons*: The evidence is the bank statement and your friend's stating the fact that she has trouble managing her checking account. What do the past 12 months' banking statements reflect in this matter?

   e. *Questions about implications and consequences*: The implications are that her credit could be ruined and she will pay more money in overdraft fees.

Review Question Answers

1. ***Answer:*** 3 (Objective: 1) ***Rationale:*** Assumptions are not used in the nursing process and are not effective in decision making. ***Nursing Process:*** Assessment ***Client Need:*** Safe, Effective Care Environment

2. ***Answer:*** 4 (Objective 3) ***Rationale:*** Trial-and-error methods lack exactness or precision because there is no guarantee any of the attempts tried will result in an optimal outcome and some attempts may cause more problems than solutions. While not an optimal method in nursing, trial-and-error can sometimes be effective, may require organization, and often requires thought to determine approaches to be tried. ***Nursing Process:*** Assessment ***Client Need:*** Safe, Effective Care Environment

3. ***Answer:*** 1 (Objective: 3) ***Rationale: The research process is most effective when used by experienced nurses.*** The research process is a formalized, logical, systematic approach to problem solving. ***Nursing Process:*** Assessment ***Client Need:*** Safe, Effective Care Environment

4. ***Answer:*** 2, 3, 4 (Objective: 2) ***Rationale:*** The nursing process involves the interaction between client and nurse as they work together. It is used to identify potential or actual health care needs, set

goals, devise a plan to meet the client's needs, and evaluate that plan's effectiveness. The nursing process is designed to work well in all environments. ***Nursing Process:*** Assessment ***Client Need:*** Safe, Effective Care Environment

5. ***Answer:*** 4 (Objective: 4) ***Rationale:*** Critical thinking enables the nurse to respond quickly even when unexpected situations arise. It enables the nurse to adapt interventions to meet specific client needs, not physician needs. While critical thinking allows the nurse to respond quickly in emergent situations, this does not necessarily allow the nurse to maintain a calm demeanor during these situations or establish teamwork with others during emergency situations. ***Nursing Process:*** Assessment ***Client Need:*** Safe, Effective Care Environment

6. ***Answer:*** 3, 4 (Objective: 4) ***Rationale:*** Implementation of client interventions requires critical thinking and creativity. The nurse is not using the scientific or modified scientific method. ***Nursing Process:*** Planning ***Client Need:*** Health Promotion and Maintenance

7. ***Answer:*** 1 (Objective: 1) ***Rationale:*** Intuition is the understanding or learning of things without the conscious use of reasoning, whereas the research process is a formalized, logical, systematic approach to problem solving. Intuition is also known as the "sixth sense." ***Nursing Process:*** Assessment ***Client Need:*** Safe, Effective Care Environment

8. ***Answer:*** 3 (Objective: 3) ***Rationale:*** Inductive reasoning generalizations are formed from a set of facts or observations. ***Nursing Process:*** Assessment ***Client Need:*** Safe, Effective Care Environment

9. ***Answer:*** 1 (Objective: 4) ***Rationale:*** Discussing any problems in a collegial way creates an environment that supports critical thinking. A nurse cannot develop or maintain critical thinking attitudes in a vacuum. Nurses should encourage colleagues to examine evidence carefully before they come to conclusions and to avoid group thinking. ***Nursing Process:*** Planning ***Client Need:*** Safe, Effective Care Environment

10. ***Answer:*** 4 (Objective: 3) ***Rationale:*** The nursing process is defined as a systematic, rational method of planning and providing individualized nursing care. ***Nursing Process:*** Assessment ***Client Need:*** Safe, Effective Care Environment

11. ***Answer:*** 1 (Objective: 2) ***Rationale:*** Nursing cognitive skills are learned through reading and applying health-related literature. The other answer choices reflect how cognitive skills are enhanced, not learned. ***Nursing Process:*** Assessment ***Client Need:*** Safe, Effective Care Environment

CHAPTER 11

Key Term Review

1.	e	2.	l	3.	k	4.	j	5.	f	6.	m
7.	p	8.	o	9.	b	10.	s	11.	c	12.	a
13.	i	14.	r	15.	t	16.	d	17.	q	18.	n
19.	h	20.	g								

Key Topic Review Answers

1. a. To identify a client's health status and actual or potential health care problems or needs.

   b. To establish plans to meet the identified needs.

   c. To deliver specific nursing interventions to meet these identified needs.

2. a

3. a

4. a. Initial assessment
   b. Problem-focused assessment
   c. Emergency assessment
   d. Time-lapsed assessment

5. 24; assessments should be completed within 24 hours according to The Joint Commission standards. It is important to note, however, that many facilities, especially acute care facilities, require assessments to be performed within the first hour after admission.

6. a. Collecting data
   b. Organizing data
   c. Validating data
   d. Documenting data

7. a. ______S______ "I feel tired all the time."

   b. ______O______ Skin warm and dry to touch

   c. ______S______ "I am itching all over."

d. O Smell of ammonia in urine

e. O Purplish discoloration on left forearm

f. O Temperature of 102 degrees orally

8. a. S "My son has vomited for three days."

b. P "I have been coughing for two weeks."

c. S "My wife is forty-five years old. "

d. P "I have a rash."

9. c

10. interview

Case Study Answers

1. *What is the objective data?* Objective data includes vital signs, appearance of the dressing, infusing IV fluids and appearance of the IV site.

2. *What is the subjective data?* Subjective data includes the comfort level of the client both when there were no complaints of pain and when he informed the nurse his pain level was increasing.

3. *Who is considered the primary source?* The client.

4. *Who is considered the secondary source?* The recovery room nurse.

Review Question Answers

1. ***Answer:*** 1, 2 (Objective: 6) ***Rationale:*** Vision and smell would be used. The color of the sputum and any smell associated with it may be important cues to the disease process. Touch is usually not useful in regards to sputum because consistency can be seen. ***Nursing Process:*** Assessment ***Client Need:*** Safe, Effective Care Environment

2. ***Answer:*** 1 (Objective: 4) ***Rationale:*** The national licensure exam does not recognize outcomes identification and diagnosis as phases of the nursing process. Analysis is recognized by the national licensure exam but is not recognized by the *Scope and Standards of Nursing Practice* and both recognize assessment and evaluation as phases of the nursing process. ***Nursing Process:*** Assessment ***Client Need:*** Safe, Effective Care Environment

3. ***Answer:*** 3, 4 (Objective: 10) ***Rationale: The seating arrangement and physical distance between the client and interviewer have cultural implications.*** The distance between the interviewer and interviewee should be neither too small nor too great because people feel uncomfortable when talking to someone who is too close or too far away. The Japanese culture has an accepted difference of 36 inches, while clients from Arab countries maintain a distance of 8 to 12 inches. ***Nursing Process:*** Assessment ***Client Need:*** Psychosocial Integrity

4. ***Answer:*** 4 (Objective: 8) ***Rationale:*** Open-ended questions are those questions that allow the interviewee to do the talking. These questions are easy to answer, are nonthreatening, and require more than a simple "yes" or "no" answer. (Refer to Table 11-6 in the text.) ***Nursing Process:*** Planning ***Client Need:*** Health Promotion and Maintenance

5. ***Answer:*** 3 (Objective: 3) ***Rationale:*** The cephalocaudal or head-to-toe approach begins the examination at the head; progresses to the neck, thorax, abdomen, and extremities; and ends at the toes. ***Nursing Process:*** Assessment ***Client Need:*** Health Promotion and Maintenance

6. ***Answer:*** 2 (Objective: 10) ***Rationale:*** Gordon's functional health pattern framework collects data about functional and dysfunctional behaviors. Orem delineates eight universal self-care requisites of humans. Roy uses the adaptation model and classifies observable behaviors into four categories: physiological, self-concept, role functions, and interdependence. ***Nursing Process:*** Assessment ***Client Need:*** Health Promotion and Maintenance

7. ***Answer:*** 3 (Objective: 4) ***Rationale:*** Validating is the act of "double-checking" or verifying data to confirm that it is accurate and factual. Validating data helps the nurse ensure that information is complete, that objective and subjective data agree, and that cues and inferences are differentiated. ***Nursing Process:*** Assessment ***Client Need:*** Safe, Effective Care Environment

8. ***Answer:*** 1 (Objective: 1) ***Rationale:*** The first step in the nursing process is assessment, the process of collecting data. The other processes rely on accurate and complete data. ***Nursing Process:*** Assessment ***Client Need:*** Safe, Effective Care Environment

9. ***Answer:*** 1 (Objective: 3) ***Rationale:*** The ongoing evaluation is done while or immediately after implementing a nursing intervention. Intermittent evaluation is performed at specified intervals, whereas terminal evaluation indicates the client's condition at the time of discharge. ***Nursing Process:*** Evaluation ***Client Need:*** Safe, Effective Care Environment

10. ***Answer:*** 2 (Objective: 5) ***Rationale:*** Data that is measurable is objective data. The client's statements and complaints of symptoms are documented as subjective data. ***Nursing Process:*** Assessment ***Client Need:*** Safe, Effective Care Environment

CHAPTER 12

Key Term Review

1. d 2. p 3. i 4. o 5. h 6. a

7. j 8. b 9. n 10. c 11. g 12. k

13. l 14. m 15. e 16. f

Key Topic Review Answers

1. Assessment

2. Diagnosis

3. taxonomy

4. a. A problem statement or diagnostic label describes the client's health problem or response for which nursing therapy is given.

   b. An etiology identifies one or more probable causes of the health problems, gives direction to the required nursing therapy, and enables the nurse to individualize the client's care.

   c. A defining characteristic is the cluster of signs and symptoms that indicate the presence of a particular diagnostic label.

5. b. only registered nurses make nursing diagnosis.

6. a

7. a. Actual

   b. Risk

   c. Wellness

   d. Possible

   e. Syndrome

8. Specific

9. a. Deficient

   b. Impaired

   c. Decreased

   d. Ineffective

   e. Compromised

10. An etiology identifies one or more probable causes of a health problem. It gives direction to the required nursing therapy and enables the nurse to individualize the client's care.

11. a

12. a

Case Study Answers

1. *What is an actual nursing diagnosis for this client? Ineffective Therapeutic Regimen Management*

2. *What is a potential nursing diagnosis for this client? Risk for Peripheral Neurovascular Dysfunction*

3. *Identify one subjective and one objective assessment to substantiate the nursing diagnosis.*

   Subjective data: "I use the bathroom about eight times per day."

   Objective data: Fingerstick blood sugar = 213 mg/dL

4. *What is the outcome goal for the client?* Effective Therapeutic Regimen Management for Type 2 diabetes

5. *What are three independent functions the nurse might perform when caring for this client?* Independent functions are functions that the nurse can perform without the order of a physician. Two examples of these functions for this patient would include medication regimen education and chronic disease management education.

Review Question Answers

1. ***Answer:*** 3 (Objectives: 2 and 4) ***Rationale:*** The identification of the actual or potential health problems of a client is the result of data collection and analysis. ***Nursing Process:*** Assessment ***Client Need:*** Safe, Effective Care Environment

2. ***Answer:*** 3 (Objective: 1) ***Rationale:*** The potential for sleep-pattern disturbances is a nursing diagnosis; the other three answer choices are considered medical diagnoses. ***Nursing Process:*** Planning ***Client Need:*** Safe, Effective Care Environment

3. ***Answer:*** 3 (Objectives: 4 and 6) ***Rationale:*** The client's problem statement consists of the diagnostic label plus etiology, which is the causal relationship between a problem and its related or risk factors. ***Nursing Process:*** Diagnosis ***Client Need:*** Safe, Effective Care Environment

4. ***Answer:*** 1, 3, 5 (Objectives: 6 and 2) ***Rationale:*** All of the listed activities are part of the diagnosing component of the nursing process except obtaining a nursing health history and reviewing the client records and nursing literature. These components are part of the patient assessment. ***Nursing Process:*** Assessment ***Client Need:*** Safe, Effective Care Environment

5. ***Answer:*** 1 (Objective: 8) ***Rationale:*** Clarifying the gaps and inconsistencies in the data is one of the three continuous and sequential activities involved in the diagnostic process. ***Nursing Process:*** Assessment ***Client Need:*** Safe, Effective Care Environment

6. ***Answer:*** 1 (Objective: 3) ***Rationale:*** Some diagnostic statements, such as wellness diagnoses and syndrome nursing diagnoses, consist of a NANDA label only. ***Nursing Process:*** Assessment ***Client Need:*** Safe, Effective Care Environment

7. ***Answer:*** 2 (Objective: 7) ***Rationale:*** This statement is considered a two-part statement and lists the diagnosis with the related factors and characteristics. ***Nursing Process:*** Diagnosis ***Client Need:*** Safe, Effective Care Environment

8. ***Answer:*** 3 (Objective: 5) ***Rationale:*** A collaborative problem is a type of potential problem that nurses manage using both independent and physician-prescribed interventions. ***Nursing Process:*** Diagnosis ***Client Need:*** Safe, Effective Care Environment

9. ***Answer:*** 1 (Objective: 5) ***Rationale:*** The basic three-part nursing diagnosis statement is called the PES format and includes the problem, etiology, and signs and symptoms. The signs and symptoms have been identified, and the PES system is ideal for beginning nursing students. ***Nursing Process:*** Diagnosis ***Client Need:*** Safe, Effective Care Environment

10. ***Answer:*** 3 (Objective: 6) ***Rationale:*** Qualifiers are words that have been added to some NANDA labels to give additional meaning to the diagnostic statement. ***Nursing Process:*** Diagnosis ***Client Need:*** Safe, Effective Care Environment

11. ***Answer:*** 1, 3, 4 (Objective: 9) ***Rationale:*** A taxonomy is a classification system or set of categories arranged based on a single principle or set of principles. The members of NANDA include staff nurses, clinical specialists, faculty, directors of nursing, deans, theorists, and researchers. The group has currently approved more than 170 nursing diagnoses labels for clinical use and testing. Physicians do not use nursing diagnoses in their practice. ***Nursing Process:*** Planning ***Client Need:*** Safe, Effective Care Environment

12. ***Answer:*** 1, 2, 3, 4, 5 (Objective: 2) ***Rationale:*** A nursing diagnoses has three components and consists of all answer choices except the medical conditions. A medical diagnosis is made by a physician and refers to a condition that only a physician can treat. ***Nursing Process:*** Planning ***Client Need:*** Safe, Effective Care Environment

CHAPTER 13

Key Term Review

1. o	2. e	3. v	4. f	5. p	6. g
7. r	8. s	9. a	10. i	11. m	12. l
13. n	14. c	15. w	16. h	17. b	18. d
19. j	20. q	21. u	22. t	23. k	

Key Topic Review Answers

1. Nursing interventions

2. Planning begins with the first client contact and continues until the nurse–client relationship ends, usually when the client is discharged from the health care agency.

3. The nurse who performs the admission assessment usually develops the initial comprehensive plan of care. Planning should be initiated as soon as possible after the initial assessment, especially because of the trend toward shorter hospital stays. The plan is then adapted according to changes in the client's condition.

4. All nurses who work with the client do ongoing planning. As nurses obtain new information and evaluate the client's responses to care, they can individualize the initial care plan further. Ongoing planning also occurs at the beginning of a shift as the nurse plans the care to be given that day. Using ongoing assessment data, the nurse carries out daily planning for the following purposes:
   a. To determine whether the client's health status has changed.
   b. To set priorities for the client's care during the shift.
   c. To decide which problems to focus on during the shift.
   d. To coordinate the nurse's activities so that more than one problem can be addressed at each client contact.

5. a. Prioritize problems/diagnosis.
   b. Formulate goals/desired outcomes.
   c. Select nursing interventions.
   d. Write nursing interventions.

6. __c__ Tailored to meet the unique needs of a specific client — needs that are not addressed by the standardized plan

   __a__ A strategy of action that exists in the nurse's mind

   __d__ A written or computerized guide that organizes information about the client's care

___b_______ A formal plan that specifies the nursing care for groups of clients with common needs

7. a. Complete list of client problems
   b. Kardex cards for client profile, basic needs, and collaborative plans
   c. Standardized plans to address client problems
   d. Critical pathways
   e. Addendum to discharge plan
   f. Addendum to teaching plan
   g. Individualized nursing care plans for nursing diagnoses

8. Standards of care are developed and accepted by the nursing staff in order to ensure that minimally acceptable standards are met and promote efficient use of nurses' time by removing the need to author common activities that are done over and over for many of the clients in a nursing unit. The advantages of standards of care are that they promote efficient use of nurse's time, they describe achievable rather than ideal nursing care, they do not contain medical interventions, and they define the interventions for which nurses are held accountable. The disadvantages are that standards of care are not individualized and communicate the minimal acceptable standards.

9. A concept map is a visual tool in which ideas or data are enclosed in circles or boxes and relationships between these are indicated by connecting lines or arrows. Concept maps are creative endeavors. They can take many different forms and encompass various categories of data, according to the creator's interpretation of the client or health condition. A rationale is the scientific principle given as the reason for selecting a particular nursing intervention. Students may also be required to cite supporting literature for their stated rationale. Students are often asked to complete pathophysiology flow sheets, concept maps, or care plans as a method of learning and demonstrating the links among disease processes, laboratory data, medications, signs and symptoms, risk factors, and other relevant data (see Figure 13–5 in the text).

10. On a care plan, the goals/desired outcomes describe, in terms of observable client responses, what the nurse hopes to achieve by implementing the nursing interventions. The terms *goal* and *desired outcome* are used interchangeably in the text, except when discussing and using standardized language. Some references also use the terms *expected outcome, predicted outcome, outcome criterion,* and *objective.* They are sometimes combined into one statement linked by the words "as evidenced by." The Nursing Outcomes Classification (NOC) is designed for describing client outcomes that respond to nursing interventions.

Case Study Answers

a. *What are the subjective and objective data?*

(O) Stage 4 pressure ulcers on the coccyx, left and right malleolus, and both heels

(O) Unable to turn himself in the bed

(S) "This happened so suddenly; he did not have these sores until he had the stroke and quit eating."

(O) Older adult

(O) Appears emaciated

(O) Immobile client

b. *What nursing diagnosis will fit this situation? Impaired Skin Integrity* related to pressure and inadequate circulation as manifested by evidence of pressure ulcer.

2c. *What are the realistic short-term and long-term goals for this client?* Some examples of short-term goals for this client are no further deterioration of the ulcer stage, reduction or elimination of the factors leading to the pressure ulcers, no development of an infection in the pressure ulcer. Some examples of long-term goals for this client are to have healing of pressure ulcers and/or no recurrence of pressure ulcers.

d. *What are four nursing orders or interventions that can be used for this client?*

1. Assess causative factors such as limited activity, limited mobility, any presence or absence of sensory deficits, altered nutrition and hydration status, oxygenation, any circulatory concerns, and incontinence issues, etc.
2. Use pressure-related devices such as foam overlays for the mattress, float the heels, etc.
3. Turn every 2 hours and have client sit up for short intervals.
4. Assess stages of wounds; measure length, width, depth and locations; assess for signs of infection, amount of granulation tissue, or other abnormal findings.

Review Question Answers

1. ***Answer:*** 2 (Objective: 8) ***Rationale:*** Short-term goals are useful for clients who require health care for a short time and for those who are frustrated by long-term goals that seem difficult to attain and who need the satisfaction of achieving a short-term goal. ***Nursing Process:*** Planning ***Client Need:*** Safe, Effective Care Environment

2. ***Answer:*** 1 (Objectives: 6 and 7) ***Rationale:*** Long-term goals are often used for clients who live at home and have chronic health problems and for clients in nursing homes, extended care facilities, and rehabilitation centers. ***Nursing Process:*** Planning ***Client Need:*** Safe, Effective Care Environment

3. ***Answer:*** 1 (Objectives: 1 and 2) ***Rationale:*** This intervention is known as an independent intervention. These are activities that nurses are licensed to initiate on the basis of their knowledge and skills. ***Nursing Process:*** Planning ***Client Need:*** Safe, Effective Care Environment

4. *Answer:* 3 (Objectives: 4, 5, and 6) ***Rationale:*** Prevention interventions prescribe the care needed to avoid complications or reduce risk factors. ***Nursing Process:*** Planning ***Client Need:*** Safe, Effective Care Environment

5. *Answer:* 2 (Objective: 5) ***Rationale:*** A licensed practical/vocational nurse has the necessary skills and training to insert Foley catheters. Unlicensed personnel, regardless of his or her experience, cannot insert a Foley catheter. It is inappropriate to delegate this intervention to the physician. The client's family member cannot perform this intervention. ***Nursing Process:*** Planning ***Client Need:*** Psychological Integrity

6. *Answer:* 3 (Objective: 7) ***Rationale:*** Selecting nursing interventions based on the assessment findings and nursing diagnosis is the next step in the nursing process. ***Nursing Process:*** Planning ***Client Need:*** Safe, Effective Care Environment

7. *Answer:* 1 (Objectives: 1 and 2) ***Rationale:*** This is a short-term nursing goal. It is useful for clients who require health care for a short period of time and clients who are frustrated by long-term goals that seem difficult for them to attain and who need the satisfaction of completing a short-term goal. The other answer choices are either not short term or are not specific goals. ***Nursing Process:*** Planning ***Client Need:*** Safe, Effective Care Environment

8. *Answer:* 4 (Objective: 2) ***Rationale: Planning begins with the first meeting, is revised throughout the hospital stay as the client's condition changes, and continues until the client is discharged. Nursing Process:*** Assessment ***Client Need:*** Safe, Effective Care Environment

9. *Answer:* 2 (Objective: 10) ***Rationale:*** The client care plan is a permanent part of the record. The protocols and procedures are not part of the permanent record. The nurse's notes are sometimes called the nurse's "brain." The nurse may write down short notes about any events that happen during the shift to help the nurse to correctly document events in the client's chart. ***Nursing Process:*** Implementation ***Client Need:*** Safe, Effective Care Environment

10. *Answer:* 3 (Objective: 2) ***Rationale:*** Implementation of the nursing care plan is part of the nursing process to achieve the goals and/or outcomes. Reassessment continues at this time to see if the interventions are working effectively. The plan of care may be altered at any time during the client's stay at the facility as needed. ***Nursing Process:*** Implementation ***Client Need:*** Safe, Effective Care Environment

11. *Answer:* 1, 2, 3, 4 (Objective: 11) ***Rationale:*** All of the selections are correct. The benefits of specific nursing interventions enable nursing professionals to provide anticipated changes in the clients. ***Nursing Process:*** Assessment ***Client Need:*** Safe, Effective Care Environment

12. *Answer:* 2 (Objective: 9) ***Rationale:*** A taxonomy of nursing outcome statements, the Nursing Outcomes Classification (NOC), has been developed to describe measurable states, behaviors, or perceptions that respond to nursing interventions. Each has a definition, a measuring scale, and indicators. ***Nursing Process:*** Assessment ***Client Need:*** Safe, Effective Care Environment

CHAPTER 14

Key Term Review

1. n 2. g 3. j 4. l 5. m 6. o

7. h 8. d 9. k 10. p 11. i 12. b

13. a 14. e 15. c 16. f

Key Topic Review Answers

1. action; client centered; outcome

2. implementing

3. Cognitive, interpersonal, technical

4. It terminates with the documentation of the nursing activities and client responses.

5. assessing, diagnosing, and planning

6. b___ "May I help you to the restroom?"

   a_____ Creativity

   a_____ Problem solving

   b___ Nurse working effectively with members of the health care team

   c__ Taking a blood pressure

   b__ Caring for a dying patient

   b____ Need self-awareness and sensitivity to others to perform this skill

   c__ Bandaging a client's leg

7. a. Reassessing the client
   b. Determining the nurse's need for assistance
   c. Implementing the nursing interventions
   d. Supervising the delegated care
   e. Documenting nursing activities

8. a

Case Study Answers

1. *List different potential nursing diagnoses for Mr. Sanchez, give an example of subjective and objective data, and list one nursing intervention for each diagnosis.*

    a. Grieving r/t terminal illness, impending death, and overwhelming grief

    b. Subjective data: "I do not want to see my family."

    c. Objective data: Client refuses to talk with family members or staff.

    d. Intervention: Provide opportunities for the client and family members to vent feelings; discuss the loss openly. Employ empathetic sharing and acknowledge the grief by sitting with client silently or talking with client during care.

2. *List other comfort measures that the nurse may implement for Mr. Sanchez.* The nurse can provide accurate information whenever the client asks questions, provide privacy during periods of acute pain, assess response to medication administration 30 minutes after the dose was given, reposition the client, splint the area of pain, employ distraction techniques, and utilize massage and music therapy.

Review Question Answers

1. ***Answer:*** 3 (Objective: 10) ***Rationale:*** An audit means the examination or review of records. A concurrent audit is the evaluation of a client's health care while the client is still receiving care from the agency. A retrospective audit is the evaluation of a client's record after discharge from an agency. Another type of evaluation is the peer review that involves other nurses reviewing the care based on preestablished standards or criteria, which are normally conducted after the client's discharge. ***Nursing Process:*** Assessment ***Client Need:*** Safe, Effective Care Environment

2. ***Answer:*** 1 (Objective: 1) ***Rationale:*** Nursing interventions are based on scientific knowledge, nursing research, and evidenced-based practice. The nurse implements the interventions and evaluates the desired outcomes. Based on this evaluation, the plan of care is modified, continued, or modified. Refer to Chapter 13 of the text. ***Nursing Process:*** Implementation ***Client Need:*** Physiological Integrity

3. ***Answer:*** 1 (Objective: 5) ***Rationale:*** Evaluating is a planned, ongoing, purposeful activity in which clients and health care professionals determine the client's progress toward achievement of goals/outcomes and the effectiveness of the nursing care plan. The steps of the nursing process in order are assessment, diagnosis, planning, implementation, and evaluation. ***Nursing Process:*** Evaluating ***Client Need:*** Safe, Effective Care Environment

4. ***Answer:*** 4 (Objective: 8) ***Rationale:*** Conclusions are drawn when the nurse uses judgments about the goal achievement status. The nurses determine whether the care plan needs to be modified. ***Nursing Process:*** Evaluation ***Client Need:*** Safe, Effective Care Environment

5. ***Answer:*** 1, 4 (Objective: 2) ***Rationale:*** One of the steps during the implementation of the plan of care is to supervise delegated care of unlicensed personnel such as nursing assistants or patient care technicians. Evaluating the client's reaction to planned interventions is an important aspect of the nursing process. The nurse does not supervise and direct care of the physician. The nurse will not perform all patient care including all baths, vital signs, and activities of daily living. These activities may be performed by unlicensed personnel and the nurse should delegate these activities. ***Nursing Process:*** Implementation ***Client Need:*** Safe, Effective Care Environment

6. ***Answer:*** 2 (Objective: 3) ***Rationale:*** Interpersonal skills are the combination of verbal and nonverbal activities individuals use when interacting with one another. ***Nursing Process:*** Implementation ***Client Need:*** Safe, Effective Care Environment

7. ***Answer:*** 4 (Objective: 2) ***Rationale:*** The nurse will need assistance during transfer of a bilateral amputee in order to provide safe care. The nurse needs to be holistic, implement safe care, adapt activities to the individual clients, and clearly understand the needed nursing interventions. ***Nursing Process:*** Implementation ***Client Need:*** Safe, Effective Care Environment

8. ***Answer:*** 4 (Objective: 6) ***Rationale: The nursing process is a dynamic, ever-changing process.*** Evaluating and assessing are two phases of the nursing process that often overlap because the nurse is continually evaluating the plan of care and assessing the client's responses to it. ***Nursing Process:*** Assessment ***Client Need:*** Safe, Effective Care Environment

9. ***Answer:*** 2 (Objective: 8) ***Rationale:*** The evaluation statement consists of two parts, conclusion and supporting data. The conclusion is a statement that the goal or desired outcome was met, partially met, or not met. Supporting data are the list of client responses that support the conclusion. Reexamining the client care plan is a process of making decisions about problem status and critiquing each phase of the nursing process. ***Nursing Process:*** Implementation ***Client Need:*** Safe, Effective Care Environment

10. ***Answer:*** 1, 2, 3 (Objective: 9) ***Rationale:*** A quality assurance program is an evaluation that includes the consideration of the structures, processes, and outcomes of nursing care. Quality improvement is a philosophy and process internal to the institution, and does not rely on inspections by an external agency. ***Nursing Process:*** Implementation ***Client Need:*** Safe, Effective Care Environment

CHAPTER 15

Key Term Review

1. r 2. d 3. s 4. t 5. f 6. o

7. q 8. l 9. n 10. g 11. c 12. e

13. u 14. j 15. i 16. a 17. b 18. k

19. v 20. m 21. p 22. h

Key Topic Review Answers

1. d

2. duty

3. (Student will choose four.)
   a. communication
   b. planning client care
   c. auditing health agencies
   d. research
   e. education
   f. reimbursement
   g. legal documentation
   h. health care analysis

4. a. timely
   b. complete
   c. accurate
   d. confidential
   e. client specific

5. The fax cover sheet should contain instructions that the faxed material is to be given only to the named recipient. Consent is needed from the client to fax information. All personally identifiable information (name, Social Security number, etc.) should be removed. Be sure to check that the fax number is correct and check the number three times.

6. b. Students or graduates are bound by a strict ethical code and legal responsibility to hold all information in confidence.

7. The traditional client record is called a source-oriented record. Each department makes notations in separate areas of the chart. Narrative charting is a traditional part of source-oriented records.

8. Advantages: It is convenient because of the forms used and it is easy to locate each department's notes regarding the client.

   Disadvantages: The information about a particular problem is scattered throughout the chart and often is not in chronological order. It can lead to decreased communication with the health care team.

9. The data in the chart are arranged according to the client's problems. The health care members contribute to the problem list, plan of care, and progress notes.

   The four basic components are the database, problem list, plan of care, and progress notes.

10. Advantages: It encourages collaboration, and the problem lists in the front of the chart alert health care members to the client's needs and make it easier to track the status of the problem.

    Disadvantages: The caregivers differ in their ability to use the required charting format, it takes vigilance to maintain the problem lists, and it is somewhat inefficient because assessments and interventions that apply to more than one problem have to be repeated.

11. SOAP is an acronym for subjective data (S), objective data (O), assessment (A), and plan (P) of care designed to resolve the stated problem.

    The SOAP format has been changed over the years to include (I) interventions, (E) evaluations of client's responses to the interventions, and (R) revision of the plan of care.

12. Charting by exception (CBE) is a documentation system in which only abnormal or significant findings or exceptions to norms are recorded. The three key elements of CBE are:
    1. Use of flow sheets
    2. Standards of nursing care
    3. Bedside access to chart forms.

    Many nurses believe the saying "not charted, not done," and they may be uncomfortable with the CBE system.

13. Advantages: The case management model emphasizes quality, cost-effective care delivered within an established length of stay. It promotes collaboration and teamwork among caregivers, helps to decrease the length of stay, and makes efficient use of time.

    Disadvantages: Clients with multiple diagnoses or those with an unpredictable course of symptoms are difficult to document on a critical path.

Case Study Answers

1. a. *What is the correct method to fix this error?* Although each institution's policies may vary in terms of what is acceptable for correcting documentation errors, the most correct method is to draw a single line through it and write the words "mistaken entry" above or next to the original entry with your name or initials.

b. *Identify an incorrect method for fixing errors in client records. Why is this method incorrect?* Any method such as using more than one single line to strike through the error, crossing out the error, or scratching out the error. These methods are incorrect because the original documentation cannot be viewed. The original documentation, even if in error, must been in plain sight for legal purposes.

2. *When preparing the change-of-shift report for this client, what kind of specific data would you want to report to the oncoming nurse assigned to Mr. Branson's care?*

Start the report by introducing the client, such as: "Mr. Michael Branson, age 47, is in room number _______. He was admitted with a medical diagnosis of alcohol withdrawal and is experiencing delirium tremens." Continue by describing the client's IV site, type of fluid infusing, rate of infusion, and whether it is infusing by pump or gravity. Describe Mr. Branson's behavior when he experiences hallucinations, vital sign measurements obtained during hallucinations compared to his baseline vital signs, what medications were administered, how long before the client responded to medications, and the type of response you assessed.

Review Question Answers

1. ***Answer:*** 4 (Objective: 4) ***Rationale:*** The Kardex is used to provide quick access to client information. It should be kept updated at all times. ***Nursing Process:*** Assessment ***Client Need:*** Safe, Effective Care Environment

2. ***Answer:*** 2, 3 (Objective: 6) ***Rationale:*** Skilled care clients require more extensive nursing with specialized nursing skills. The intermediate care focus is on clients with chronic illnesses. ***Nursing Process:*** Assessment ***Client Need:*** Physiological Integrity

3. ***Answer:*** 4 (Objective: 6) ***Rationale:*** The client with an MI would require more frequent charting due to the unstable changes occurring after a major MI. ***Nursing Process:*** Implementation ***Client Need:*** Physiological Integrity

4. ***Answer:*** 2 (Objective: 7) ***Rationale:*** Draw a line through it and write the words "mistaken entry" above or next to the original entry with your name or initials. Do not erase, blot out, or use correction fluid. Avoid writing the word "error" when recording that a mistake has been made. ***Nursing Process:*** Implementation ***Client Need:*** Physiological Integrity

5. ***Answer:*** 1 (Objective: 7) ***Rationale:*** The documentation is complete and states that education was given informing the client of the consequences of refusal. ***Nursing Process:*** Implementation ***Client Need:*** Physiological Integrity

6. ***Answer:*** 2, 3, 5 (Objective: 2) ***Rationale:*** The main purposes of charting are to communicate care, help identify patterns of responses and changes in status, provide a basis for evaluation, provide a legal document, and supply validation for insurance purposes. The purpose of charting is not to fill up the nurse's spare time or to demonstrate what the nurse did every moment of the shift. ***Nursing Process:*** Assessment ***Client Need:*** Safe, Effective Care Environment

7. ***Answer:*** 4 (Objective: 3) ***Rationale:*** The student nurse needs to read the charts and ask questions such as "What are the diagnoses?" "What are they doing to treat the client?" "How is the client responding?" ***Nursing Process:*** Assessment ***Client Need:*** Safe, Effective Care Environment

8. ***Answer:*** 1 (Objective: 7) ***Rationale:*** The charting is specific, concise, descriptive, nonjudgmental, and objective. The other three examples are vague and subjective. ***Nursing Process:*** Implementation ***Client Need:*** Physiological Integrity

9. ***Answer:*** 2 (Objective: 8) ***Rationale:*** When giving the change-of-shift report, the nurse should use a guide, begin by giving background information of the client, be specific, describe abnormal findings and provide supporting evidence. ***Nursing Process:*** Implementation ***Client Need:*** Safe, Effective Care Environment

10. ***Answer:*** 4 (Objective: 1) ***Rationale:*** Flow sheet charting allows nurses to record nursing data quickly and concisely. It provides an easy-to-read record of the client's condition over time. ***Nursing Process:*** Implementation ***Client Need:*** Physiological Integrity

11. ***Answer:*** 1, 2, 3 (Objective: 1) ***Rationale:*** The nurse has a legal and ethical duty to maintain confidentiality of the client's record. Personal passwords should not be shared, the nurse should never leave the computer unattended, and paperwork should not be left unattended in an unsecured location. Client records should never be discarded into a trash can; they should be shredded or disposed of per the facility policies. ***Nursing Process:*** Assessment ***Client Need:*** Safe, Effective Care Environment

12. ***Answer:*** 1, 3, 4 (Objective: 5) ***Rationale:*** The client's status or care should never be discussed in situations where other persons may overhear the privileged information. Nurses have a legal and ethical duty to maintain confidentiality of the client's record, personal information, and any other information that relates to that individual's health care. Appropriate use of sharing client information includes during change-of-shift report, contacting the physician, and during care plan conferences. ***Nursing Process:*** Assessment ***Client Need:*** Safe, Effective Care Environment

CHAPTER 16

Key Term Review

1. d 2. x 3. v 4. h 5. q 6. k

7. s 8. r 9. c 10. m 11. t 12. l

13. n 14. g 15. f 16. p 17. a 18. i

19. u 20. e 21. y 22. b 23. o 24. w

25. j

Key Topic Review Answers

1. a. They are self-regulating.
   b. They are compensatory.
   c. They tend to be regulated by negative feedback systems.
   d. They may require several feedback mechanisms to correct only one physiological imbalance.

2. a. Health promotion
   b. Health maintenance
   c. Health education
   d. Illness prevention
   e. Restorative-rehabilitation care

3. a. Physiological needs—Air, food, H_2O, shelter, rest, sleep, activity, and temperature maintenance are crucial for survival.
   b. Safety and security needs—Client needs to feel safe in both physical environments and in relationships.
   c. Love and belonging needs—Giving and receiving affection, attaining a place in a group, and maintaining the feeling of belonging.
   d. Self-esteem needs—Feelings of independence, competence, and self-respect and esteem from others such as recognition, respect, and appreciation.
   e. Self-actualization—When self-esteem is satisfied, the individual strives for the innate need to develop one's maximum potential and realize one's abilities and qualities.

4. Richard Kalish added an additional category between the physiological needs and the safety and security needs. This level includes sex, activity, exploration, manipulation, and novelty.

5. a

6. a. "Increase quality and years of healthy life" indicates the aging of the population.
   b. "Eliminate health disparities" reflects the diversity of the population.

   These two goals reflect the nation's changing demographics.

7. a

8. The health promotion plan needs to fit the desires and priorities of the client.

9. The nurse acts as a resource person in a nonjudgmental manner.

10. All of the selections except the marital status would be relevant to the lifestyle assessment. Assessment of marital status falls under the sociocultural domain.

Case Study Answers

1. *What health promotion education will you provide?* Health promotion education may include encouraging group support and social support, providing health education, enhancing behavior change, and modeling wellness. The nurse will encourage the client to quit smoking and join a support group to help in doing so. The nurse will provide the client health education regarding the client's acute symptoms, as well as education on prevention of disease.

2. *When providing education to Mr. Conner, what type of prevention will you be demonstrating?* Tertiary prevention. This type of prevention begins after an illness, when a defect or disability is fixed, stabilized, or determined to be irreversible.

Review Question Answers

1. ***Answer:*** 4 (Objective: 10) ***Rationale:*** In the precontemplation stage, the person does not change his/her behavior during the next 6 months. In this stage, the client tends to avoid reading, talking, or thinking about his or her high-risk behaviors. ***Nursing Process:*** Assessment ***Client Need:*** Psychosocial Integrity

2. ***Answer:*** 1, 4 (Objective: 11) ***Rationale:*** Information dissemination is the most basic type of health promotion program. Examples are billboards, posters, brochures, newspapers, books, and health fairs. It raises the level of knowledge and awareness of individuals and groups about healthy behaviors. ***Nursing Process:*** Implementation ***Client Need:*** Health Promotion and Maintenance

3. ***Answer:*** 3 (Objective: 8) ***Rationale:*** Tertiary care begins after an illness, when a disability is fixed, stabilized, or determined to be irreversible. The focus is to assist rehabilitation and restore clients

to the highest level of functioning. ***Nursing Process:*** Implementation ***Client Need:*** Health Promotion and Maintenance

4. ***Answer:*** 1 (Objective: 11) ***Rationale:*** Primary prevention is generalized health promotion and specific protection against diseases or specific accidents targeted to a specific group. This intervention precedes disease or dysfunction and is applied to generally healthy individuals or groups. Secondary prevention emphasizes early detection of disease, prompt intervention, and health maintenance for individuals experiencing health problems. Tertiary prevention begins after an illness, when a defect or disability is fixed, stabilized, or determined to be irreversible. Its focus is to help the client rehabilitate and be restored to an optimum level of functioning within the constraints of disability. Limited prevention is not a type of prevention. ***Nursing Process:*** Implementation ***Client Need:*** Health Promotion and Maintenance

5. ***Answer:*** 3 (Objective: 13) ***Rationale:*** Primary prevention is generalized health promotion and specific protection against diseases or specific accidents targeted to a specific group. This intervention precedes disease or dysfunction and is applied to generally healthy individuals or groups. Secondary prevention emphasizes early detection of disease, prompt intervention, and health maintenance for individuals experiencing health problems. Tertiary prevention begins after an illness, when a defect or disability is fixed, stabilized, or determined to be irreversible. Its focus is to help the client rehabilitate and be restored to an optimum level of functioning within the constraints of disability. Limited prevention is not a type of prevention. ***Nursing Process:*** Implementation ***Client Need:*** Health Promotion and Maintenance

6. ***Answer:*** 2 (Objective: 11) ***Rationale:*** Primary prevention is generalized health promotion and specific protection against diseases or specific accidents targeted to a specific group. This intervention precedes disease or dysfunction and is applied to generally healthy individuals or groups. Secondary prevention emphasizes early detection of disease, prompt intervention, and health maintenance for individuals experiencing health problems. Tertiary prevention begins after an illness, when a defect or disability is fixed, stabilized, or determined to be irreversible. Its focus is to help the client rehabilitate and be restored to an optimum level of functioning within the constraints of disability. Limited prevention is not a type of prevention. ***Nursing Process:*** Implementation ***Client Need:*** Health Promotion and Maintenance

7. ***Answer:*** 1, 2, 3 (Objective: 6) ***Rationale:*** All of the individuals listed are engaging in health promotion activities. However, the overweight 29-year-old who engages in risky behaviors is not engaged in health promotion activity. ***Nursing Process:*** Assessment ***Client Need:*** Health Promotion and Maintenance

8. ***Answer:*** 1 (Objective: 10) ***Rationale:*** The maintenance stage is when the person is striving to prevent relapse by integrating newly adopted behaviors into his or her lifestyle. The action stage occurs when the person actively implements the changes needed to interrupt the previous risky behaviors. The preparation stage occurs when the person intends to take action in the immediate future. The termination stage is when the individual has complete confidence that the problem is no longer a temptation or threat. ***Nursing Process:*** Evaluation ***Client Need:*** Health Promotion and Maintenance

9. ***Answer:*** 1 (Objective: 10) ***Rationale:*** The maintenance stage is when the person is striving to prevent relapse by integrating newly adopted behaviors into his or her lifestyle. The action stage occurs when the person actively implements the changes needed to interrupt the previous risky behaviors. The preparation stage occurs when the person intends to take action in the immediate future. The termination stage is when the individual has complete confidence that the problem is no longer a temptation or threat. ***Nursing Process:*** Assessment ***Client Need:*** Health Promotion and Maintenance

10. ***Answer:*** 3 (Objective: 11) ***Rationale:*** The client develops his or her own plan with some assistance from the other team members as needed. ***Nursing Process:*** Assessment ***Client Need:*** Health Promotion and Maintenance

CHAPTER 17

Key Term Review

1.	g	2.	i	3.	h	4.	k	5.	a	6.	j
7.	n	8.	r	9.	m	10.	p	11.	o	12.	f
13.	e	14.	c	15.	b	16.	q	17.	d	18.	l

Key Topic Review Answers

1. Illness is usually associated with disease, but may occur independently of it. Illness is a highly personal state in which the person feels unhealthy or ill. Disease alters body functions and results in a reduction of capacities or a shortened life span.

2. ______b___ Outlined five stages of illness

   ______a___ Described four aspects of the sick role

3. An individual's usual pattern of behavior changes with illness and hospitalization, which disrupt a person's privacy, autonomy, lifestyle, roles, and finances. Nurses need to be aware that the illness of one member of a family affects all other members.

4. Internal variables include biologic, psychological, and cognitive dimensions. The biologic dimension includes genetic makeup, sex, age, and developmental level. The psychological dimension includes

mind–body interactions and self-concept. The cognitive dimension includes lifestyle choices and spiritual and religious beliefs.

5. Well-being is a subjective perception of vitality and feeling well that can be described, experienced, and measured. Wellness is an active, seven-dimensional process of becoming aware of and making choices toward a higher level of well-being.

6. External variables influencing health include: (Student will choose three.)

   a. Physical environment

   b. Standards of living

   c. Family and cultural beliefs

   d. Social support networks

7. The seven dimensions of wellness include:

   a. Physical

   b. Social

   c. Emotional

   d. Intellectual

   e. Spiritual

   f. Occupational

   g. Environmental dimensions

8. etiology

9. a. Clients are not held responsible for their condition.

   b. Clients are excused from certain social roles and tasks.

   c. Clients are obliged to try to get well as quickly as possible.

   d. Clients or their families are obliged to seek competent help.

10. a. Locus of control (LOC): A concept from social learning theory that nurses can use to determine whether clients are likely to take action regarding health—that is, whether clients believe that their health status is under their own or others' control.

   b. Exacerbation: An increase in the severity of a disease or any of its signs or symptoms.

   c. Health behaviors: The actions people take to understand their health state, maintain an optimal state of health, prevent illness and injury, and reach their maximum physical and mental potential.

   d. Health beliefs: Concepts about health that an individual believes are true.

   e. Health status: Level of health of an individual, a group, or a population as assessed by that individual or by objective measures.

   f. Acute illness: Typically characterized by severe symptoms of relatively short duration, for example, appendicitis.

   g. Remission: Abatement or lessening in severity of the symptoms of a disease.

   h. Risk factors: Practices that have potentially negative effects on health, for example, overeating.

Case Study Answers

1. *With consideration of the goals of* Healthy People 2020, *how can the nurse assist the client?* The goals of *Healthy People 2020* are to increase the length and quality of life and to eliminate health disparities within populations. When the client decides to quit smoking, she will reduce her risks of many of the diseases associated with smoking. The nurse could supply the client with smoking cessation information, refer her to social support groups, and notify the physician of the client's desires.

Review Question Answers

1. ***Answer:*** 3 (Objective: 3) ***Rationale:*** The role performance model identifies health as the ability of an individual to fulfill societal roles, such as performing his or her own work. People are viewed as physiological systems with related functions, and health is identified by the absence of signs and symptoms of disease or injury, in the clinical model. In the adaptive model, health is a creative process; disease is a failure in adaptation, or maladaption. The eudemonistic model incorporates a comprehensive view of health. Health is seen as a condition of actualization or realization of a person's potential. In this model the highest aspiration of people is fulfillment and complete development, which is actualization. Illness, in this model, is a condition that prevents self-actualization. ***Nursing Process:*** Assessment ***Client Need:*** Health Promotion and Maintenance

2. ***Answer:*** 4 (Objective: 3) ***Rationale:*** The eudemonistic model incorporates a comprehensive view of health. Health is seen as a condition of actualization or realization of a person's potential. Actualization is the apex of the fully developed personality, described by Abraham Maslow. In this model the highest aspiration of people is fulfillment and complete development, which is actualization. Illness, in this model, is a condition that prevents self-actualization. People are viewed as physiological systems with related functions, and health is identified by the absence of signs and symptoms of disease or injury, in the clinical model. In the adaptive model, health is a creative process; disease is a failure in adaptation, or maladaption. The role performance model identifies

health as the ability of an individual to fulfill societal roles, such as performing his or her own work. ***Nursing Process:*** Evaluation ***Client Need:*** Health Promotion and Maintenance

3. ***Answer:*** 2 (Objective: 4) ***Rationale:*** Gender influences the distribution of disease. Certain acquired and genetic diseases are more common in one gender than the other. Genetic makeup influences biologic characteristics, innate temperament, activity level, and intellectual potential. Age is also a significant factor. The distribution of disease varies with age. Developmental level has a major impact on health status. ***Nursing Process:*** Assessment ***Client Need:*** Health Promotion and Maintenance

4. ***Answer:*** 4 (Objective: 5) ***Rationale:*** Developmental level has a major impact on health status. Genetic makeup influences biologic characteristics, innate temperament, activity level, and intellectual potential. Gender influences the distribution of disease. Certain acquired and genetic diseases are more common in one gender than the other. Age is also a significant factor. The distribution of disease varies with age. ***Nursing Process:*** Assessment ***Client Need:*** Health Promotion and Maintenance

5. ***Answer:*** 1, 2 (Objective: 9) ***Rationale:*** Role changes often occur when a family member becomes ill. The client may become dependent on the health care provider, may distance from the family, or may no longer be able to work. The change is not usually one of becoming more outgoing although that is possible. Self-esteem tends to be reduced by illness. ***Nursing Process:*** Evaluation ***Client Need:*** Health Promotion and Maintenance

6. ***Answer:*** 2, 3, 4 (Objective: 6) ***Rationale: Exercise, regular oral care, and use of seat belts have been shown to have a positive effect on health. Use of tobacco is a lifestyle choice known to have a negative effect on health. Nursing Process:*** Assessment ***Client Need:*** Health Promotion and Maintenance

7. ***Answer:*** 1 (Objective: 3) ***Rationale: The locus of control is a concept nurses can use to determine whether clients are likely to take action regarding health. People who believe that they have a major influence on their own health status are more likely than others to take the initiative on their own health care, be more knowledgeable about their health, make and keep appointments with primary care providers, and give up smoking. Nursing Process:*** Assessment ***Client Need:*** Health Promotion and Maintenance

8. ***Answer:*** *1* (Objective: 4) ***Rationale:*** Physical wellness is the ability to carry out daily tasks and practice positive lifestyle habits. Social wellness is the ability to interact successfully with people and within the environment. Emotional wellness is the ability to manage stress and express emotions appropriately. Intellectual wellness is the ability to learn and use that information positively. ***Nursing Process:*** Assessment ***Client Need:*** Health Promotion and Maintenance

9. ***Answer:*** 2 (Objective: 5) ***Rationale:*** Many factors influence adherence to healthy practices. Role modeling by the nurse is a very important aspect when teaching clients about healthier choices. ***Nursing Process:*** Implementation ***Client Need:*** Health Promotion and Maintenance

10. ***Answer:*** 3 (Objective: 6) ***Rationale: Diabetes mellitus is a chronic illness.*** A chronic illness is one that lasts for an extended period, usually 6 months or longer, and often for the person's life. Acute illness is typically characterized by symptoms of relatively short duration. The symptoms often appear abruptly and subside quickly and, depending on the cause, may or may not require intervention by health care professionals. Adherence and exacerbations are not types of illnesses and diabetes mellitus would not be categorized by these terms. ***Nursing Process:*** Assessment ***Client Need:*** Health Promotion and Maintenance

CHAPTER 18

Key Term Review

1. w 2. p 3. m 4. j 5. t 6. y

7. d 8. g 9. a 10. q 11. f 12. l

13. o 14. n 15. e 16. i 17. v 18. u

19. b 20. k 21. x 22. r 23. c 24. h

25. s

Key Topic Review Answers

1. Culture can be defined as the nonphysical traits, such as values, beliefs, attitudes, and customs, that are shared by a group of people and passed from one generation to the next. It is also considered the thoughts, communications, actions, customs, beliefs, values, and institutions of racial, ethnic, religious, or social groups. Culture defines how health is perceived, how health care information is received, how rights and protections are exercised, how a health problem is defined, how concerns are expressed, who should provide treatment, and how and what kind of treatment should be given.

2. heritage

3. The U.S. Department of Health and Human Services (USDHHS) houses the Office of Minority Health "to improve and protect the health of racial and ethnic minority populations through the development of health policies and programs that will eliminate health disparities." In collaboration with other organizations, it developed the *National Standards for Culturally and Linguisti-*

cally Appropriate Services in Health Class (CLAS). Culture and language have a considerable impact on how clients access and respond to health care services.

4. The Centers for Disease Control (CDC) has an Office of Minority Health to "promote health and quality of life by preventing and controlling the disproportionate burden of disease, injury and disability among racial and ethnic minority populations."

5. The purpose of the National Center on Minority Health and Health Disparities (NCMHD) within the National Institutes of Health (NIH) is to promote minority health and to lead, coordinate, support, and assess the NIH effort to reduce and ultimately eliminate health disparities.

6. The nursing profession plays a major role in REACH by striving to eliminate racial and ethnic disparities in infant mortality; in screening and management of breast and cervical cancer, cardiovascular diseases, diabetes, and HIV infections/AIDS; and in child and adult immunizations.

7. One of the major goals of *Healthy People 2010* is to eliminate health disparities by gender, race or ethnicity, education, income, disability, geographic location, and sexual orientation.

8. It influences nursing because it includes a comprehensive overview of disparities in health care among racial, ethnic, and socioeconomic groups in the general U.S. population and among priority populations.

9. Culturally sensitive nursing implies basic knowledge of and constructive attitudes toward the health traditions observed among the diverse cultural group found in the setting in which the nurse is practicing.

   Culturally appropriate nursing implies that nurses apply the underlying background knowledge that must be possessed to provide the client with the best possible health care.

   Culturally competent nursing implies that the nurse understands and attends to the total content of the client's situation and uses a complex combination of knowledge, attitudes, and skills. Providing nursing care within these three parameters is critical.

10. Madeline Leininger

Case Study Answers

1a. *If the nurse is culturally competent, what would be an appropriate comment?* "Are these areas from using traditional treatments to aid in healing your illness?"

1b. *If the nurse has xenophobia, what comment might the nurse make regarding the coining or cupping that occurred?* "You appear to be too smart to believe cupping will actually cure you!"

1c. *Give an example of an ethnocentric statement from the nurse.* "An antibiotic would treat you quicker than these bruises. We have a better success rate with antibiotics, and it's less painful!"

1d. *What nursing action would be considered discrimination?* Denying the client basic care or any medical treatment that one might offer other clients.

2a. *If the client does not return direct eye contact, is this indicative of a cultural difference or a result of a "shifty," evasive client?* Hispanic culture does not always use direct eye contact. The nurse must treat all clients with a nonjudgmental attitude.

2b. *The client's family desires to spend as much time with him as possible, including staying after hours. How does the nurse handle this situation?* The nurse should use her own judgment and see if the family members are hindering the client's recovery process. It may be necessary to obtain a physician's order or the supervisor's permission for the family to remain after hours. If the family members are disturbing other clients, they may need to leave, or have only one or two family members remain with the client.

2c. *The client does not want to take his preventive medication to prevent stress ulcers. He states that his life and recovery status are in God's hands, and that he has "no need of pharmaceutical medications." What action should the nurse take at this time?* Notify the physician of the client's wishes to decline the medication and explain the consequences of the medication refusal to the client.

Review Question Answers

1. ***Answer:*** 3. (Objective 3) ***Rationale:*** There is an ongoing shift in the U.S. population that includes a decreasing number of White Americans (formerly the majority population) and increasing numbers of other cultural groups. The birth rate is actually decreasing; limited access to health care is a complex issue that is not the major factor here; and immigration has increased. ***Client Need:*** Psychosocial Integrity.

2. ***Answer:*** 1 (Objective: 9) ***Rationale:*** The term *bicultural* is used to describe a person with dual patterns of identification who crosses two cultures, lifestyles, and sets of values. Diversity refers to the fact or state of being different. ***A subculture is usually composed of people who have a distinct identity and yet are related to a larger cultural group.. Acculturation occurs when people incorporate traits from another culture. Nursing Process:*** Assessment ***Client Need:*** Psychosocial Integrity

3. ***Answer:*** 3 (Objective: 8) ***Rationale:*** Diversity refers to the fact or state of being different. Many factors account for diversity: race, gender, sexual orientation, culture, ethnicity, socioeconomic status, educational attainment, religious affiliation, and so on. ***Nursing Process:*** Assessment ***Client Need:*** Psychosocial Integrity

4. ***Answer:*** 2 (Objective: 8) ***Rationale:*** Acculturation is the involuntary process that occurs when people adapt to or borrow traits from another culture. ***Nursing Process:*** Assessment ***Client Need:*** Psychosocial Integrity

5. ***Answer:*** 3 (Objective: 9) ***Rationale:*** Assimilation is the process by which an individual develops a new cultural identity. It means the person becomes similar to the members of the dominant culture. ***Nursing Process:*** Assessment ***Client Need:*** Psychosocial Integrity

6. ***Answer:*** 3 (Objective: 5) ***Rationale:*** Stereotyping is assuming that all members of a culture or ethnic group are alike, instead of unique individuals. ***Nursing Process:*** Assessment ***Client Need:*** Psychosocial Integrity

7. ***Answer:*** 4 (Objective: 2) ***Rationale:*** Healing rituals are considered both a mental and spiritual method of maintaining health, protecting health, and restoring health. The other answer choices are not outlined in this model. ***Nursing Process:*** Assessment ***Client Need:*** Psychosocial Integrity

8. ***Answer:*** 4 (Objective: 3) ***Rationale:*** An interpreter is "an individual who mediates spoken or signed communication between people speaking different languages, without adding, omitting, or distorting material from one language to another. ***Nursing Process:*** Planning ***Client Need:*** Safe, Effective Care Environment

9. ***Answer:*** 1 (Objective: 6) ***Rationale:*** Stereotyping is assuming that all members of a culture or ethnic group are alike. Stereotyping that is unrelated to reality may be based on racism or discrimination. ***Nursing Process:*** Assessment ***Client Need:*** Safe, Effective Care Environment

10. ***Answer:*** 2, 3, 5 (Objective: 9) ***Rationale: The nurse should speak slowly, use nonverbal communication, and address the client when communicating with a client who has limited knowledge of the English language. The nurse should*** avoid slang words and should not use a member of the client's family to act as an interpreter because the client may not want the family to know about his condition. ***Nursing Process:*** Assessment ***Client Need:*** Safe, Effective Care Environment

11. ***Answer:*** 1, 3, 4 (Objective: 7) ***Rationale:*** Nurses are encouraged to integrate cultural skills, encounters, desires, awareness, and knowledge. Methods to obtain the integration include attending in-services, participating in community events that entertain other cultures, and reviewing professional nursing journals that include cultural awareness topics. ***Nursing Process:*** Assessment ***Client Need:*** Safe, Effective Care Environment.

CHAPTER 19

Key Term Review

1. w	2. g	3. y	4. d	5. e	6. i
7. n	8. b	9. p	10. q	11. u	12. l
13. t	14. c	15. a	16. x	17. j	18. s
19. f	20. v	21. h	22. k	23. o	24. r
25. m					

Key Topic Review Answers

1. Holism

2. The vision statement of the AHNA states "…a world in which nursing nurtures wholeness and inspires peace and healing" and has a purpose to "promote the education of nurses, other health care professionals and the public in all aspects of holistic caring and healing."

3. Healing environments are created when nurses empower clients by providing the knowledge, skills, and support that allow them to tap into their inner wisdom and make healthy decisions for themselves.

4. Methods of self-healing include: (Student will choose three.)
   a. Identify behaviors that indicate overinvolvement (example = saying yes instead of no, feeling selfish when you do say no).
   b. Perform relaxation exercises on a regular basis.
   c. Maintain and enhance your physical health.
   d. Develop support networks with other nurses or health care workers.

5. a, d, e

6. Energy

7. chiropractic

8. __b__ No specific outcome is requested during prayer time

   __d__ An informal talk with God—like talking with a good friend

   __e__ Individual who is praying asks for a specific outcome

   __a__ Asking God for things for oneself or others

____c____ The use of formal prayers or rituals such as prayers from a prayer book or Jewish siddur

____f____ Contemplative prayer

9. Contraindications include pregnancy, pacemakers, implanted defibrillators, aneurysm clips in the brain, cochlear implants, or other implanted electric devices. Magnetic therapy works on the principle that every animal, plant, and mineral has an electromagnetic field that enables organic beings and inorganic objects, such as crystals, to communicate and interact as part of a single, unified energy system. Magnetic fields are able to penetrate the body and affect the functioning of cells, tissues, organs, and systems. These therapies work best in combination with other healing modalities and are considered to be adjunct treatments to conventional medicine.

10. Chelation therapy is the introduction of chemicals into the bloodstream that bind with heavy minerals in the body.

Case Study Answers

1a. *What type of questions should the nurse ask to investigate Ms. Sinclair's use of complementary and alternative therapies?* "What alternative therapies have you used, such as acupuncture, touch therapies, herbs, or dietary supplements?" "Tell me about any teas, herbs, vitamins, or other natural products you use to improve your health."

2a. *Which popular herbal preparations could interfere with Mr. Santos's current medication regimen?* Feverfew, ginger, gingko, and garlic may increase the anticoagulant effects of aspirin and anticoagulant medications.

2b. *Which additional complementary and alternative healing modalities might the nurse suggest to Mr. Santos to help treat his hypertension?* Yoga and meditation have been shown to improve hypertension and these modalities are appropriate for this client.

Review Question Answers

1. ***Answer:*** 1, 2, 3 (Objective: 1) ***Rationale:*** Holism, balance, and spirituality are concepts common to all alternative practices. Alternative practices do not generally involve prescription medications. While technology and instrumentation may be used, these are not common to most alternative practices. ***Nursing Process:*** Assessment ***Client Need:*** Safe, Effective Care Environment

2. ***Answer:*** 1 (Objective: 4) ***Rationale:*** Naturopathic medicine places an emphasis on client responsibility, client education, health maintenance, and disease prevention. Nutritional therapy consists of the consumption of several kinds of diets. Homeopathy is a self-healing system, assisted by small doses of remedies or medicines, which is useful in a variety of acute and chronic disorders. Chiropractic practitioners believe that health is a state of balance, especially of the nervous and musculoskeletal systems. ***Nursing Process:*** Assessment ***Client Need:*** Health Promotion and Maintenance

3. ***Answer:*** 3 (Objective: 7) ***Rationale:*** Nurses should encourage all clients to discuss any use of complementary and alternative medicine use. Hydrotherapy may not be appropriate for all older adult clients. Nurse's will not encourage or suggest colonics to a client with Crohn's disease. Acupuncture and yoga may not be appropriate for all populations. ***Nursing Process:*** Implementation ***Client Need:*** Safe, Effective Care Environment

4. ***Answer:*** 3 (Objective: 3) ***Rationale:*** Pilates is a method of physical movement and exercise designed to stretch, strengthen, and balance the body. Increased lung capacity, improved flexibility and joint health, improved muscular coordination, increased bone density, and better posture and balance are possible benefits. Pilates may not necessarily decrease boredom or increase spirituality in the client. Pilates does not cleanse the colon. ***Nursing Process:*** Planning ***Client Need:*** Health Promotion and Maintenance

5. ***Answer:*** 4 (Objective: 10) ***Rationale: Humor and laughter in nursing are defined as helping the client "to acknowledge and express what is funny, amusing, or ludicrous in order to establish relationships, relieve tension, release anger, facilitate learning, or cope with painful feelings or emotions." Nursing Process:*** Planning ***Client Need:*** Psychosocial Integrity

6. ***Answer:*** 3 (Objective: 10) ***Rationale: The program consists of 108 hours of in-depth, hands-on training to provide nurses with training in relaxation and therapeutic imagery skills. This program does not provide certification in music therapy or hypnotherapy. Humor therapy may be used by all nurses and does not require a separate certification. Nursing Process:*** Assessment ***Client Need:*** Physiological Integrity.

7. ***Answer:*** 1 (Objective: 7) ***Rationale:*** Physical resting and rhythmic breathing are used in all three modalities of CAM. Meditation is a general term for a wide range of practices that involve relaxing the body and easing the mind. Guided imagery is a two-way communication between the conscious and unconscious mind and involves the whole body and all of its senses. It is a state of focused attention that encourages changes in attitudes, behaviors, and physiological reactions. Biofeedback is a method for learned control of physiological responses of the body. ***Nursing Process:*** Planning ***Client Need:*** Physiological Integrity

8. ***Answer:*** 3 (Objectives: 2 and 3) ***Rationale:*** Music without words is often used to relax and distract clients in a variety of settings, such as operating rooms and birthing rooms. The other genres of music have not been shown effective in relaxation and distraction

of clients. ***Nursing Process:*** Implementation ***Client Need:*** Physiological Integrity

9. ***Answer:*** 3, 5, 6 (Objective: 2) ***Rationale:*** Massage aids in the relief of muscle tension, reduces muscle spasms, and increases relaxation. Music without words is often used to relax and distract clients in a variety of settings. Guided imagery is a two-way communication between the conscious and unconscious mind and involves the whole body and all of its senses. It is a state of focused attention that encourages changes in attitudes, behaviors, and physiological reactions. Administering medication is a pharmacologic intervention. The client is on bed rest and should not be assisted to a chair. Telling the client that the health care provider will see him tomorrow does not ease the client's discomfort. ***Nursing Process:*** Implementation ***Client Need:*** Physiological Integrity

CHAPTER 20

Key Term Review

1. r	2. s	3. i	4. p	5. v	6. g
7. q	8. w	9. o	10. a	11. t	12. n
13. u	14. b	15. x	16. j	17. m	18. e
19. f	20. l	21. h	22. c	23. d	24. k

Key Topic Review Answers

1. Growth is defined as physical change and increase in size. Some indicators of growth include height, weight, bone size, and dentition.

2. Development is an increase in the complexity of function and skill progression. It is the capacity and skill of a person to adapt to the environment and is the behavior aspect of growth.

3. Four factors that influence growth and development include: (Student will choose four.)

   a. genetics

   b. temperament

   c. family influence

   d. adequate nutrition

   e. environmental conditions

   f. the individual's state of health

   g. cultural influences

4. Psychosocial development refers to the development of personality.

5. Defense mechanisms, or adaptive mechanisms, as they are more commonly called today, are the result of conflicts between the id's impulses and the anxiety created by the conflicts due to social and environmental restrictions. The third aspect of the personality, according to Freud, is the superego. The superego contains the conscience and the ego ideal. The conscience consists of society's "do nots," usually as a result of parental and cultural expectations. The ego ideal comprises the standards of perfection toward which the individual strives. Freud proposed that the underlying motivation to human development is a dynamic, psychic energy, which he called libido.

6. Social learning theory states that learning can occur by observation. Role modeling and learning from watching role models are a part of social learning theory. Attention and cognitive function, in which the individual thinks about the behavior of self and others, as well as the expected rewards and punishments for certain behaviors, are important to social learning.

7. Moral development—a complex process not fully understood—involves learning what ought not to be done. Kohlberg's theory focuses on the reason an individual makes a decision.

8. Behaviorist learning theory emphasizes stimulus-response and either positive or negative reinforcement as the basis for learning and behavior change.

9. Fowler and Westerhoff are two theorists who describe stages of spiritual development or faith. The spiritual component of growth and development refers to individuals' understanding of his or her relationship with the universe and his or her perceptions about the direction and meaning of life.

10. a. Accommodation: A process of change whereby cognitive processes mature sufficiently to allow the person to solve problems that were unsolvable before.

    b. Adaptation: The ability to handle the demands made by the environment. Also known as coping behavior.

    c. Assimilation: The process through which humans encounter and react to the new situations by using the mechanisms they already possess.

    d. Developmental task: A task that arises at or about a certain period in the life of an individual, successful achievement of which leads to her or his happiness and to success with later tasks, while failure leads to unhappiness in the individual, disapproval by society, and difficulty with later tasks.

Case Study Answers

1. *What primary abilities will the infant use in this phase of cognitive development? In each phase of Piaget's phases of cognitive development, the individual uses three primary abilities: assimilation, accommodation, and adaptation.*

2. *Describe the significant behavior noted in this phase of cognitive development. The infant is in stage 3 of the sensorimotor phase, secondary circular reaction. The significant behavior in this phase is that the infant begins to discover and rediscover the external environment.*

Review Question Answers

1. ***Answer:*** 4 (Objective: 2) ***Rationale:*** The cephalocaudal direction of growth starts at the head and moves to the trunk, legs, and the feet. This pattern is very obvious at birth, when the head of the infant is larger than the body. Proximodistal describes growth from the center of the body outward. Simple to complex and peripheral to medial are not patterns of growth. ***Nursing Process:*** Assessment ***Client Need:*** Physiological Integrity

2. ***Answer:*** 3 (Objective: 10) ***Rationale:*** The preconceptual phase is from ages 2 to 4 years. The significant behavior at this phase is when toddlers associate words with objects and everything relates to "me." The toddler associates the nurse with the needle and pain. Primary circular reaction is stage 2 from ages 1–4 months where the significant behavior is perception that events are centered on the body and objects are extension of self. Intuitive versus guilt phase is an aspect of Erikson's theory, not Piaget's. The concrete operations phase is ages 7–11 years and the significant behaviors include solving concrete problems. Refer to Table 20–5n the text. ***Nursing Process:*** Assessment ***Client Need:*** Physiological Integrity

3. ***Answer:*** 2 (Objective: 9) ***Rationale:*** According to Peck, preoccupation with declining body functions reduces happiness and satisfaction with life. The individual is adjusting to decreasing physical capacities and maintaining feelings of well-being. Body transcendence versus body preoccupation and this task calls for the individual to adjust to decreasing physical capacities and at the same time maintain feelings of well-being. Ego differentiation versus work-role perception is when an adult's identity and feelings of worth are highly dependent on that person's work role. Ego transcendence versus ego preoccupation is the acceptance without fear of one's death as inevitable. Integrity versus despair is Erikson's stage of development that deals with maturity. ***Nursing Process:*** Assessment ***Client Need:*** Physiological Needs

4. ***Answer:*** 1 (Objective: 8) ***Rationale:*** Adolescents are achieving new and mature relations. The other answers apply to other stages of development that take place after adolescence. Havighurst believed learning is basic to life and that people continue to learn throughout life. His developmental tasks provide a framework that the nurse can use to evaluate a person's general accomplishments. ***Nursing Process:*** Assessment ***Client Need:*** Health Promotion and Maintenance

5. ***Answer:*** 1 (Objective: 11) ***Rationale:*** Morals means relating to "both right and wrong." Spirituality and religion are not indicated by the client's behavior and statement. The client's moral development, not psychological development, is demonstrated in the question. ***Nursing Process:*** Assessment ***Client Need:*** Health Promotion and Maintenance

6. ***Answer:*** 4 (Objective: 9) ***Rationale:*** Peck's theory believes mental and social capacities tend to increase in the later part of life. In Freud's theory of psychosexual development, the personality develops in five overlapping stages from birth to adulthood. Piaget's theory deals with the child's cognitive ability. Kohlberg's theory deals with males and is not applicable. ***Nursing Process:*** Assessment ***Client Need:*** Safe, Effective Care Environment

7. ***Answer:*** 3 (Objective: 9) ***Rationale:*** Stage 4 is when marriages and careers are established. The other answers apply to other stages. ***Nursing Process:*** Assessment ***Client Need:*** Health Promotion and Maintenance

8. ***Answer:*** 2 (Objective: 11) ***Rationale:*** In stage 2, women feel the need for a caring relationship. Stage 1 is when women feel more isolated and selfish. Stage 3 is when women identify the need for balance between caring for self and others. There is an increased awareness of responsibility. ***Nursing Process:*** Assessment ***Client Need:*** Psychosocial Integrity

CHAPTER 21

Key Term Review

1. h	2. f	3. m	4. o	5. r	6. k
7. j	8. c	9. w	10. a	11. v	12. b
13. d	14. x	15. t	16. p	17. n	18. s
19. e	20. l	21. i	22. u	23. q	24. g

Key Topic Review Answers

1. Prenatal or intrauterine development lasts approximately 9 calendar months (10 lunar months) or 38 to 40 weeks, depending on the method of calculation.

2. Trimesters; 3

3. a. Embryonic phase is the first semester—the fertilized ovum develops into an organism.
   b. Fetal phase is the second trimester—rapid growth of fetus occurs and it resembles a small baby.
   c. Third trimester—the baby is approximately 20 inches in length and approximately 7 pounds in weight.

4. a. Underweight before pregnancy
   b. Less than 21 pounds gained during pregnancy
   c. Low socioeconomic level
   d. High stress levels, including physical or emotional abuse
   e. Smoking cigarettes during pregnancy

5. doubles; 5th; triples; 12th

6. In the infant, cognitive development occurs due to interactions between individual and environment.

7. a. Learning to walk and speak, and increased voluntary control
   b. Learning to control their bladder and bowels
   c. Learning about their environment

8. initiative versus guilt task

9. a

10. a, c, e

Case Study Answers

1a. *What reflex disappears after 8 months?* The plantar reflex disappears after 8 months.

1b. *If the Babinski reflex persists after 1 year and remains positive, what does that indicate?* If the Babinski reflex persists after 1 year, it could indicate possible upper motor neuron damage.

2a. *What explanation might the nurse give this mother to explain the adolescent's behavior? As girls become adolescents they shift their focus to establishing their own identity. Their peers take on increased importance and they question the values and beliefs of what they have been taught by their family as a means of developing their own values and beliefs that they will take with them into adulthood. Independence becomes increasingly more important as they learn to be an adult.*

2b. *What anticipatory guidance will the nurse provide this mother to prepare her for future changes she is likely to see in her daughter?* Health promotion regarding sexual practices, substance use, diet, and physical activity are important to discuss with not only the mother but also the adolescent. Preparing the parent and child for driving and the importance of safety belts, traffic regulations, and careful monitoring of the child's ability to be trusted with an automobile are essential types of information to share. The nurse might teach the mother about signs and symptoms of substance abuse. Helping the mother to promote an open relationship that encourages communication and sharing may be the most important anticipatory guidance the nurse can provide.

3a. *At what time(s) will the nurse perform the Apgar score?* Apgar scoring occurs at 1 minute and 5 minutes after birth. The scoring provides an indication of the newborn's physiological adaptation to extrauterine life.

3b. *What is the newborn's current Apgar score?* 9. The APGAR score is based on heart rate, respirations, muscle tone, reflex irritability, and color. The newborn's presentation adds up to a score of 9. (See Table 21–2 in the text for an in-depth representation of the Apgar score.)

Review Question Answers

1. ***Answer:*** 1 (Objectives: 8 and 10) ***Rationale:*** Significant changes in maternal temperature can alter the amniotic fluid and fetus, which may result in birth defects. Temperature maintenance is one of the areas of health promotion. Oxygen, nutrition and fluids, rest, safe activities, and safety are also areas of instruction for pregnant mothers in order to promote a safe pregnancy and delivery of a healthy child. The other statements indicate that the prenatal client understands nursing teaching. ***Nursing Process:*** Assessment ***Client Needs: Health*** Promotion and Maintenance

2. ***Answer:*** 4 (Objective: 4) ***Rationale:*** According to Piaget, school-age children begin the phase of concrete operations. Children learn about cause and effect during this time and learn to distinguish fantasy from fact. The other answer choices reflect different age groups, according to Piaget. ***Nursing Process:*** Assessment ***Client Need:*** Psychosocial Integrity

3. ***Answer:*** 2 (Objective: 8) ***Rationale:*** The increasing number of overweight children contributes to an increasing incidence of hypertension and type 2 diabetes. Falls occur more often in the late adult stage, while colic is seen in infants. Unprotected sex occurs more often in the adolescence period. ***Nursing Process:*** Assessment ***Client Need:*** Health Promotion and Maintenance

4. ***Answer:*** 2 (Objective: 1) ***Rationale:*** Fetal movements may be felt by the mother around 5 months of gestation. All the other responses are incorrect based on normal prenatal development. The fetal heartbeat may also be heard around this time. ***Nursing Process:*** Assessment ***Client Need:*** Physiological Integrity

5. ***Answer:*** 2, 3, 4, 5 (Objective: 7) ***Rationale:*** The Denver Developmental Screening Test (DDST-II) is used to screen children from birth to 6 years of age. The test compares the abilities of the child

with an average group of children of the same age. Four main areas of development screened are personal-social, fine motor adaptive, language, and gross motor skills. Growth and weight, as well as fine motor skills, are not assessed in the DDST-II. ***Nursing Process:*** Assessment ***Client Need:*** Physiological Integrity

6. ***Answer:*** 3 (Objective: 2) ***Rationale:*** The heads of many newborn babies are misshapen because of head molding that occurs during vaginal deliveries. Fontanels are unossified membranous gaps in the bone structure of the skull. Sutures are junction lines of the skull bones that override to provide flexibility for molding of the head. The head usually regains its symmetry in approximately 1 week. All other responses are incorrect responses to the new mother. ***Nursing Process:*** Implementation ***Client Need:*** Physiological Integrity

7. ***Answer:*** 3 (Objective: 7) ***Rationale: Stroking the sole of the foot elicits the Babinski reflex.*** The stepping reflex can be elicited by holding the baby upright so that the feet touch a flat surface. The legs move up and down as if walking. This reflex disappears around 2 months. ***Touching or stroking the baby's cheek causes the rooting reflex, in which the head turns to the touched side. It will disappear after 4 months.*** The plantar reflex occurs when an object is placed just beneath the toes and causes the toes to curl around it. This reflex disappears after 8–10 months. ***Nursing Process:*** Assessment ***Client Need:*** Physiological Integrity

8. ***Answer:*** 1 (Objectives: 2 and 7) ***Rationale:*** The toddler can walk, stand, dress self, and recognize and delay elimination. By 3 years of age, most children are toilet trained, although they may still have the occasional "accident." The other answer choices do not reflect a readiness for toilet training. ***Nursing Process:*** Planning ***Client Need:*** Physiological Integrity

9. ***Answer:*** 4 (Objectives: 1 and 3) ***Rationale:*** Teenagers respond more readily if they know they are not alone and other teens have the same issues. Adolescents do not routinely want their parents present. Any instructional material should be age appropriate. ***Nursing Process:*** Implementation ***Client Need:*** Psychosocial Integrity

10. ***Answer:*** 2 (Objectives: 6 and 8) ***Rationale:*** The parents have the right to request that the child be circumcised on that date. The nurse needs to inform the health care provider and obtain orders to carry out the request. ***Nursing Process:*** Implementation ***Client Need:*** Safe, Effective Care Environment

CHAPTER 22

Key Term Review

1. d 2. h 3. c 4. e 5. g 6. b

7. j 8. i 9. a 10. f

Key Topic Review Answers

1. Adulthood is categorized into emerging adulthood (ages 18–25), young adulthood (ages 25–40), and middle (ages 40–65).

2. a. Baby boomers

   b. Generation X

   c. Generation Y

3. lifestyle; behaviors

4. Maturity

5. Generativity

6. a. Adjusting to aging parents

   b. Valuing work as a central theme

   c. Achieving social and civic responsibility

   d. Establishing and maintaining an economic standard of living

7. a. Cancer

   b. Heart disease

8. a

9. Generativity versus stagnation; middle-aged adults look back for a sense of successfully having met goals they developed earlier in life.

10. a. Marry or remain single/rearing children
    b. Employment
    c. Starting a home
    d. Education

Case Study Answers

1a. *What health problem could Lou be at risk for, especially since Mary reported to you that he has been staying out late and arrives home with alcohol on his breath?* Lou could be at risk for alcoholism.

1b. *How can the nurse help Mary, Lou, and their families in dealing with this concern?* The nurse can provide information about the dangers of excessive alcohol use, help the client clarify values about health, and refer the client and/or family to special groups such as Alcoholics Anonymous.

1c. *What other resources might help the couple resolve their other issues?* Marriage counseling, pastor counseling, or a support group could be beneficial, among other options.

Review Question Answers

1. ***Answer:*** 4 (Objective: 7) ***Rationale:*** *Unintentional injuries (primarily motor vehicle crashes) are the fifth leading cause of death for the total population, but the leading cause of death for individuals 1 to 44 years of age. Suicide, cancer, and STIs are not the leading cause of death in individuals 1 to 44 years of age.* ***Nursing Process:*** Assessment ***Client Need:*** Physiological Integrity

2. ***Answer:*** 1 (Objective: 1) ***Rationale: High divorce and unemployment rates are factors that influence "boomerang kids" to move back in with their parents. Additional contributing factors include*** high housing costs, maladaptive behaviors, and substance abuse issues. Fear of intimacy, lack of supervision, and parental requests are not factors that typically influence the decision of "boomerang kids" to move back in with their parents. ***Nursing Process:*** Evaluation ***Client Need:*** Psychosocial Integrity

3. ***Answer:*** 3 (Objective: 7) ***Rationale: Young African American adults, especially men, have increased incidence of hypertension.*** Many of the causes of hypertension are unknown. Contributing factors include smoking, obesity, high-sodium diet, and high stress levels. Although hypertension occurs within the other population groups, these groups are not associated with the highest incidence of hypertension. ***Nursing Process:*** Assessment ***Client Need:*** Physiological Integrity

4. ***Answer:*** 1 (Objective: 9) ***Rationale: Testicular cancer is*** the most common neoplasm in men ages 20 to 34. Young men should be instructed in how to perform testicular self-examination. The other types of cancer listed are not the most common neoplasm among this population. ***Nursing Process:*** Assessment ***Client Need:*** Physiological Integrity

5. ***Answer:*** 2 (Objective: 2) ***Rationale:*** The average age for menopause is 47 years. Menopause refers to the so-called change-of-life in women. The other responses would not be relevant to the symptoms the client reported. ***Nursing Process:*** Assessment ***Client Need:*** Physiological Integrity

6. ***Answer:*** 1 (Objective: 2) ***Rationale:*** Decreased metabolic and physical activity means a decrease in caloric need. The nurse should counsel clients about reducing caloric intake and exercising regularly. ***Nursing Process:*** Implementation ***Client Need:*** Health Promotion and Maintenance

7. ***Answer:*** 1 (Objective: 8) ***Rationale:*** According to Havighurst, achieving adult civic and social responsibility is a developmental milestone for middle-aged adults. Civic and social responsibility is not a developmental milestone for any of the other populations. ***Nursing Process:*** Assessment ***Client Need:*** Psychosocial Integrity

8. ***Answer:*** 2 (Objective: 8) ***Rationale:*** The young adult group has several psychosocial development tasks to meet, such as feeling independent from parents yet interacting well with the family. Young adults should like their lives and demonstrate emotional, social, and economic responsibility for their own lives. ***Nursing Process:*** Assessment ***Client Need:*** Psychosocial Integrity

9. ***Answer:*** 3 (Objective: 1) ***Rationale:*** Baby boomers were born from 1945 to 1964; Generation X individuals were born from 1965 to 1978; Generation Y individuals were born from 1979 to 2000; and boomerang kids are young adults who have returned home to live. ***Nursing Process:*** Assessment ***Client Need:*** Psychosocial Integrity

10. ***Answer:*** 1 (Objective: 3) ***Rationale:*** Generativity is concern for establishing and guiding the next generation. Ageism is discrimination against an individual based on the individual's age. Generation gap is the difference of opinions among various generations. Generativity is not the concern for one's own generation. ***Nursing Process:*** Assessment ***Client Need:*** Psychosocial Integrity

11. ***Answer:*** 1, 4, 5 (Objectives: 5 and 6) ***Rationale: According to Erikson, the middle-aged adult is in the generativity versus stagnation phase of Erikson's stages of development.*** . The middle-aged adult feels the need to achieve adult civic and social responsibility and is also adjusting to aging parents. ***The*** middle-aged adult has work as a central theme instead of leisure time activities. Kohlberg is a moral developmental theorist and that answer does not address the psychosocial development. ***Nursing Process:*** Assessment ***Client Needs:*** Psychosocial Integrity, Health Promotion and Maintenance

CHAPTER 23

Key Term Review

1.	q	2.	f	3.	u	4.	h	5.	s	6.	g
7.	i	8.	b	9.	w	10.	n	11.	o	12.	d
13.	t	14.	m	15.	e	16.	l	17.	y	18.	c
19.	x	20.	v	21.	r	22.	p	23.	k	24.	j
25.	a										

Key Topic Review Answers

1. With advancements in disease control, living conditions, and health technology, people are living longer.

2. older adult; young

3. Individuals 85 years and older are the fastest growing of all age groups in the country, numbering 4.6 million in 2002 and projected to reach 9.6 million by the year 2030.

4. a. 60; 74
   b. old; 75; 100
   c. 100

5. a. Reduce the proportion of older adults who have moderate to severe functional limitations.
   b. Increase the proportion of older adults with one or more chronic health conditions who report confidence in managing their conditions.

6. b. Disease often occurs with aging; however, it is not a guarantee and individuals may have "successful aging" in that the client will age without disease.

7. b. Ageism is a term used to describe negative attitudes toward aging or older adults.

8. a

9. Gerontology; Geriatrics

10. Gerontological nursing involves advocating for the health of older persons at all levels of prevention (<BIB>Mauk, 2014</BIB>). Practicing gerontological nurses can obtain gerontological nursing certification through the American Nurses Association. Advanced practice in gerontological nursing requires a master's degree in nursing, of which there are two options: the gerontological clinical nurse specialist and the gerontological nurse practitioner.

11. Long-term care facilities support clients and maintain their optimal level of functioning. Long-term care includes many different levels of care; e.g., assisted living, intermediate care, skilled care, and Alzheimer's units.

12. Many long-term care facilities offer specialized units for clients with Alzheimer's disease (AD), which is characterized by progressive dementia, memory loss, and inability to care for oneself. The gerontological nurses working in Alzheimer's units have specialized knowledge and help family members understand and cope with the disease process affecting their loved ones.

13. a. Humans, like automobiles, have vital parts that run down with time, leading to aging and death.
    b. The faster an organism lives, the quicker it dies.
    c. Cells wear out through exposure to internal and external stressors, including trauma, chemicals, and buildup of natural wastes.

Case Study Answers

1a. *What age category of the aging population is this client currently in?* The client belongs in the old-old age population.

1b. *What is the myth of aging that the client's children are subscribing to? What is the reality?* The myth is that older adults are depressed and should be allowed to withdraw from society. The reality of that myth is that only about one third of older adults exhibit depressive symptoms.

1c. *According to Erikson, what developmental task occurs at this phase?* The developmental task at this time is ego integrity versus despair.

Review Question Answers

1. ***Answer:*** 2 (Objective: 8) ***Rationale:*** By age 80, nearly all older adults have some lens opacity or cataracts that reduce visual acuity. Presbyopia is the inability to focus or accommodate due to loss of flexibility in the lens, causing a decrease in near vision. Presbycusis is vision loss, and glaucoma is a different visual concern. ***Nursing Process:*** Assessment ***Client Need:*** Physiological Integrity

2. ***Answer:*** 1, 3, 4, 5 (Objective: 15) ***Rationale:*** The working capacity of the heart diminishes with age. The heart rate at normal rest may decrease with age and is slower to respond to stress or after physical activity. There is reduced arterial elasticity in the arteries. Orthostatic hypotension may place the older adult client at risk for falls due to sudden changes in position. ***Nursing Process:*** Assessment ***Client Need:*** Physiological Integrity

3. ***Answer:*** 2 (Objective: 9) ***Rationale: The activity theory suggests that the best way to age healthily is to stay active physically and mentally.*** The disengagement theory states that older adults withdraw from others. The continuity theory states that individuals continue practicing their values, behaviors, and habitats in older age. The growth and development theory is not an aging theory. ***Nursing Process:*** Assessment ***Client Need:*** Psychosocial Integrity

4. ***Answer:*** 1 (Objective: 6) ***Rationale:*** Many nursing homes offer respite care for caregivers. Assisted living, adult day care , and home health care do not provide around-the-clock supervision and the type of assistance a client with Alzheimer's would need. ***Nursing Process:*** Planning ***Client Need:*** Safe, Effective Care Environment

5. ***Answer:*** 3 (Objective: 15) ***Rationale: Falls are the leading cause of morbidity and mortality among older adults (<BIB>Edelman & Mandle, 2010</BIB>, pg. 635). Motor vehicle crashes, drownings, and homicides are not the leading cause of morbidity and mortality among older adults. Nursing Process:*** Planning ***Client Need:*** Health Promotion and Maintenance

6. ***Answer:*** 4 (Objective: 2) ***Rationale:*** Older adults are the fastest growing population group in the United States today. All other responses are incorrect. ***Nursing Process:*** Assessment ***Client Need:*** Health Promotion and Maintenance

7. ***Answer:*** 2, 3 (Objective: 15) ***Rationale:*** Older adult mistreatment may affect either gender; however, the victims most often are women over 75 years of age, those with physical or mental impairments, and those who are dependent on care from the abuser. The abuse may involve physical, psychological, or emotional abuse; sexual abuse; financial abuse; violation of human or civil rights; and active or passive neglect. Others are beaten and even raped by family members. Most victims experience two or more forms of abuse. Older adult abuse or neglect may occur in private homes, senior citizens homes, nursing homes, hospitals, and long-term care facilities. ***Nursing Process:*** Assessment ***Client Need:*** Safe, Effective Care Environment

8. ***Answer:*** 1 (Objective: 15) ***Rationale:*** By increasing roughage and fluids in the diet, constipation may be prevented. The other answers do not take priority for this particular diagnosis. ***Nursing Process:*** Implementation ***Client Need:*** Physiological Integrity

9. ***Answer: 4*** (Objective: 7) ***Rationale:*** The endocrine theory states that the hypothalamus and pituitary are responsible for changes in hormone production and response, then the organism's decline. The idea that the faster an organism lives, the faster it dies is a proposal of the wear-and-tear theory. The genetic theory proposes that organisms are programmed for a predetermined number of cell divisions, after which the cells die. The immunologic theory suggests that the immune system declines with age. ***Nursing Process:*** Assessment ***Client Need:*** Physiological Integrity

10. ***Answer:*** 1, 2, 3, 5 (Objective: 16) ***Rationale:*** All of the measures listed except for removing the carpet and waxing the floors are measures to prevent falls. With aging comes the gradual reduction in the speed and power of skeletal or voluntary muscle contractions and sustained muscular effort. The client's reaction time slows with aging. ***Nursing Process:*** Implementation ***Client Need:*** Safe, Effective Care Environment

CHAPTER 24

Key Term Review

1. e 2. d 3. a

4. c 5. f 6. b

Key Topic Review Answers

1. family

2. system

3. systems theory

4. The purpose of a family assessment is to determine the level of family functioning, to clarify family interaction patterns, to identify family strengths and weaknesses, and to describe the health status of the family and its individual members.

5. affordable child care

6. genogram

7. 13; 10.5; 2.5

8. a. Child care concerns

   b. Financial concerns

   c. Role overload and fatigue in managing daily tasks,

   d. Social isolation

9. Feedback

10. structural–functional theory

Case Study Answers

1a. *What would be the best interventions by the nurse in this situation?* The nurse could attempt to talk with the client alone by sending her husband on an errand or insisting that he step out of the room while she is being examined, and then perform a thorough physical examination, attempting to ascertain the extent of the current injuries and also looking for any previous injuries (scarring, old bruising, prior injuries). The nurse needs to verbalize concerns to the health care provider so that he or she can evaluate for signs of abuse. The nurse could also place a small brochure about battered women's shelters within reach of the client so she might place the item in her purse or pocket.

1b. *What should the nurse be observing during the interactions between herself, the client, and the spouse?* Communications between all three individuals should be observed, including nonverbal communications.

Review Question Answers

1. ***Answer: 1,*** 3, 4 (Objective: 6) ***Rationale: Due to the mother's substance abuse, the family is experiencing interrupted family***

processes. The mother is demonstrating the inability to create, maintain, or regain an environment that promotes the optimum growth and development of children. The parent is also displaying caregiver role strain because she is having difficulty performing the family caregiver role. The scenario does not describe the mother as wanting or seeking care, so the diagnosis of *Readiness for Enhanced Family Coping* is not appropriate. ***Nursing Process:*** Diagnosis ***Client Need:*** Health Promotion and Maintenance

2. ***Answer:*** 2 (Objective: 5) ***Rationale:*** Individuals born into families with a history of certain diseases, such as diabetes or cardiovascular disease, are at greater risk of developing these conditions, due to hereditary factors. The other answer choices are factors that may lead to health problems; however, these are not the types of factors identified in the question. ***Nursing Process:*** Assessment ***Client Need:*** Health Promotion and Maintenance

3. ***Answer:*** 4 (Objective: 6) ***Rationale:*** Many diseases are preventable, the effects of some diseases can be minimized, or the onset of disease can be delayed through lifestyle modifications. The other answer choices are factors that may lead to health problems; however, these are not the types of factors identified in the question. ***Nursing Process:*** Assessment ***Client Need:*** Health Promotion and Maintenance

4. ***Answer:*** 3 (Objective: 2) ***Rationale:*** In this case, the grandparents live with and care for their grandchild, but the child's parents are not a part of this family. Foster families contain children who can no longer live with their birth parents and require placement with a family that has agreed to include them temporarily. Traditional families are viewed as an autonomous unit in which both parents reside in the home with their children, the mother often assuming the nurturing role and the father providing the necessary economic resources. Cohabiting (or communal) families consist of unrelated individuals or families who live under one roof. ***Nursing Process:*** Assessment ***Client Need:*** Health Promotion and Maintenance

5. ***Answer:*** 3 (Objective: 4) ***Rationale:*** Family assessment includes family structure, roles and functions, physical health status, interaction patterns, family values, and coping resources. When the nurse is observing the ways the family expresses affection, love, sorrow, and anger, the nurse is assessing the interaction patterns of the family. Family assessment gives an overview of the family process and helps the nurse identify areas that need further investigation. The purpose of family assessment is to determine the level of family functioning, clarify family interaction patterns, identify family strengths and weaknesses, and describe the health status of the family and its individual members. ***Nursing Process:*** Assessment ***Client Need:*** Psychosocial Integrity

6. ***Answer:*** 1 (Objective: 4) ***Rationale:*** Family assessment includes family structure, roles and functions, physical health status, interaction patterns, family values, and coping resources. When the nurse is evaluating how the family members handle stressful situations and conflicting goals, the concept of coping resources is being assessed. Family assessment gives an overview of the family process and helps the nurse identify areas that need further investigation. The purpose of family assessment is to determine the level of family functioning, clarify family interaction patterns, identify family strengths and weaknesses, and describe the health status of the family and its individual members. ***Nursing Process:*** Assessment ***Client Need:*** Psychosocial Integrity

7. ***Answer:*** 1 (Objective: 7) ***Rationale:*** Late manifestations of family violence often seen are depression, alcohol and substance abuse, and suicide attempts. Early symptoms are evident in burns, cuts, fractures, and even death. Nurses should be alert to the symptoms of family violence and take appropriate measures to report it and obtain resources for the family. ***Nursing Process:*** Assessment ***Client Need:*** Health Promotion and Maintenance

8. ***Answer:*** 2 (Objective: 6) ***Rationale:*** Nurses committed to family-centered care involve both the ailing individual and the family in the nursing process. Through their interaction with families, nurses can give support and information. Nurses make sure that not only the individual but also each family member understands the disease, its management, and the effect of these two factors on family functioning. The nurse will not leave out treatment information for the client. While the nurse will assess the treatment effects on the client, this does not represent family-centered care. Family-centered care does not involve discussing with the primary care provider how the treatment is affecting the family unit. ***Nursing Process:*** Assessment ***Client Need:*** Health Promotion and Maintenance

9. ***Answer:*** 4 (Objective: 4) ***Rationale:*** Nurses assess and plan health care for three types of clients: the individual, the family, and the community. The beliefs and values of each person and the support he or she receives come in large part from the family and are reinforced by the community. Thus, an understanding of family dynamics and the context of the community assists the nurse in planning care. When a family is the client, the nurse determines the health status of the family and its individual members, the level of family functioning, family interaction patterns, and family strengths and weaknesses. Political values are not an aspect of the family assessment. ***Nursing Process:*** Assessment ***Client Need:*** Health Promotion and Maintenance

10. ***Answer:*** 1, 3 (Objective: 6) ***Rationale:*** Hand washing and knowledge of personal hygiene are age-appropriate classes and this information will keep students from sharing illnesses with family members. Other topics are not age appropriate and these programs are best directed toward parents, rather than third graders. ***Nursing Process:*** Planning ***Client Need:*** Health Promotion and Maintenance

CHAPTER 25

Key Term Review

1. c 2. e 3. a 4. g

5. b 6. d 7. f

Key Topic Review Answers

1. Caring; central
2. a. Connection between individuals
   b. Mutual recognition
   c. Involvement of both client and nurse
3. a. Compassion,
   b. Competence
   c. Confidence
   d. Commitment
   e. Comportment
   f. Conscience
4. a
5. e
6. a
7. b
8. d
9. f
10. c
11. Aesthetic knowing
12. Personal knowing
13. Reflection
14. b. Caring in nursing always takes place in a relationship. Mutuality within this relationship involves a partnership between the nurse and client. This cannot be taught in nursing school.

Case Study Answers

1a. *What are two additional interventions the nurse may implement to provide comfort measures?* Any of the following are appropriate responses: (1) Turn every 2 hours while in bed if client is immobile; (2) offer fluids/refreshments every 2–4 hours unless contraindicated; (3) provide privacy to the client during care.

2a. *As a student nurse assigned to this client, which of the six C's of caring in nursing do you want to incorporate in your interventions?* You would want to incorporate compassion, competence, confidence, conscience, commitment, and comportment—all six of the six C's.

2b. *If you are using the caring processes from Swanson's theory of caring, on what five processes would you base your nursing interventions for this client?*The processes are knowing, being with, doing for, enabling, and maintaining belief.

2c. *What type of knowing would you demonstrate if you are observing and documenting phenomena as they occur in this case?* This would demonstrate empirical knowing—the science of nursing.

Review Question Answers

1. ***Answer:*** 4 (Objective: 2) ***Rationale:*** Leininger's theory of culture care diversity and universality is based on the assumption that nurses must understand different cultures in order to function effectively. Watson views caring as the moral ideal of nursing. Miller believes that caring validates the humanness of both client and caregiver. Swanson focuses on caring processes as nursing interventions. ***Nursing Process:*** Assessment ***Client Need:*** Safe, Effective Care Environment

2. ***Answer:*** 3 (Objective: 2) ***Rationale:*** Compassion is showing individuals that one cares. The nurse is sharing herself with the client. Nursing implementation and competence are not types of caring. The nurse's actions are not empowering the client. ***Nursing Process:*** Implementation ***Client Need:*** Safe, Effective Care Environment

3. ***Answer:*** 1, 2, 3, (Objective: 3) ***Rationale:*** Caring for self is defined as helping oneself grow and actualize one's possibilities and it means taking the time to nurture oneself. Eating a balanced diet, performing regular exercise, and obtaining adequate rest and sleep all help when caring for self. Taking medication is not an action that promotes caring for self. While hours per week may contribute to caring for self, an individual does not need to work part-time in order to care for self. ***Nursing Process:*** Assessment ***Client Need:*** Psychosocial Integrity

4. ***Answer:*** 1, 3, 4 (Objective: 5) ***Rationale:*** All of the responses are interventions to promote a healthier lifestyle, except for delaying

exercise. ***Nursing Process:*** Implementation ***Client Need:*** Health Promotion and Maintenance

5. ***Answer:*** 1 (Objective: 6) ***Rationale:*** Personal knowing is developed through critical reflection on one's actions and feelings in practice. The other choices are examples of ethical knowing, empirical knowing, and aesthetic knowing. ***Nursing Process:*** Evaluation ***Client Need:*** Physiological Adaptation

6. ***Answer:*** 2 (Objective: 1) ***Rationale:*** Physical presence combined with the promise of availability, especially at a time of need, demonstrates caring in the form of nursing presence. The other answer choices do not reflect the nurse's actions. ***Nursing Process:*** Implementation ***Client Need:*** Psychosocial Integrity

7. ***Answer:*** 3 (Objective: 4) ***Rationale:*** There are times when the nurse "enables" and "empowers" the client in order to enhance and encourage self-care. The other answer choices do not reflect the nurse's actions. ***Nursing Process:*** Implementation ***Client Need:*** Psychosocial Integrity

8. ***Answer:*** 1, 4 (Objective: 4) ***Rationale:*** The nurse demonstrates both competence and compassion by providing the actions listed in the question. The other answer choices do not reflect the nurse's actions. ***Nursing Process:*** Implementation ***Client Need:*** Safe, Effective Care Environment

9. ***Answer:*** 2 (Objective: 3) ***Rationale:*** Guided imagery uses the power of imagination as a therapeutic tool. Music therapy involves listening, singing, rhythm, and body movement. Yoga utilizes various postures and breathing practices to relax and tone the muscles and improve function of the internal organs. Storytelling assists individuals to move toward wholeness. ***Nursing Process:*** Implementation ***Client Need:*** Health Promotion and Maintenance

10. ***Answer:*** 1 (Objective: 1) ***Rationale:*** Caring means that people, relationships, and things matter. The nurse best demonstrates caring when holding and rocking an infant so the mother can rest quietly for a few hours after being up all night. The nurse will administer pain medications as the client needs them, not necessarily by schedule. Enforcing the hospital's visitations hours and performing the newborn assessment in a timely manner do not best demonstrate caring. ***Nursing Process:*** Implementation ***Client Need:*** Psychosocial Integrity

CHAPTER 26

Key Term Review

1. r 2. o 3. k 4. h 5. u 6. b

7. s 8. e 9. n 10. a 11. w 12. q

13. c 14. t 15. f 16. y 17. p 18. m

19. d 20. i 21. l 22. g 23. x 24. j

25. v

Key Topic Review Answers

1. In nursing, communication is a dynamic process used to gather assessment data, to teach and persuade, and to express caring and comfort. It is an integral part of the helping relationship.

2. c, d, e, f

3. a. Failure to listen

   b. Improperly decoding the client's intended message

   c. Placing the nurse's needs above the client's needs

4. a. Face the client squarely in an open posture.

   b. Lean into the client.

   c. Maintain good eye contact.

   d. Try to be relatively relaxed.

5. a, c, d

6. Elderspeak

7. congruent communication

8. a

9. Teaching groups impart information to the participants, whereas self-help groups are voluntary organizations composed of people who share similar health, social, or daily living problems.

Case Study Answers

1a. *What could the nurse do in order to create a more positive environment for the health interview?* Explaining what the client can expect with the health care provider visit, as well as answering any of the client's questions may help to reduce anxiety before proceeding with the interview. The nurse could make sure the interview and exam take place in a private and nonthreatening environment. Also, attentive listening could be used as well as open-ended questions.

1b. *If the nurse shares a similar experience with the client, then what communication technique is the nurse using?* The nurse is using the therapeutic communication of offering self by empathetic listening and responding to the client and of being genuine in her desire to place the client at ease.

1c. *What are three therapeutic responses the nurse could employ in this situation?* The nurse could use several therapeutic communication techniques such as offering self, giving information about procedures, acknowledging the client's apprehension, and using therapeutic touch.

Review Question Answers

1. ***Answer:*** 1 (Objective: 3) ***Rationale:*** Proxemics is the study of distance between people in their interactions. Intimate distance is 0 to 1.5 feet, such as observing a client's wound. While the other answer choices represent distances according to proxemics, these do not best describe the clinical scenario in the question. ***Nursing Process:*** Assessment ***Client Need:*** Safe, Effective Care Environment

2. ***Answer:*** 3 (Objective: 6) ***Rationale: The verbal message in this case is incongruent with the nonverbal message.*** The sender, receiver, and feedback are not the areas that are incongruent. ***Nursing Process:*** Assessment ***Client Need:*** Psychosocial Integrity

3. ***Answer:*** 2 (Objective: 3) ***Rationale:*** The nurse who is establishing an intravenous infusion is best demonstrating personal distance. The nurse who is positioning an immobile client is demonstrating intimate space. The nurse making rounds on all the clients in the unit is demonstrating social distance. Finally, the nurse who is speaking at a conference is demonstrating public distance. ***Nursing Process:*** Assessment ***Client Need:*** Psychological Integrity

4. ***Answer:*** 3 (Objective: 1) ***Rationale:*** Congruent communication is when the words and actions are focused in the same direction. Nonverbal communications are actions without verbal expression. Process recording is a word-for-word account of a conversation. Incongruent communication is when actions and words do not match or focus in the same direction. ***Nursing Process:*** Assessment ***Client Need:*** Psychosocial Integrity

5. ***Answer:*** 1 (Objective: 3) ***Rationale:*** For nurses, professional boundaries are crucial in the context of the nurse–client relationship. To keep clear boundaries, the nurse keeps the focus on the client and avoids sharing personal information or meeting his or her own needs through the nurse–client relationship. The nurse will demonstrate empathy, not sympathy. ***Nursing Process:*** Implementation ***Client Need:*** Psychosocial Integrity

6. ***Answer:*** 1, 3 (Objective: 6) ***Rationale:*** Using open-ended questions and restating or paraphrasing the client's comments are the most therapeutic communication techniques. The other answer choices are not therapeutic communication techniques. ***Nursing Process:*** Implementation ***Client Need:*** Psychosocial Integrity

7. ***Answer:*** 3 (Objective: 6) ***Rationale:*** There are situations when appropriate use of touch reinforces caring feelings. However, the nurse must be sensitive to the differences in attitudes and practices of clients and self. The other answers are not acceptable uses of touch. ***Nursing Process:*** Implementation ***Client Need:*** Psychosocial Integrity

8. ***Answer:*** 1 (Objective: 8) ***Rationale:*** During the initial parts of the introductory phase, the client may display some resistant behaviors that inhibit involvement, cooperation, or change. It may be because of difficulty in asking for assistance. All of the other answers are not correct. ***Nursing Process:*** Assessment ***Client Need:*** Psychosocial Integrity

9. ***Answer:*** 2 (Objective: 6) ***Rationale:*** The introductory phase includes a mutual nurse–client agreement about the overall purpose of the relationship. The other answer choices do not reflect this aspect of the helping relationship. ***Nursing Process:*** Planning ***Client Need:*** Safe, Effective Care Environment

10. ***Answer:*** 4 (Objective: 7) ***Rationale:*** While giving expert advice is therapeutic, giving common advice is nontherapeutic and acts as a barrier to communication. Common advice is telling the client what to do, denying the client the right to an equal partnership. The other answer choices do not reflect the scenario presented. ***Nursing Process:*** Implementation ***Client Need:*** Psychosocial Integrity

CHAPTER 27

Key Term Review

1.	l	2.	k	3.	q	4.	j	5.	r	6.	f
7.	n	8.	p	9.	o	10.	m	11.	i	12.	c
13.	s	14.	t	15.	b	16.	g	17.	d	18.	a
19.	h	20.	e								

Key Topic Review Answers

1. a

2. a

3. a

4. b. Active learning promotes critical thinking, enabling learners to problem solve more effectively. Also, listening to a lecture or watching a film is passive, not active learning.

5. a

6. E-health

7. anxiety

8. concepts

9. cultural

10. avoid

11. ___g_ The term used to describe the process involved in stimulating and helping elders to learn

___a___ A system of activities intended to produce learning

___i___ The art and science of teaching adults

___b___ A desire or a requirement to know something that is presently unknown to the learner

___f___ A change in human disposition or capability that persists and that cannot be solely accounted for by growth

___j___ A commitment or attachment to a regimen

___h___ The discipline concerned with helping children learn

___e___ The process by which a person learns by observing the behavior of others

___d___ Means to learn is the desire to learn

____c__ The process by which individuals copy or reproduce what they have observed

12. Andragogy

13. Cognitivism

14. psychomotor

15. a, b, c

16. a

Case Study Answers

1a. *How will you be able to determine if Ms. Whitman is ready to learn?* Readiness to learn is the demonstration of behaviors or cues that reflect the learner's motivation to learn at a specific time. Readiness reflects not only the desire or willingness to learn, but also the ability to learn at a specific time. For example, a client may want to learn self-care during a dressing change, but if the client experiences pain or discomfort, he or she may not be able to learn. The nurse can provide pain medication to make the client more comfortable and more able to learn. The nurse's role is often to encourage the development of readiness.

1b. *Identify three ways you could facilitate Ms. Whitman's learning.* Use of video or audio may help the client learn despite difficulty reading. Explaining to the client why the material is important to learn may help to supply motivation for learning. Reducing the client's anxiety by developing a trusting relationship with the nurse may also improve her ability to learn. Information should be presented in short quantities.

1c. *Discuss various teaching aids to help foster Ms Whitman's learning.*

- Keep language level at or below the fifth-grade level.
- Use active, not passive, voice.
- Use easy, common words of one or two syllables (e.g., *use* instead of *utilize* or *give* instead of *administer*).
- Use the second person (*you*) rather than the third person (*client*).
- Use a large type size (14 to 16 point).
- Write short sentences.
- Avoid using all capital letters.

Review Question Answers

1. ***Answer:*** 2 (Objective: 3) ***Rationale:*** Andragogy is the art and science of teaching adults. Geragogy is the term used to describe the process involved in stimulating and helping elders to learn. Pedagogy is the discipline concerned with helping children learn. Adherence is commitment or attachment to a regimen. ***Nursing Process:*** Assessment ***Client Need:*** Health Promotion and Maintenance

2. ***Answer:*** 1 (Objective: 2) ***Rationale:*** Modeling is the process by which an individual learns by observing the behavior of others. Imitation is the process by which individuals copy or reproduce what they have observed. Trial and error is the process of experimenting with various techniques until finding the best method. Positive reinforcement (e.g., a pleasant experience such as praise and encouragement) is fostering repetition of an action. ***Nursing Process:*** Planning ***Client Need:*** Health Promotion and Maintenance

3. ***Answer:*** 2 (Objective: 5) ***Rationale:*** Teaching a client how to self-administer insulin is in the psychomotor domain, one of Piaget's five major phases of cognitive development. The sensorimotor phase is the first of Piaget's cognitive development phases. This phase is from birth to age 2, and would not be used when teaching the client to self-administer insulin. The cognitive domain, the "thinking" domain, includes six intellectual abilities and thinking processes be-

ginning with knowing, comprehending, and applying to analysis, synthesis, and evaluation. The affective domain, known as the "feeling" domain, is divided into categories that specify the degree of a "person's depth of emotional response to tasks." ***Nursing Process:*** Assessment ***Client Need:*** Health Promotion and Maintenance

4. ***Answer:*** 1 (Objective: 4) ***Rationale:*** The nurse is applying the humanistic theory by encouraging the learner to establish goals and promote self-directed learning. The nurse would be applying cognitive theory when encouraging a positive teacher–learner relationship; providing a social, emotional, and physical environment conducive to learning; and selecting multisensory teaching strategies, because perception is influenced by the senses. ***Nursing Process:*** Implementation ***Client Need:*** Health Promotion and Maintenance

5. ***Answer:*** 3 (Objective: 1) ***Rationale:*** In teaching a client about heart disease who may need to know the effects of smoking before recognizing the need to stop smoking, motivation is the factor that can facilitate client learning. Readiness, active involvement, and allotted time are not the best choices for this clinical scenario. ***Nursing Process:*** Implementation ***Client Need:*** Health Promotion and Maintenance

6. ***Answer:*** ***1, 2,*** 3 (Objective: 6) ***Rationale:*** Fear, sensory deficits, and muscle weakness are barriers to learning. Chronic illness and medication use are not specific barriers to learning. ***Nursing Process:*** Assessment ***Client Need:*** Health Promotion and Maintenance

7. ***Answer:*** ***3,***4 (Objective: 8) ***Rationale:*** If the client displays a pattern of excuses for not reading the instructions, the nurse may have reason to suspect a literacy problem. A pattern of noncompliance in client behaviors may cause a nurse to suspect a literacy problem. A client reading the information slowly does not always indicate a literacy problem. A client insisting that he or she already knows the information could sometimes be an indication of a literacy problem. The client who is able to read the instructions but is unable to repeat the instructions in medical terms is not displaying a literacy problem. ***Nursing Process:*** Planning ***Client Need:*** Health Promotion and Maintenance

8. ***Answer:*** 2 (Objective: 9) ***Rationale:*** "The client selects low-fat foods from a menu" is a learning outcome for a teaching plan. Avoid using words such as *knows, understands, believes*, and *appreciates* because they are neither observable nor measurable. State the client (learner) behavior or performance, not the nurse behavior. The other answer choices are not correct. ***Nursing Process:*** Planning ***Client Need:*** Health Promotion and Maintenance

9. ***Answer:*** 4 (Objective: 7) ***Rationale:*** Sending a computer-generated billing statement to the client's home address is not part of e-health. E-health includes many aspects, such as online appointment access, e-mail access between the client and health care provider, and online health information. ***Nursing Process:*** Planning ***Client Need:*** Health Promotion and Maintenance

10. ***Answer:*** 4 (Objective: 1) ***Rationale: The sexual orientation is not an element in the nursing history that provides clues to learning needs.*** Several elements in the nursing history provide clues to learning needs: (a) age, (b) the client's understanding and perceptions of the health problem, (c) health beliefs and practices, (d) cultural factors, (e) economic factors, (f) learning style, and (g) the client's support systems. ***Nursing Process:*** Planning ***Client Need:*** Health Promotion and Maintenance

11. ***Answer:*** 1 (Objective 4) ***Rationale:*** Skinner introduced the concept of positive reinforcement. Imitation and modeling are concepts developed by Bandura. Behaviorism is a concept introduced by Thorndike. ***Nursing Process:*** Assessment ***Client Need:*** Psychosocial Integrity

12. ***Answer:*** 1, 3, 5 (Objective: 4) ***Rationale:*** Having the client write down information, giving handouts on the information, and having the client be active in the learning process all promote retention. Reading the information several times to the client does not promote retention, nor does speaking very slowly. ***Nursing Process:*** Implementation ***Client Need:*** Health Promotion and Maintenance

CHAPTER 28

Key Term Review

1. q 2. a 3. e 4. x 5. b 6. n

7. c 8. r 9. f 10. y 11. v 12. h

13. i 14. s 15. t 16. k 17. l 18. p

19. m 20. j 21. d 22. o 23. g 24. u

25. w

Key Topic Review Answers

1. a

2. b. The formal leader, or appointed leader, is selected by an organization and given official authority to make decisions and take action.

3. a

4. a

5. b. A manager is an employee of an organization who is given authority, power, and responsibility for planning, organizing, coordinating, and directing the work of others, and for establishing and evaluating standards.

6. democratic

7. laissez-faire

8. bureaucratic

9. situational

10. charismatic

11. Organizing

12. Authority

13. Networking

14. Efficiency

15. Delegation

Case Study Answers

1a. *Is Mr. Thomas assuming the role of a leader or manager?*
Mr. Thomas is assuming the role of a leader, as evidenced by the following: influencing others to work together to accomplish a specific goal and demonstrating initiative, ability, and confidence to innovate change, motivate, facilitate, and mentor others.

1b. *Compare and contrast the role of a leader and manager.* A leader influences others to work together to accomplish a specific goal. Leaders are often visionary; they are informed, articulate, confident, and self-aware. Leaders also usually have outstanding interpersonal skills and are excellent listeners and communicators.

Leaders have initiative, ability, and confidence to innovate change, motivate, facilitate, and mentor others. Within their organizations, nurse leaders participate in and guide teams that assess the effectiveness of care, implement evidence-based practice, and construct process improvement strategies. They may be employed in a variety of positions—from shift team leader to institutional president. Leaders may also hold volunteer positions such as chairperson of a professional organization or community board of directors.

A manager is an employee of an organization who is given authority, power, and responsibility for planning, organizing, coordinating, and directing the work of others, and for establishing and evaluating standards. Managers understand organizational structure and culture. They control human, financial, and material resources. Managers set goals, make decisions, and solve problems. They initiate and implement change.

1c. *What particular leadership style has Mr. Thomas developed?*
Mr. Thomas has developed a democratic (participative, consultative) leadership style. This type of leader encourages group discussion and decision-making. This type of leader acts as a catalyst or facilitator, actively guiding the group toward achieving group goals. Group productivity and satisfaction are high as group members contribute to the work effort. The democratic leader assumes individuals are internally motivated (their driving force is intrinsic; they desire self-satisfaction), capable of making decisions, and value independence. This leadership style can be extremely effective in the health care setting.

Review Question Answers

1. ***Answer:*** 3 (Objective: 1) ***Rationale:*** The democratic leadership style demands that the leader have faith in the group members to accomplish the goals. In the laissez-faire leadership style, the leader assumes a "hands-off" approach. Under the autocratic leadership style, the group may feel secure because procedures are well defined and activities are predictable. The bureaucratic leader does not trust self or others to make decisions and instead relies on the organization's rules, policies, and procedures to direct the group's work efforts. ***Nursing Process:*** Assessment ***Client Need:*** Safe, Effective Care Environment

2. ***Answer:*** 3 (Objective: 3) ***Rationale:*** A transformational leader fosters creativity, risk taking, commitment, and collaboration by empowering the group to share in the organization's vision. A charismatic leader is rare and is characterized by an emotional relationship with group members. The charming personality of the leader evokes strong feelings of commitment to both the leader and the leader's cause and beliefs. The transactional leader has a relationship with followers based on an exchange for some resource valued by the follower. These incentives are used to promote loyalty and performance. Shared leadership recognizes that a professional workforce is made up of many leaders. No one individual is considered to have knowledge or ability beyond that of other members of the work group. ***Nursing Process:*** Assessment ***Client Need:*** Safe, Effective Care Environment

3. ***Answer:*** 3 (Objective: 5) ***Rationale:*** Upper-level (top-level) managers are organizational executives who are primarily responsible for establishing goals and developing strategic plans. First-level managers are responsible for managing the work of nonmanagerial personnel and the day-to-day activities of a specific work group or groups. Middle-level managers supervise a number of first-level managers and are responsible for the activities in the departments they supervise. Middle-level managers serve as liaisons between first-level managers and upper-level managers. They may be called supervisors, nurse managers, or head nurses. Supervising managers are not a category of organizational executives. ***Nursing Process:*** Assessment ***Client Need:*** Safe, Effective Care Environment

4. ***Answer:*** 1 (Objective: 4) ***Rationale:*** The management principle being demonstrated is accountability. Accountability is the ability and

willingness to assume responsibility for one's actions and to accept the consequences of one's behavior. Authority is defined as the legitimate right to direct the work of others. It is an integral component of managing. Responsibility is an obligation to complete a task. Coordinating is the process of ensuring that plans are carried out and evaluating outcomes. ***Nursing Process:*** Assessment ***Client Need:*** Safe, Effective Care Environment

5. ***Answer:*** 4 (Objective: 11) ***Rationale:*** Planned change is an intended, purposeful attempt by an individual, group, organization, or larger social system to influence its own current status. Unplanned change is an alteration imposed by external events or persons; it occurs when unexpected events force a reaction. It is usually haphazard, and the results can be unpredictable. Drift is a type of unplanned change in which change occurs without effort on anyone's part. Natural, or situational, change also may be considered unplanned and occurs without any control by the person or group impacted. ***Nursing Process:*** Assessment ***Client Need:*** Safe, Effective Care Environment

6. ***Answer:*** 1 (Objective: 2) ***Rationale:*** The leader role influences others toward goal setting, either formally or informally. The manager role carries out predetermined policies, rules, and regulations; maintains an orderly, controlled, rational, and equitable structure; relates to people according to their roles; and feels rewarded when fulfilling the organizational mission or goals. ***Nursing Process:*** Planning ***Client Need:*** Safe, Effective Care Environment

7. ***Answer:*** 2 (Objective: 10) ***Rationale:*** The nurse who is initiating, motivating, and implementing change is acting in the role of change agent. The other answer choices do not apply to this nursing role. ***Nursing Process:*** Assessment ***Client Need:*** Safe, Effective Care Environment

8. ***Answer:*** 3 (Objective: 11) ***Rationale:*** Perception that the change will improve the situation is considered a driving force. Restraining forces include low tolerance for change related to intellectual or emotional insecurity; misunderstanding of the change and its implications; and lack of time or energy. ***Nursing Process:*** Assessment ***Client Need:*** Safe, Effective Care Environment

9. ***Answer:*** 2 (Objective: 7) ***Rationale:*** Guidelines for dealing with resistance to change include the following: Emphasize the positive consequences of the change and how the individual or group will benefit. Clarify information and provide accurate information. Maintain a climate of trust, support, and confidence. Communicate with those who oppose the change. Get to the root of their reasons for opposition. ***Nursing Process:*** Planning ***Client Need:*** Safe, Effective Care Environment

10. ***Answer: 1,*** 2, 3, 4 (Objective: 1) ***Rationale:*** The situational leader flexes task and relationship behaviors, considers the staff members' abilities, knows the nature of the task to be done, and is sensitive to the context or environment in which the task takes place. The transactional leader has a relationship with followers based on an exchange for some resource valued by the follower. ***Nursing Process:*** Assessment ***Client Need:*** Safe, Effective Care Environment

CHAPTER 29

Key Term Review

1. g 2. i 3. b 4. m 5. n 6. c

7. l 8. f 9. v 10. k 11. e 12. w

13. r 14. d 15. s 16. h 17. u 18. y

19. t 20. x 21. q 22. o 23. j 24. p

25. a

Key Topic Review Answers

1. b 2. a 3. a 4. b 5. b 6. b

7. Vital signs

8. exhaustion

9. Compliance

10. deficit

11. Hypothermia

12. i, e, a, c, h, g, f, d, b

13. d

14. b

15. c

16. a

17. c

Case Study Answers

1. *What are the normal vital signs for a 20-year-old male client?*
A typical blood pressure for a healthy adult is 120/80 mmHg (pulse pressure of 40).

Oral temperature = 37°C (98.6°F)

Pulse average (range) = 80 beats/min (60–100 beats/min)

Respiration average (range) = 16/min (12–20/min)

2. *What type of fever is the client most likely experiencing?* A temperature that rises to fever level rapidly following a normal temperature and then returns to normal within a few hours is called a fever spike.

3. *Why has the doctor ordered blood work?* A temperature that rises to fever level rapidly following a normal temperature and then returns to normal within a few hours is called a fever spike. Bacterial blood infections often cause fever spikes.

Review Question Answers

1. ***Answer:*** 1 (Objective: 1) ***Rationale:*** Conduction is the transfer of heat from one molecule to a molecule of lower temperature. Radiation is the transfer of heat from the surface of one object to the surface of another without contact between the two objects, mostly in the form of infrared rays. Vaporization is continuous evaporation of moisture from the respiratory tract and from the mucosa of the mouth and from the skin. Convection is the dispersion of heat by air currents. ***Nursing Process:*** Assessment ***Client Need:*** Physiological Integrity

2. ***Answer:*** 1 (Objective: 3) ***Rationale:*** With intermittent fever, the body temperature alternates at regular intervals between periods of fever and periods of normal or subnormal temperatures. During a remittent fever such as with a cold or influenza, a wide range of temperature fluctuations (more than 2°C [3.6°F]) occurs over the 24-hour period, all of which are above normal. In a relapsing fever, short febrile periods of a few days are interspersed with periods of 1 or 2 days of normal temperature. During a constant fever, the body temperature fluctuates minimally but always remains above normal. ***Nursing Process:*** Assessment ***Client Need:*** Physiological Integrity

3. ***Answer:*** 3 (Objective: 4) ***Rationale:*** Individuals experiencing heatstroke generally have been exercising in hot weather, have warm, flushed skin, and often do not sweat. They usually have a temperature of 41°C (106°F) or higher, and may be delirious, unconscious, or having seizures. Hypothermia is a core body temperature below the lower limit of normal. Heat exhaustion is a result of excessive heat and dehydration. Signs of heat exhaustion include paleness, dizziness, nausea, vomiting, fainting, and a moderately increased temperature (38.3–38.9°C [101–102°F]). A blood pressure that is persistently above normal is a condition called hypertension. ***Nursing Process:*** Assessment ***Client Need:*** Physiological Integrity

4. ***Answer:*** 4 (Objective: 3) ***Rationale:*** When the Celsius reading is 40:

$$F = (40 \times 9/5) + 32 = (72) + 32 = 104$$

Nursing Process: Assessment ***Client Need:*** Physiological Integrity

5. ***Answer:*** 1 (Objective: 5) ***Rationale:*** The posterior tibial site is on the medial surface of the ankle where the posterior tibial artery passes behind the medial malleolus. The popliteal site is where the popliteal artery passes behind the knee. The femoral site is where the femoral artery passes along side the inguinal ligament. The radial site is where the radial artery runs along the radial bone, on the thumb side of the inner aspect of the wrist. ***Nursing Process:*** Assessment ***Client Need:*** Physiological Integrity

6. ***Answer:*** 3 (Objective: 12) ***Rationale:*** Having the arm above the level of the heart can cause an erroneously low blood pressure result. Having the cuff wrapped too loosely or unevenly, having the bladder cuff too narrow, and assessing immediately after a meal or while the client smokes or has pain can cause an erroneously high blood pressure result. ***Nursing Process:*** Implementation ***Client Need:*** Physiological Integrity

7. ***Answer:*** 3 (Objective: 3) ***Rationale:*** Pull the pinna straight back and upward for children over age 3. Pull the pinna slightly downward and backward for an adult patient. Insert the probe slowly using a circular motion until snug. Point the probe slightly anteriorly, toward the eardrum. Presence of cerumen can affect the reading. ***Nursing Process:*** Implementation ***Client Need:*** Physiological Integrity

8. ***Answer:*** 4 (Objective: 9) ***Rationale:*** Dyspnea, not stridor, is difficult and labored breathing during which the individual has a persistent, unsatisfied need for air and feels distressed. Stridor is a shrill, harsh sound heard during inspiration with laryngeal obstruction. Stertor is a snoring or sonorous respiration, usually due to a partial obstruction of the upper airway. Wheeze is a continuous, high-pitched musical squeak or whistling sound occurring on expiration and sometimes on inspiration when air moves through a narrowed or partially obstructed airway. Bubbling is a gurgling sound heard as air passes through moist secretions in the respiratory tract. ***Nursing Process:***Assessment ***Client Need:*** Physiological Integrity

9. ***Answer:*** 1 (Objective: 9) ***Rationale:*** Hemoptysis is the presence of blood in the sputum. Productive cough is a cough accompanied by expectorated secretions. Nonproductive cough is a dry, harsh cough without secretions. Orthopnea is the ability to breathe only in upright sitting or standing positions. ***Nursing Process:*** Planning ***Client Need:*** Physiological Integrity

10. ***Answer:*** 4 (Objective: 11) ***Rationale:*** Phase 1—The pressure level at which the first faint, clear tapping or thumping sounds are heard. These sounds gradually become more intense. The first tapping sound heard during deflation of the cuff is the systolic blood pressure. Phase 2—The period during deflation when the sounds have a muffled, whooshing, or swishing quality. Phase 4—The time when

the sounds become muffled and have a soft, blowing quality. Phase 5—The pressure level when the last sound is heard. Nursing Process: Evaluation ***Client Need:*** Physiological Integrity

CHAPTER 30

Key Term Review

1. k 2. t 3. b 4. r 5. j 6. p

7. h 8. v 9. f 10. g 11. m 12. w

13. s 14. q 15. c 16. x 17. d 18. a

19. u 20. y 21. i 22. o 23. n 24. l

25. e

Key Topic Review Answers

1. a

2. b. Palpation is the examination of the body using the sense of touch.

3. a

4. a

5. b. Percussion is the act of striking the body surface to elicit sounds that can be heard or vibrations that can be felt.

6. Bruit

7. aphasia

8. reflex

9. hernia

10. Discrimination

11. ___i___ The process of listening to sounds produced within the body

___h___ Nearsightedness

___j__ Loss of elasticity of the lens and thus loss of ability to see close objects

___d__ An uneven curvature of the cornea that prevents horizontal and vertical rays from focusing on the retina; is a common problem that may occur in conjunction with myopia and hyperopia

__f______ A disturbance in the circulation of aqueous fluid, which causes an increase in intraocular pressure; is the most frequent cause of blindness in people over age 40

___g___ Constricted pupils that may indicate an inflammation of the iris or result from such drugs as morphine or pilocarpine

___b___ An instrument for examining the interior of the ear, especially the eardrum, consisting essentially of a magnifying lens and a light

___e_____ A part of the middle ear that connects the middle ear to the nasopharynx

___c___ Earwax that lubricates and protects the canal

___a___ Farsightedness

12. b

13. d

14. d

15. c

16. c

Case Study Answers

1a. *Discuss the purposes of the physical examination.* Some of the purposes of the physical examination are to:

- Obtain baseline data about the client's functional abilities.
- Supplement, confirm, or refute data obtained in the nursing history.
- Obtain data that will help establish nursing diagnoses and plans of care.
- Evaluate the physiological outcomes of health care and thus the progress of a client's health problem.
- Make clinical judgments about a client's health status.
- Identify areas for health promotion and disease prevention.

1b. *Several client positions are frequently required during the physical assessment. List six client positions used during the physical assessment and provide a description of each one.*

Dorsal recumbent: back-lying position with knees flexed and hips externally rotated; small pillow under the head; soles of feet on the surface

Supine (horizontal recumbent): back-lying position with legs extended; with or without pillow under the head

Sitting: a seated position; back unsupported and legs hanging freely

Lithotomy: back-lying position with feet supported in stirrups; the hips should be in line with the edge of the table

Sims: side-lying position with lowermost arm behind the body, uppermost leg flexed at hip and knee, upper arm flexed at shoulder and elbow

Prone: lying on abdomen with head turned to the side, with or without a small pillow

1c. *List the equipment and supplies used for a health examination.*

Flashlight or penlight

Nasal speculum

Ophthalmoscope

Otoscope

Percussion (reflex) hammer

Tuning fork

Vaginal speculum

Cotton applicators

Gloves

Lubricant

Tongue blades (depressors)

Review Question Answers

1. ***Answer:*** 1, 2, 3, 4 (Objective: 1) ***Rationale:*** The following statements would be correct responses by the nurse regarding purposes for a physical examination:

"To obtain baseline data about a client's functional abilities."

"To obtain data that will help establish nursing diagnoses and plans of care."

"To identify areas for health promotion and disease prevention."

"To supplement, confirm, or refute data obtained in the nursing history."

Implementing appropriate, individualized care is an important aspect of the nursing process; however, this is achieved in the implementation phase, after the assessment of the client.

Nursing Process: Assessment ***Client Need:*** Physiological Integrity

2. ***Answer:*** 4 (Objective: 2) ***Rationale:*** Auscultation is the process of listening to sounds produced within the body. Inspection is the visual examination—that is, assessing by using the sense of sight. Palpation is the examination of the body using the sense of touch. Percussion is the act of striking the body surface to elicit sounds that can be heard or vibrations that can be felt. ***Nursing Process:*** Assessment ***Client Need:*** Physiological Integrity

3. ***Answer:*** 3 (Objective: 3) ***Rationale:*** Jaundice (a yellowish tinge) may first be evident in the sclera of the eyes and then in the mucous membranes and the skin. Pallor is the result of inadequate circulating blood or hemoglobin and subsequent reduction in tissue oxygenation. Cyanosis (a bluish tinge) is most evident in the nail beds, lips, and buccal mucosa. Cyanosis is the result of tissue hypoxia. Erythema is a redness associated with a variety of rashes. ***Nursing Process:*** Assessment ***Client Need:*** Physiological Integrity

4. ***Answer:*** 1 (Objective: 3) ***Rationale:*** Myopia means nearsightedness; hyperopia means farsightedness; presbyopia means loss of elasticity of the lens and thus loss of ability to see close objects; and stigmatism means an uneven curvature of the cornea that prevents horizontal and vertical rays from focusing on the retina. ***Nursing Process:*** Assessment ***Client Need:*** Physiological Integrity

5. ***Answer:*** 2 (Objective: 3) ***Rationale:*** Sound transmission and hearing are complex processes. In brief, sound can be transmitted by air conduction or bone conduction. Air-conducted transmission occurs by this process:

- A sound stimulus enters the external canal and reaches the tympanic membrane.
- The sound waves vibrate the tympanic membrane and reach the ossicles.
- The sound waves travel from the ossicles to the opening in the inner ear (oval window).
- The cochlea receives the sound vibrations.
- The stimulus travels to the auditory nerve (the eighth cranial nerve) and the cerebral cortex.

Nursing Process: Assessment ***Client Need:*** Physiological Integrity

6. ***Answer:*** 4 (Objective: 3) ***Rationale:*** The left hypochondriac, not lumbar, region includes the stomach, the spleen, the tail of the pancreas, the splenic flexure of the colon, the upper half of the left kidney, and the suprarenal gland. The epigastric region includes the aorta, the pyloric end of the stomach, part of the duodenum, and the pancreas. The umbilical region includes the omentum, the mesentery, the lower part of the duodenum, and part of the jejunum and ileum. The right lumbar region includes the ascending colon, the lower half of the right kidney, and part of the duodenum and jejunum. ***Nursing Process:*** Assessment ***Client Need:*** Physiological Integrity

7. ***Answer:*** 2 (Objective: 5) ***Rationale:*** Cranial nerve II, not IV, is assessed by asking the client to read a Snellen-type chart. Cranial nerve I is assessed by asking the client to close his/her eyes and identify different mild aromas, such as coffee, vanilla, peanut but-

ter, orange/lemon, or chocolate. Cranial nerve VI is assessed by observing the client's directions of gaze. Cranial nerve VII is assessed by asking the client to smile, raise the eyebrows, frown, puff out cheeks, close eyes tightly. ***Nursing Process:*** Assessment ***Client Need:*** Physiological Integrity

8. ***Answer:*** 1 (Objective: 3) ***Rationale:***

A friction rub is a superficial grating or creaking sounds heard during inspiration and expiration; this is not relieved by coughing. Crackles (rales) are fine, short, interrupted crackling sounds; alveolar rales are high pitched. Their sound can be simulated by rolling a lock of hair near the ear. Crackles are best heard on inspiration, but can be heard on both inspiration and expiration. Crackles may not be cleared by coughing. A wheeze is a continuous, high-pitched, squeaky musical sound. This is best heard on expiration and is not usually altered by coughing. Gurgles (rhonchi) are continuous, low-pitched, coarse, gurgling, harsh, louder sounds with a moaning or snoring quality. Rhonchi is best heard on expiration, but can be heard on both inspiration and expiration. Rhonchi may be altered by coughing. ***Nursing Process:*** Assessment ***Client Need:*** Physiological Integrity

9. ***Answer:*** 3 (Objective: 4) ***Rationale:***

The lithotomy position is used for assessing the female genitals, rectum, and female reproductive tract. The prone position is used for assessing the posterior thorax and hip joint movement. The supine position is used for assessing the head, neck, axillae, anterior thorax, lungs, breasts, heart, vital signs, heart, abdomen, extremities, and peripheral pulses. The sitting position is used for assessing the head, neck, posterior and anterior thorax, lungs, breasts, axillae, heart, vital signs, upper and lower extremities, and reflexes. ***Nursing Process:*** Assessment ***Client Need:*** Physiological Integrity

10. ***Answer:*** 2 (Objective: 4) ***Rationale:*** Assessment of peripheral perfusion of toes, capillary blanch test, pedal pulse if able, and vital signs is most appropriate for a client who has a cast to the lower extremity. This type of assessment assesses the neurovascular patency of the client's lower extremity. Assessment of tissue turgor as well as input and output is most appropriate for the client with alterations to fluid volume. While assessment of apical pulse is an important nursing assessment, this is not the most important assessment after a new cast is applied to an extremity. Assessment of neurovascular patency is more important. Assessment of the client's level of consciousness is also an important assessment; however, this is not the most important assessment after a new cast is applied to an extremity. Assessment of neurovascular patency is more important.

Nursing Process: Assessment ***Client Need:*** Physiological Integrity

CHAPTER 31

Key Term Review

1. s 2. n 3. a 4. b 5. v 6. f

7. h 8. i 9. e 10. c 11. j 12. k

13. m 14. y 15. w 16. o 17. p 18. q

19. r 20. g 21. l 22. t 23. d 24. u

25. x

Key Topic Review Answers

1. b. An infection is an invasion of body tissue by microorganisms and their growth within that tissue.

2. a

3. a

4. b. Surgical asepsis, or sterile technique, refers to those practices that keep an area or object free of all microorganisms; it includes practices that destroy all microorganisms and spores (microscopic dormant structures formed by some pathogens that are very hardy and often survive common cleaning techniques). Surgical asepsis is used for all procedures involving the sterile areas of the body.

5. a

6. communicable

7. opportunistic

8. Asepsis

9. Bacteria

10. dirty

11. _____j__ Consist primarily of nucleic acid and therefore must enter living cells in order to reproduce

_____h_____ Include yeasts and molds

_____f__ Live on other living organisms

____d__ The process by which strains of microorganisms become resident flora ___b___ The direct result of diagnostic or therapeutic procedures

___i___ A person or animal reservoir of a specific infectious agent that usually does not manifest any clinical signs of disease

___a___ Any substance that serves as an intermediate means to transport and introduces an infectious agent into a susceptible host through a suitable portal of entry

___g___ An animal or flying or crawling insect that serves as an intermediate means of transporting the infectious agent

__c____ A person at increased risk, an individual who for one or more reasons is more likely than others to acquire an infection

___e___ Protect the person against all microorganisms, regardless of prior exposure

12. d

13. b

14. c

15. a

16. b

Case Study Answers

1a. *What is the difference between asepsis and sepsis, and between medical asepsis and surgical asepsis?* Asepsis is the freedom from disease-causing microorganisms. To decrease the possibility of transferring microorganisms from one place to another, aseptic technique is used. There are two basic types of asepsis: medical and surgical. Medical asepsis includes all practices intended to confine a specific microorganism to a specific area, limiting the number, growth, and transmission of microorganisms. In medical asepsis, objects are referred to as clean, which means the absence of almost all microorganisms, or dirty (soiled, contaminated), which means likely to have microorganisms, some of which may be capable of causing infection. Surgical asepsis, or sterile technique, refers to those practices that keep an area or object free of all microorganisms; it includes practices that destroy all microorganisms and spores (microscopic dormant structures formed by some pathogens that are very hardy and often survive common cleaning techniques). Surgical asepsis is used for all procedures involving the sterile areas of the body. Sepsis is a state of infection and can take many forms, including septic shock.

1b. *What four major categories of microorganisms cause infection in humans?* Four major categories of microorganisms cause infection in humans: bacteria, viruses, fungi, and parasites. Bacteria are by far the most common infection-causing microorganisms. Several hundred species can cause disease in humans and can live and be transported through air, water, food, soil, body tissues and fluids, and inanimate objects. Most of the microorganisms listed in Table 31–1 in the text are bacteria. Viruses consist primarily of nucleic acid and therefore must enter living cells in order to reproduce. Common virus families include the rhinovirus (causes the common cold), hepatitis, herpes, and human immunodeficiency (HIV) virus. Fungi include yeasts and molds. *Candida albicans* is a yeast considered to be normal flora in the human vagina. Parasites live on other living organisms. They include protozoa such as the one that causes malaria, helminths (worms), and arthropods (mites, fleas, ticks).

1c. *Explain the difference between standard precautions and transmission-based precautions.* Standard precautions: These precautions are used in the care of all hospitalized persons regardless of their diagnosis or possible infection status. They apply to blood, all body fluids, secretions, excretions except sweat (whether or not blood is present or visible), nonintact skin, and mucous membranes. Thus they combine the major features of UP and BSI.

Transmission-based precautions: These precautions are used in addition to standard precautions for clients with known or suspected infections that are spread in one of three ways: by airborne or droplet transmission, or by contact. The three types of transmission-based precautions may be used alone or in combination but always in addition to standard precautions. They encompass all of the conditions or diseases previously listed in the category-specific or disease-specific classifications developed by the CDC in 1983.

Review Question Answers

1. ***Answer:*** 2 (Objective: 1) ***Rationale:*** Asepsis is the freedom from disease-causing microorganisms. Medical asepsis includes all practices intended to confine a specific microorganism to a specific area, limiting the number, growth, and transmission of microorganisms. Surgical asepsis, or sterile technique, refers to those practices that keep an area or object free of all microorganisms; it includes practices that destroy all microorganisms and spores (microscopic dormant structures formed by some pathogens that are very hardy and often survive common cleaning techniques). Sepsis is a state of infection and can take many forms, including septic shock. ***Nursing Process:*** Assessment ***Client Need:*** Physiological Integrity

2. ***Answer:*** 3 (Objective: 1) ***Rationale:*** Viruses consist primarily of nucleic acid and therefore must enter living cells in order to reproduce. Fungi include yeasts and molds. Bacteria are by far the most common infection-causing microorganisms. Parasites live on other living organisms. ***Nursing Process:*** Assessment ***Client Need:*** Physiological Integrity

3. ***Answer:*** 4 (Objective: 3) ***Rationale:*** Fatigue is not a sign of inflammation. Inflammation is a local and nonspecific defensive response of the tissues to an injurious or infectious agent. It is an adaptive mechanism that destroys or dilutes the injurious agent,

prevents further spread of the injury, and promotes the repair of damaged tissue. It is characterized by five signs: (a) pain, (b) swelling, (c) redness, (d) heat, and (e) impaired function of the part, if the injury is severe. ***Nursing Process:*** Assessment ***Client Need:*** Physiological Integrity

4. ***Answer:*** 4 (Objective: 8) ***Rationale:*** Boiling water: This is the most practical and inexpensive method for sterilizing in the home. The main disadvantage is that spores and some viruses are not killed by this method. Boiling a minimum of 15 minutes is advised for disinfection of articles in the home. Gas: Ethylene oxide gas destroys microorganisms by interfering with their metabolic processes. It is also effective against spores. Its advantages are good penetration and effectiveness for heat-sensitive items. Its major disadvantage is its toxicity to humans. Moist heat: To sterilize with moist heat (such as with an autoclave), steam under pressure is used because it attains temperatures higher than the boiling point. Radiation: Both ionizing (such as alpha, beta, and x-rays) and nonionizing (ultraviolet light) radiation are used for disinfection and sterilization. The main drawback to ultraviolet light is that the rays do not penetrate deeply. Ionizing radiation is used effectively in industry to sterilize foods, drugs, and other items that are sensitive to heat. Its main advantage is that it is effective for items difficult to sterilize; its chief disadvantage is that the equipment is very expensive. ***Nursing Process:*** Assessment ***Client Need:*** Physiological Integrity

5. ***Answer:*** 3 (Objective: 6) ***Rationale:*** Acute infections generally appear suddenly or last a short time. A chronic infection may occur slowly, over a very long period, and may last months or years. A local infection is limited to the specific part of the body where the microorganisms remain. In a systemic infection, the microorganisms spread and damage different parts of the body. Nosocomial infections are classified as infections that are associated with the delivery of health care services in a health care facility. ***Nursing Process:*** Assessment ***Client Need:*** Physiological Integrity

6. ***Answer:*** 3 (Objective: 9) ***Rationale:*** Six links make up the chain of infection: the etiologic agent, or microorganism; the place where the organism naturally resides (reservoir); a portal of exit from the reservoir; a method (mode) of transmission; a portal of entry into a host; and the susceptibility of the host. ***Nursing Process:*** Planning ***Client Need:*** Physiological Integrity

7. ***Answer:*** 2 (Objective: 4) ***Rationale:*** An antigen is a substance that induces a state of sensitivity or immune responsiveness (immunity). With active immunity, the host produces antibodies in response to natural antigens (e.g., infectious microorganisms) or artificial antigens (e.g., vaccines). With passive (or acquired) immunity, the host receives natural (e.g., from a nursing mother) or artificial (e.g., from an injection of immune serum) antibodies produced by another source. Antibodies, also called immunoglobulins, are part of the body's plasma proteins. ***Nursing Process:*** Assessment ***Client Need:*** Physiological Integrity

8. ***Answer:*** 1 (Objective: 11) ***Rationale:*** The CDC recommends antimicrobial hand cleansing agents in the following situations:

   - When there are known multiple resistant bacteria
   - Before invasive procedures
   - In special care units, such as nurseries and ICUs
   - Before caring for severely immunocompromised clients

   Nursing Process: Assessment ***Client Need:*** Physiological Integrity

9. ***Answer:*** 3 (Objective: 11) ***Rationale:*** Disinfectants and antiseptics often have similar chemical components, but the disinfectant is a more concentrated solution. A disinfectant is a chemical preparation, such as phenol or iodine compounds, used on inanimate objects. Disinfectants are frequently caustic and toxic to tissues. An antiseptic is a chemical preparation used on skin or tissue. A disinfectant is an agent that destroys pathogens other than spores. ***Nursing Process:*** Assessment ***Client Need:*** Physiological Integrity

10. ***Answer:*** 2 (Objective: 10) ***Rationale:*** Droplet precautions are used for clients known or suspected to have serious illnesses transmitted by particle droplets larger than 5 microns. Airborne precautions are used for clients known to have or suspected of having serious illnesses transmitted by airborne droplet nuclei smaller than 5 microns. Contact precautions are used for clients known or suspected to have serious illnesses easily transmitted by direct client contact or by contact with items in the client's environment. Connection precautions do not exist. ***Nursing Process:*** Assessment ***Client Need:*** Physiological Integrity

CHAPTER 32

Key Term Review

1. g 2. k 3. i 4. l 5. a 6. c
7. e 8. b 9. m 10. f 11. h 12. j
13. d

Key Topic Review Answers

1. a

2. b. Restraints are never used for staff convenience or client punishment.

3. a

4. b. Partial seizures (also called focal) involve electrical discharges from one area of the brain.

5. a

6. Terrorism

7. homicide

8. scald

9. Radiation

10. Risk

11. ______h______ An intentional attack using weapons of viruses, bacteria, and other infectious agents

______f______ A bed or chair ________ has a position-sensitive switch that triggers an audio alarm when the client attempts to get out of the bed or chair

______a______ A sudden onset of excessive electrical discharges in one or more areas of the brain

______i______ Safety measures taken by the nurse to protect clients from injury should they have a seizure

______j______ An odorless, colorless, tasteless gas that is very toxic

______b______ Suffocation, or ________, is lack of oxygen due to interrupted breathing

____g____ The emergency response is the ________, or abdominal thrust, which can dislodge the foreign object and reestablish an airway

____e____ Protective devices used to limit the physical activity of the client or a part of the body

____c____ Occurs when a current travels through the body to the ground rather than through electric wiring, or from static electricity that builds up on the body

____d____ Medications such as neuroleptics, anxiolytics, sedatives, and psychotropic agents used to control socially disruptive behavior.

12. c

13. b

14. d

15. d

16. c

Case Study Answers

1a. *What preventive measures do you need to teach the couple?*

- Keep emergency numbers near the telephone, or stored for speed dialing.
- Be sure to install smoke alarms that are operable and appropriately located.
- Change the batteries in smoke alarms annually on a special day, such as a birthday or January 1.
- Have a family "fire drill" plan. Every member needs to know the plan for the nearest exit from different locations of the home.
- Keep fire extinguishers available and in working order.
- Close windows and doors if possible; cover the mouth and nose with a damp cloth when exiting through a smoke-filled area; and avoid heavy smoke by assuming a bent position with the head as close to the floor as possible.

1b. *Explain the three categories of fires.*

Class A: paper, wood, upholstery, rags, ordinary rubbish

Class B: flammable liquids and gases

Class C: electrical

Review Question Answers

1. ***Answer:*** 1, 3 (Objective: 3) ***Rationale:*** The 2014 National Patient Safety Goals (NPSGs) include a goal to improve accuracy of patient information. Aspects of this goal include using at least two patient identifiers when providing care, treatment, and services; and eliminating transfusion errors related to patient misidentification. The other answer choices are appropriate goals of the NPSGs, however, these are not aspects of the goal to improve patient information. ***Nursing Process:*** Planning ***Client Need:*** Safe, Effective Care Environment

2. ***Answer:*** 4 (Objective: 4) ***Rationale:*** A common accident during infancy is suffocation. Trash bags or any type of plastic bag must be kept out of an infant's reach. All of the other responses by the parent are correct in preventing safety hazards in children. ***Nursing Process:*** Evaluation ***Client Need:*** Safe, Effective Care Environment

3. ***Answer:*** 2 (Objective: 4) ***Rationale:*** Obtaining a driver's license is an important event in the life of a U.S. adolescent, but the privilege is not always wisely handled. Teenagers may use driving as an outlet for stress, as a way to assert independence, or as a way to impress peers. When setting limits on automobile use, parents need to assess the teenager's level of responsibility, common sense, and ability to resist peer pressure. The age of the teenager alone does not determine readiness to handle this responsibility.

Adolescents have better coordination skills than toddlers. It is not necessary for an adolescent to sleep in a low bed. Lead poisoning (plumbism) is a risk for children exposed to lead paint chips, fumes from leaded gasoline, or any "leaded" substances. The ingestion of lead-based paint chips is the most common cause of lead poisoning in children, not adolescents. Adolescents would need safety training about driving an automobile, not a tricycle. ***Nursing Process:*** Planning ***Client Need:*** Safe, Effective Care Environment

4. ***Answer:*** 2 (Objective: 4) ***Rationale:*** Suicide and homicide are two leading causes of death among teenagers. Adolescent males commit suicide at a higher rate than adolescent females, and African Americans commit homicide at a higher rate than European Americans. Strong emotions towards friendships may be positive or negative and do not directly increase the rate of suicide among teenagers. Suicides by firearms, drugs, and automobile exhaust gases are the most common. Factors influencing the high suicide and homicide rates include economic deprivation, family breakup, and the availability of firearms, which are the most frequently used weapons. ***Nursing Process:*** Planning ***Client Need:*** Psychosocial Integrity

5. ***Answer:*** 1 (Objective: 4) ***Rationale:*** Accidents are the leading cause of death in school-age children. Natural disasters are not one of the leading causes of death among school-age children. The most frequent causes of fatalities, in descending order, are motor vehicle crashes, drownings, fires, and firearms. School-age children are also involved in many minor accidents, frequently resulting from outdoor activities and recreational equipment such as swings, bicycles, skateboards, and swimming pools. ***Nursing Process:*** Implementation ***Client Need:*** Health Promotion and Maintenance

6. ***Answer:*** 3, 4 (Objective: 7) ***Rationale:*** Falls are the leading cause of accidents among older adults. They are also a major cause of hospital and nursing home admissions. Most falls occur in the home and are a major threat to the independence of older adults. Suicide is a leading cause of death among teenagers and older adults. The incidence of suicide in older adults is increasing and often goes unnoticed when the causes are due to hidden self-destructive behaviors, such as starvation, overdosing with medications, and noncompliance with medical care, treatments, and medications. In older individuals, the suicide attempt is usually more serious, because it is truly intended to end the life, not just to get attention as is often seen in other age groups. Also, the method of suicide is generally more violent in the older person, such as a gunshot wound to the head, or hanging. Natural disasters are not the leading cause of death among older adults. ***Nursing Process:*** Planning ***Client Need:*** Health Promotion and Maintenance

7. ***Answer:*** 2 (Objective: 2) ***Rationale:*** During the nursing assessment, all of the following should be assessed: the behavior indicating the possible need for a restraint; underlying cause for assessed behavior; other protective measures that may be implemented before applying a restraint; status of skin to which restraint is to be applied; circulatory status distal to restraints and of extremities; effectiveness of other available safety precautions. ***Nursing Process:*** Assessment ***Client Need:*** Safe, Effective Care Environment

8. ***Answer:*** 1 (Objective: 6) ***Rationale:*** Avoid storing toxic liquids or solids in food containers, such as soft drink bottles, peanut butter jars, or milk cartons. Display the phone number of the poison control center near or on all telephones in the home so that it is available to babysitters, family, and friends. Teach children never to eat any part of an unknown plant or mushroom and not to put leaves, stems, bark, seeds, nuts, or berries from any plant into their mouths. Do not refer to medicine as candy or pretend false enjoyment when taking medications in front of children; allow them to see the necessity of the medicine without glamorizing it. ***Nursing Process:*** Evaluation ***Client Need:*** Safe, Effective Care Environment

9. ***Answer:*** 1 (Objective: 8) ***Rationale:*** If clients have frequent or recurrent seizures or take anticonvulsant medications, they should wear a medical identification tag (bracelet or necklace) and carry a card delineating any medications they take. Assist the client in determining which persons in the community should/must be informed of their seizure disorder (e.g., employers, health care providers such as dentists, motor vehicle department if driving, companions). Discuss safety precautions for inside and out of the home. If seizures are not well controlled, activities that may require restriction or direct supervision by others include tub bathing, swimming, cooking, using electric equipment or machinery, and driving. Discuss with the client and family factors that may precipitate a seizure. ***Nursing Process:*** Planning ***Client Need:*** Safe, Effective Care Environment

10. ***Answer:*** 3 (Objective: 6) ***Rationale:*** All of the following would be a preventive measure for an older client with poor vision: ensuring eyeglasses are functional, ensuring appropriate lighting, marking doorways and edges of steps as needed, and keeping the environment tidy. ***Nursing Process:*** Planning ***Client Need:*** Safe, Effective Care Environment

CHAPTER 33

Key Term Review

1. y	2. d	3. m	4. u	5. s	6. e
7. h	8. b	9. v	10. j	11. n	12. l
13. o	14. c	15. p	16. i	17. t	18. f
19. w	20. q	21. r	22. a	23. g	24. k
25. x					

Key Topic Review Answers

1. a

2. b. Most dentists recommend that dental hygiene should begin when the first tooth erupts and be practiced after each feeding.

3. a

4. a

5. b. Water used for the shampoo should be 40.5°C (105°F) for an adult or child to be comfortable and not injure the scalp.

6. Pediculosis

7. Scabies

8. hirsutism

9. Lanugo

10. Plaque

11. ___h___ Personal ______ is the self-care by which people attend to such functions as bathing, toileting, general body hygiene, and grooming

    _____i_____ Are on all body surfaces except the lips and parts of the genitals

    _____d___ The ________, located largely in the axillae and anogenital areas, begin to function at puberty under the influence of androgens

    _____c_____ Given for physical effects, such as to soothe irritated skin or to treat an area (e.g., the perineum)

    ____e____ Thickened portion of epidermis, a mass of keratotic material

    ____j__A keratosis caused by friction and pressure from a shoe

    _____f____ Deep grooves that frequently occur between the toes as a result of dryness and cracking of the skin

    ____a____ Athlete's foot, or ________ (ringworm of the foot), is caused by a fungus

    ____b____ The growing inward of the nail into the soft tissues around it; most often results from improper nail trimming

    ____g____ A visible, hard deposit of plaque and dead bacteria that forms at the gum lines

12. a

13. b

14. b

15. c

16. c

Case Study Answers

1a. *What is the proper water temperature for the client's bath?* The temperature of the bath water should be between 43°C and 46°C (110°C and 115°F).

1b. *List two reasons why a nurse should check the temperature of the bath water.* The nurse must check the water temperature to avoid burning the client with water that is too hot. The water for a bath should be changed when it becomes dirty or cold.

1c. *Why is it important to verify the temperature of the water for this client?* Clients with decreased cognitive problems will not be able to verify the temperature.

Review Question Answers

1. ***Answer:*** 2, 3, 5 (Objective: 10) ***Rationale:*** When stripping and making the client's bed, it is important to avoid shaking soiled linen in the air because shaking can disseminate secretions and excretions and the microorganisms they contain. When stripping and making a bed, the nurse can conserve time and energy by stripping and making up one side as much as possible before working on the other side. The nurse should raise the bed to a comfortable working height when stripping and making the bed to avoid back strain. To avoid contamination from soiled linens, the nurse should avoid holding the linens close to his or her uniform, and should never place linens on another client's bed. ***Nursing Process:*** Implementation ***Client Need:*** Safe, Effective Care Environment

2. ***Answer:*** 3 (Objective: 6) ***Rationale:*** The water for a bath should feel comfortably warm to the client. People vary in their sensitivity to heat. The bath water temperature is generally included in the order; 37.7°C to 46°C (100°F to 115°F) may be ordered for adults. All other bath water temperatures listed are too cold or too hot. ***Nursing Process:*** Implementation ***Client Need:*** Physiological Integrity

3. ***Answer:*** 1 (Objective: 1) ***Rationale:*** Dental caries occur frequently during the toddler period, often as a result of the excessive intake of sweets or prolonged use of the bottle during naps and at bedtime. The nurse should give parents the following

instructions to promote and maintain dental health: Beginning at about 18 months of age, brush the child's teeth with a soft toothbrush. Use only a toothbrush moistened with water at first and introduce toothpaste later. Use one that contains fluoride. Give a fluoride supplement daily or as recommended by the physician or dentist, unless the drinking water is fluoridated. Schedule an initial dental visit for the child at about 2 or 3 years of age or as soon as all 20 primary teeth have erupted. Some dentists recommend an inspection type of visit when the child is about 18 months old to provide an early pleasant introduction to the dental examination. Seek professional dental attention for any problems such as discoloring of the teeth, chipping, or signs of infection such as redness and swelling. ***Nursing Process:*** Evaluation ***Client Need:*** Health Promotion and Maintenance

4. ***Answer:*** 1 (Objective: 4) ***Rationale:*** During discharge planning for preventing dry skin the nurse should review the following with the client: Use cleansing creams to clean the skin rather than soap or detergent, which cause drying and, in some cases, allergic reactions. Use bath oils, but take precautions to prevent falls caused by slippery tub surfaces. Humidify the air with a humidifier or by keeping a tub or sink full of water. Use moisturizing or emollient creams that contain lanolin, petroleum jelly, or cocoa butter to retain skin moisture. ***Nursing Process:*** Implementation ***Client Need:*** Safe, Effective Care Environment

5. ***Answer:*** 1 (Objective: 4) ***Rationale:*** While washing the feet, the nurse should inspect the skin of the feet for breaks or red or swollen areas. Use a mirror if needed to visualize all areas. The nurse should cover the feet—except between the toes—with creams or lotions to moisten the skin. Lotion will also soften calluses. A lotion that reduces dryness effectively is a mixture of lanolin and mineral oil. When providing foot care for a client, the nurse should check the water temperature before immersing the feet to prevent any burns. The nurse should wash the feet daily, and dry them well, especially between the toes. ***Nursing Process:*** Implementation ***Client Need:*** Physiological Integrity

6. ***Answer:*** 4 (Objective: 4) ***Rationale:*** The client's nail should be cut or filed straight across beyond the end of the finger or toe. Healthy nail care practices are reflected in clean, short nails with smooth edges and intact cuticles. The client should avoid trimming or digging into nails at the lateral corners. This predisposes the client to ingrown toenails. ***Nursing Process:*** Evaluation ***Client Need:*** Physiological Integrity

7. ***Answer:*** 4 (Objective: 7) ***Rationale:*** The nurse must evaluate the client's understanding of measures to prevent tooth decay. Brushing the teeth thoroughly after meals and at bedtime, flossing the teeth daily, avoiding sweet foods and drinks between meals, and having a checkup by a dentist every 6 months are just some of the measures that must be understood by the client. ***Nursing Process:*** Evaluation ***Client Need:*** Physiological Integrity

8. ***Answer:*** 4 (Objective: 7) ***Rationale:*** The student nurse should perform all of the following when shaving a client with a safety razor: The student nurse holds the skin taut, particularly around creases, to prevent cutting the skin. The student nurse wears gloves in case facial nicks occur and she comes in contact with blood. The student nurse applies shaving cream or soap and water to soften the bristles and make the skin more pliable. The student nurse holds the razor so that the blade is at a 45° angle to the skin, and shaves in short, firm strokes in the direction of hair growth. ***Nursing Process:*** Implementation ***Client Need:*** Safe, Effective Care Environment

9. ***Answer:*** 1 (Objective: 6) ***Rationale:*** Appropriate actions must be followed by the nurse bathing a person with dementia. The following are just a few of the actions that must be followed: Move slowly and let the person know when you are going to move him or her. Use a supportive, calm approach and praise the person often. Gather everything that you will need for the bath (e.g., towels, washcloths, clothes) before approaching the person. Help the person feel in control. ***Nursing Process:*** Implementation ***Client Need:*** Physiological Integrity

10. ***Answer:*** 2 (Objective: 10) ***Rationale:*** Before a nurse inserts a hearing aid into a patient's ear it is very important to perform the following steps: Determine from the client if the earmold is for the left or the right ear. Gently press the earmold into the ear while rotating it backward. Inspect the earmold to identify the ear canal portion. Check that the earmold fits snugly by asking the client if it feels secure and comfortable. ***Nursing Process:*** Implementation ***Client Need:*** Physiological Integrity

CHAPTER 34

Key Term Review

1. u	2. h	3. w	4. v	5. r	6. d
7. s	8. i	9. c	10. k	11. q	12. a
13. m	14. t	15. b	16. x	17. p	18. l
19. n	20. j	21. g	22. f	23. c	24. o
25. y					

Key Topic Review Answers

1. a

2. a

3. b. Decreased RBC counts are indicative of anemia.

4. a

5. a

6. organisms

7. biopsy

8. manometer

9. Aspiration

10. Hematocrit

11. ___a___ A person from a laboratory who performs venipuncture to collect a blood specimen for the ordered by a physician

_____e_____ The number of RBCs per cubic millimeter of whole blood

_____c_____ The main intracellular protein of erythrocytes

___f___ Produced in relatively constant quantities by the muscles and is excreted by the kidneys

___h___ Substance used in a chemical reaction to detect a specific substance

___i___ A measure of the solute concentration of urine and a more exact measurement of urine concentration than specific gravity

___j___ An indicator of urine concentration, or the amount of solutes (metabolic wastes and electrolytes) present in the urine

___g___ A measure of the solute concentration of the blood

___d___ Measures the percentage of red blood cells in the total blood volume

___b___ Includes hemoglobin and hematocrit measurements, erythrocyte (RBC) count, leukocyte (WBC) count, red blood cell (RBC) indices, and a differential white cell count

12. c

13. a

14. b

15. d

16. c

Case Study Answers

1a. *Why did the health care provider order sputum specimens?* The health care provider ordered an AFB to identify the presence of tuberculosis (TB).

1b. *How will you collect the sputum specimens?* To collect a sputum specimen, the nurse follows these steps:

- Offer mouth care so that the specimen will not be contaminated with microorganisms from the mouth.
- Ask the client to breathe deeply and then cough up 1 to 2 tablespoons, or 15 to 30 mL (4 to 8 fluid drams), of sputum.
- Ask the client to expectorate (spit out) the sputum into the specimen container. Make sure the sputum does not contact the outside of the container. If the outside of the container does become contaminated, wash it with a disinfectant.
- Following sputum collection, offer mouthwash to remove any unpleasant taste.

1c. *What PPE should you wear when you collect the sputum specimens?* Wear gloves and PPE to avoid direct contact with the sputum. Follow special precautions if tuberculosis is suspected, obtaining the specimen in a room equipped with a special airflow system or ultraviolet light, or outdoors. If these options are not available, wear a mask capable of filtering droplet nuclei.

1d. *What information should you document in the client medical record after collecting the sputum specimens?* Document the collection of the sputum specimens on the client's chart. Include the amount, color, odor, and consistency (thick, tenacious, watery) of the sputum, the presence of hemoptysis (blood in the sputum), any measures needed to obtain the specimen (e.g., postural drainage), and any discomfort experienced by the client.

1e. *How should the specimens be stored until they are transported to the laboratory?* Ensure that the specimen labels and the laboratory requisitions contain the correct information. Arrange for the specimens to be sent to the laboratory immediately or refrigerated. Bacterial cultures must be started immediately before any contaminating organisms can grow, multiply, and produce false results.

Review Question Answers

1. ***Answer:*** 3 (Objective: 2) ***Rationale:*** The normal hematocrit finding for an adult female is 36%–46%. The normal hemoglobin finding for an adult female is 12–16 g/dL. The normal RBC finding for an adult female is 4.1–5.1 million/mm^3. The normal MCV finding for an adult female is 78–102 μm^3. ***Nursing Process:*** Assessment ***Client Need:*** Physiological Integrity

2. ***Answer:*** 2 (Objective: 2) ***Rationale:*** The normal potassium serum level is 3.5–5.0 mEq/L. The normal sodium serum level is 135–145 mEq/L. The normal chloride level is 95–105 mEq/L. The normal magnesium level is 1.5–2.5 mEq/L or 1.6–2.5 mg/dL. ***Nursing Process:*** Assessment ***Client Need:*** Physiological Integrity

3. ***Answer:*** 1 (Objective: 2) ***Rationale:*** The normal hematocrit level for an adult male is 37%–49%. The normal hemoglobin level for an adult male is 13.8–18 g/dL. ***Nursing Process:*** Assessment ***Client Need:*** Physiological Integrity

4. ***Answer:*** 3 (Objective: 7) ***Rationale:*** For a male client, using a circular motion to clean the urinary meatus is the correct technique. For a female client, the perineal area should be cleaned from front to back. Always explain to the client that a urine specimen is required, give the reason, and explain the method to be used to collect it. A nurse should always perform hand hygiene and observe other appropriate infection control procedures. The nurse must ensure that the specimen label is attached to the specimen cup, not the lid, and that the laboratory requisition provides the correct information. ***Nursing Process:*** Implementation ***Client Need:*** Physiological Integrity

5. ***Answer:*** 2 (Objective: 11) ***Rationale:*** A bone marrow biopsy is the removal of a specimen of bone marrow for laboratory study. The biopsy is used to detect specific diseases of the blood, such as pernicious anemia and leukemia. The bones of the body commonly used for a bone marrow biopsy are the sternum, iliac crests, anterior or posterior iliac spines, and proximal tibia in children. The posterior superior iliac crest is the preferred site with the client placed prone or on the side. The knee–chest, lithotomy, and dorsal recumbent positions are incorrect positions for a bone marrow biopsy. ***Nursing Process:*** Implementation ***Client Need:*** Physiological Integrity

6. ***Answer:*** 4 (Objective: 11) ***Rationale:*** Assist the client to a dorsal recumbent position with only one head pillow. The client remains in this position for 1 to 12 hours, depending on the health care provider's orders. The knee–chest, lithotomy, and prone positions are incorrect positions for recovery after a lumbar puncture. ***Nursing Process:*** Implementation ***Client Need:*** Physiological Integrity

7. ***Answer:*** 3 (Objective: 11) ***Rationale:*** After a client returns from a thoracentesis the nurse should have the client lie on the unaffected side with the head of the bed elevated 30 degrees for at least 30 minutes because this position facilitates expansion of the affected lung and eases respirations. If the head of bed is elevated at a position other than 30 degrees, the client will not have ease of respiration and will not achieve proper expansion of the lungs. ***Nursing Process:*** Implementation ***Client Need:*** Physiological Integrity

8. ***Answer:*** 1 (Objective: 11) ***Rationale:*** An abdominal paracentesis is carried out to obtain a fluid specimen for laboratory study and to relieve pressure on the abdominal organs due to the presence of excess fluid. A health care provider performs the procedure with the assistance of a nurse. Strict sterile technique is followed. Normally about 1,500 mL is the maximum amount of fluid drained at one time to avoid hypovolemic shock. The fluid is drained very slowly for the same reason. ***Nursing Process:*** Implementation ***Client Need:*** Physiological Integrity

9. ***Answer:*** 1 (Objective: 4) ***Rationale:*** Taking the sample from the center of a formed stool to ensure a uniform sample is a correct technique for a fecal occult blood test. Using a ballpoint pen to label the specimens with your name, address, age, and date of specimen is a correct technique for a fecal occult blood test. Avoiding contamination of the specimen with urine or toilet tissue is a correct technique for a fecal occult blood test. The nurse should state "Avoid collecting specimens during your menstrual period and for 3 days afterward, and while you have bleeding hemorrhoids or blood in your urine." Either of these situations would give a false positive to the fecal occult blood tests. ***Nursing Process:*** Implementation ***Client Need:*** Physiological Integrity

10. ***Answer:*** 2 (Objective: 8) ***Rationale:*** Sterile gloves are not necessary for obtaining a throat culture. Wearing sterile gloves during this procedure is considered an unnecessary expense. To obtain a throat culture specimen, the nurse puts on clean gloves, then inserts the swab into the oropharynx and runs the swab along the tonsils and areas on the pharynx that are reddened or contain exudate. The gag reflex, active in some clients, may be decreased by having the client sit upright if health permits, open the mouth, extend the tongue, and say "ah," and by taking the specimen quickly. The sitting position and extension of the tongue help expose the pharynx; saying "ah" relaxes the throat muscles and helps minimize contraction of the constrictor muscle of the pharynx (the gag reflex). If the posterior pharynx cannot be seen, use a light and depress the tongue with a tongue blade. ***Nursing Process:*** Implementation ***Client Need:*** Physiological Integrity

CHAPTER 35

Key Term Review

1. j	2. a	3. g	4. t	5. b	6. c
7. h	8. d	9. l	10. e	11. f	12. i
13. k	14. m	15. n	16. o	17. r	18. p
19. q	20. u	21. v	22. w	23. s	24. x
25. y					

Key Topic Review Answers

1. b. Medications may have natural (e.g., plant, mineral, and animal) sources, or they must be synthesized in the laboratory.

2. a

3. a

4. b. The action of a drug in the body can be described in terms of its half-life, the time interval required for the body's elimination processes to reduce the concentration of the drug in the body by 50%.

5. b. Oral administration is the most common, least expensive, and most convenient route for most clients.

6. eyes

7. intramuscular

8. vial

9. bevel

10. plunger

11. _____a_____ The written direction for the preparation and administration of a drug

_____d_____ A drug's name given by the drug manufacturer

_____e_____ The study of the effect of drugs on living organisms

_____g_____ A book containing a list of products used in medicine, with descriptions of the product, chemical tests for determining identity and purity, and formulas and prescriptions

____i____ A secondary effect of a drug, one that is unintended

_____j_____ Deleterious effects of a drug on an organism or tissue that results from overdosage, ingestion of a drug intended for external use, and buildup of the drug in the blood because of impaired metabolism or excretion (cumulative effect)

_____h_____ The _______ of a drug, also referred to as the desired effect, is the primary effect intended, that is, the reason the drug is prescribed.

____f____ The art of preparing, compounding, and dispensing drugs

_____c_____ Given before a drug officially becomes an approved medication

_____b_____ A substance administered for the diagnosis, cure, treatment, or relief of a symptom or for prevention of disease.

12. b

13. d

14. d

15. a

16. c

Case Study Answers

1a. *What are the 10 "rights" of medication administration?*

1. Right medication
2. Right dose
3. Right time
4. Right route
5. Right client
6. Right client education
7. Right documentation
8. Right to refuse
9. Right assessment
10. Right evaluation

1b. *The Compazine is available in an ampule. How will you properly prepare the Compazine from the ampule?*

a. Check the label on the ampule carefully against the MAR to make sure that the correct medication is being prepared.

b. Perform drug calculations as necessary to determine amount of medication to prepare.

c. Follow the three checks for administering medications: Read the label on the medication (1) when it is taken from the medication cart, (2) before withdrawing the medication, and (3) after withdrawing the medication.

d. Organize the equipment.

e. Perform hand hygiene and observe other appropriate infection control procedures.

f. Flick the upper stem of the ampule several times with a fingernail.

g. Use an ampule opener or place a piece of sterile gauze or alcohol wipe between your thumb and the ampule neck or around the ampule neck, and break off the top by bending it toward you to ensure the ampule is broken away from yourself and away from others or place the antiseptic wipe packet over the top of the ampule before breaking off the top.

h. Dispose of the top of the ampule in the sharps container.

i. Place the ampule on a flat surface.

j. Attach the filter needle/straw to the syringe.

k. Remove the cap from the filter needle and insert the needle into the center of the ampule. Do not touch the rim of the ampule with the needle tip or shaft.

l. With a single-dose ampule, hold the ampule slightly on its side, if necessary, to obtain more than the ordered amount of medication.

m. Dispose of the filter needle by placing it in a sharps container.

n. Replace the filter needle with a regular needle, tighten the cap at the hub of the needle, and push solution into the needle, to the prescribed amount.

1c. *Describe the process of administering Compazine by intramuscular injection.*

a. Check the label on the medication carefully against the MAR to make sure that the correct medication is being prepared.

b. Follow the three checks for administering the medication and dose: Read the label on the medication (1) when it is taken from the medication cart, (2) before withdrawing the medication, and (3) after withdrawing the medication.

c. Confirm that the dose is correct.

d. Perform hand hygiene and observe other appropriate infection control procedures (e.g., clean gloves).

e. Provide for client privacy.

f. Prior to performing the procedure, introduce self and verify the client's identity using agency protocol.

g. Assist the client to a supine, lateral, prone, or sitting position, depending on the chosen site. If the target muscle is the gluteus medius (ventrogluteal site), have the client in the supine position flex the knee(s); in the lateral position, flex the upper leg; and in the prone position, toe in.

h. Obtain assistance in immobilizing an uncooperative client.

i. Explain the purpose of the medication and how it will help, using language that the client can understand. Include relevant information about effects of the medication.

j. Select a site free of skin lesions, tenderness, swelling, hardness, or localized inflammation and one that has not been used frequently.

k. If injections are to be frequent, alternate sites. Avoid using the same site twice in a row.

l. Locate the exact site for the injection.

m. Apply clean gloves.

n. Clean the site with an antiseptic swab using circular motions and beginning in the center moving about 5 cm outward.

o. Transfer and hold the swab between the third and fourth fingers of your nondominant hand in readiness for needle withdrawal, or position the swab on the client's skin above the intended site. Allow skin to dry prior to injecting medication.

p. Remove the needle cover and discard without contaminating the needle.

q. Use the ulnar side of the nondominant hand to pull the skin approximately 2.5 cm (1 in.) to the side. Under some circumstances, such as for an emaciated client or an infant, the muscle may be pinched.

r. Holding the syringe between the thumb and forefinger (as if holding a pen), pierce the skin quickly and smoothly at a 90° angle, in a dart-like motion, and insert the needle into the muscle.

s. Hold the barrel of the syringe steady with your nondominant hand and aspirate by pulling back on the plunger with your dominant hand. Aspirate for 5 to 10 seconds. If blood appears in the syringe, withdraw the needle, discard the syringe, and prepare a new injection.

t. If blood does not appear, inject the medication steadily and slowly (approximately 10 seconds per milliliter) while holding the syringe steady.

u. After injection, wait 10 seconds to permit the medication to disperse into the muscle tissue, thus decreasing the client's discomfort.

v. Withdraw the needle smoothly at the same angle of insertion.

w. Apply gentle pressure at the site with a dry sponge.

x. It is not necessary to massage the area at the site of injection.

y. If bleeding occurs, apply pressure with a dry sterile gauze until it stops.

z. Activate the needle safety device or discard the uncapped needle and attached syringe into the proper receptacle.

aa. Remove and dispose of gloves. Perform hand hygiene.

bb. Document all relevant information. Include the time of administration, drug name, dose, route, and the client's reactions.

cc. Assess effectiveness of the medication at the time it is expected to act.

Review Question Answers

1. ***Answer:*** 1 (Objective: 16) ***Rationale:*** The type of syringe used for subcutaneous injections depends on the medication to be given. Generally a 2-mL syringe is used for most subcutaneous injections. Needle sizes and lengths are selected based on the client's

body mass, the intended angle of insertion, and the planned site. Generally a #25-gauge, 5/8-inch needle is used for adults of normal weight and the needle is inserted at a 45° angle; a 3/8-inch needle is used at a 90° angle. A child may need a 1/2-inch needle inserted at a 45° angle. One method nurses use to determine length of needle is to pinch the tissue at the site and select a needle length that is half the width of the skinfold. To determine the angle of insertion, a general rule to follow relates to the amount of tissue that can be bunched or grasped at the site. A 45° angle is used when 1 inch of tissue can be grasped at the site; a 90° angle is used when 2 inches of tissue can be grasped. ***Nursing Process:*** Implementation ***Client Need:*** Physiological Integrity

2. ***Answer:*** 1 (Objective: 1) ***Rationale:*** A drug that produces the same type of response as the physiological or endogenous substance is called an agonist. Conversely, a drug that inhibits cell function by occupying receptor sites is called an antagonist. The antagonist prevents natural body substances or other drugs from activating the functions of the cell by occupying the receptor sites. A receptor, usually a protein, is located on the surface of a cell membrane or within the cell. A cell membrane contains receptors for physiological or endogenous substances such as hormones and neurotransmitters. Biotransformation, also called detoxification or metabolism, is a process by which a drug is converted to a less active form. Most biotransformation takes place in the liver, where many drug-metabolizing enzymes in the cells detoxify the drugs. ***Nursing Process:*** Assessment ***Client Need:*** Physiological Integrity

3. ***Answer:*** 2 (Objective: 3) ***Rationale:*** Drug habituation denotes a mild form of psychological dependence. The individual develops the habit of taking the substance and feels better after taking it. The habituated individual tends to continue the habit even though it may be injurious to health. Drug dependence is a person's reliance on or need to take a drug or substance. The two types of dependence, physiological and psychological, may occur separately or together. Physiological dependence is due to biochemical changes in body tissues, especially the nervous system. These tissues come to require the substance for normal functioning. A dependent person who stops using the drug experiences withdrawal symptoms. Psychological dependence is emotional reliance on a drug to maintain a sense of well-being, accompanied by feelings of need or cravings for that drug. There are varying degrees of psychological dependence, ranging from mild desire to craving and compulsive use of the drug. ***Nursing Process:*** Planning ***Client Need:*** Psychosocial Integrity

4. ***Answer:*** 2 (Objective: 7) ***Rationale:*** When converting pounds to kilograms: The pound is a smaller unit than the kilogram, and the nurse converts by dividing or multiplying by 2.2:

$$2.2 \text{ lb} = 1 \text{ kg}$$

$$110 \text{ lb} = x \text{ kg}$$

$$2.2 \text{ lb} = 1 \text{ kg}$$

$$110 \text{ lb} = x \text{ kg}$$

$$x = \frac{110 \times 1}{2.2}$$

$$= 50 \text{ kg}$$

Any other amount listed is incorrect. ***Nursing Process:*** Implementation ***Client Need:*** Physiological Integrity

5. ***Answer:*** 1 (Objective: 7) ***Rationale:*** Erythromycin 500 mg is ordered. It is supplied in a liquid form containing 250 mg in 5 mL. To calculate the dosage, the nurse uses the formula

$$\frac{\text{Dose on hand (250 mg)}}{\text{Quantity on hand (5 mL)}} = \frac{\text{desired dose (500 mg)}}{\text{quantity desired (x)}}$$

Then the nurse cross multiplies:

$$250\,x = 5 \text{ mL} \times 500 \text{ mg}$$

$$x = \frac{5 \text{ mL} \times 500 \text{ mg}}{250 \text{ mg}}$$

$$x = 10 \text{ mL}$$

Therefore, the dose ordered is 10 mL. The nurse can also use this formula to calculate dosages:

$$\text{Amount to administer } (x) = \frac{\text{desired dose}}{\text{dose on hand}} \times \text{quantity on hand}$$

Nursing Process: Implementation ***Client Need:*** Physiological Integrity

6. ***Answer:*** 1 (Objective: 14) ***Rationale:*** When handling a syringe, the nurse may touch the outside of the barrel and the handle of the plunger; however, the nurse must avoid letting any unsterile object touch the tip or inside of the barrel, the shaft of the plunger, or the shaft or tip of the needle. ***Nursing Process:*** Implementation ***Client Need:*** Physiological Integrity

7. ***Answer:*** 4 (Objective: 17) ***Rationale:*** The client should remain in the left lateral or supine position for at least 5 minutes to help retain the suppository. Assist the client to a left lateral or left Sims' position, with the upper leg flexed. Unwrap the suppository and lubricate the smooth, rounded end, or see manufacturer's instructions. The rounded end is usually inserted first and lubricant reduces irritation of the mucosa. Press the client's buttocks together for a few minutes. ***Nursing Process:*** Implementation ***Client Need:*** Physiological Integrity

8. *Answer:* 1 (Objective: 17) ***Rationale:*** Explain that the client may experience a feeling of fullness, warmth, and, occasionally, discomfort when the fluid comes in contact with the tympanic membrane. Insert the tip of the syringe into the auditory meatus, and direct the solution gently upward against the top of the canal. The solution will flow around the entire canal and out at the bottom. The solution is instilled gently because strong pressure from the fluid can cause discomfort and damage the tympanic membrane. Straighten the ear canal prior to inserting the tip of the syringe and during the procedure. After the procedure the nurse should place a cotton ball, not a cotton-tipped applicator, in the auditory meatus to absorb the excess fluid. ***Nursing Process:*** Implementation ***Client Need:*** Physiological Integrity

9. *Answer:* 2 (Objective: 17) ***Rationale:*** The client needs to remain lying in the supine position for 5 to 10 minutes following the insertion. Gently insert the applicator into the vagina about 5 cm (2 in.). Slowly push the plunger until the applicator is empty. Remove the applicator and place it on the towel. The applicator is put on the towel to prevent the spread of microorganisms. Discard the applicator if disposable or clean it according to the manufacturer's directions. ***Nursing Process:*** Implementation ***Client Need:*** Physiological Integrity

10. *Answer:* 3 (Objective: 17) ***Rationale:*** When applying a transdermal patch the nurse must select a clean, dry area that is free of hair and matches the manufacturer's recommendations. The nurse should then remove the patch from its protective covering, holding it without touching the adhesive edges, and apply it by pressing firmly with the palm of the hand for about 10 seconds. ***Nursing Process:*** Implementation ***Client Need:*** Physiological Integrity

CHAPTER 36

Key Term Review

1. h 2. n 3. u 4. i 5. v 6. a

7. c 8. x 9. e 10. s 11. b 12. r

13. p 14. o 15. f 16. q 17. j 18. k

19. t 20. l 21. g 22. m 23. y 24. d

25. w

Key Topic Review Answers

1. a

2. b. Hypoproteinemia is an abnormally low protein content in the blood.

3. a

4. b. Because an inadequate intake of calories, protein, vitamins, and iron is believed to be a risk factor for pressure ulcer development, nutritional supplements should be considered for nutritionally compromised clients.

5. a

6. health

7. maceration

8. cleaning

9. piston

10. skin

11. _____i_____ A force acting parallel to the skin surface

_____j_____ A reduction in the amount and control of movement a person has

_____a_____ Renewal of tissues

_____b_____ The cessation of bleeding that results from vasoconstriction of the larger blood vessels in the affected area, retraction (drawing back) of injured blood vessels, the deposition of fibrin (connective tissue), and the formation of blood clots in the area

_____h_____ A whitish protein substance that adds tensile strength to the wound

_____c_____ A material, such as fluid and cells, that has escaped from blood vessels during the inflammatory process and is deposited in tissue or on tissue surfaces

_____f_____ The washing or flushing out of an area

_____d_____ A strip of cloth used to wrap some part of the body

_____g_____ Any lesion caused by unrelieved pressure (a compressing downward force on a body area) that results in damage to underlying tissue, as defined by the U.S. Public Health Service's Panel for the Prediction and Prevention of Pressure Ulcers in Adults

_____e_____ A deficiency in the blood supply to the tissue

12. b

13. a

14. b

15. a

16. c

Case Study Answers

1a. *Explain the local effects of cold.* The physiological effects of cold are opposite to the effects of heat. Cold lowers the temperature of the skin and underlying tissues and causes vasoconstriction. Vasoconstriction reduces blood flow to the affected area and thus reduces the supply of oxygen and metabolites, decreases the removal of wastes, and produces skin pallor and coolness. Prolonged exposure to cold results in impaired circulation, cell deprivation, and subsequent damage to the tissues from lack of oxygen and nourishment. The signs of tissue damage due to cold are a bluish-purple mottled appearance of the skin, numbness, and sometimes blisters and pain. Cold is most often used for sports injuries (e.g., sprains, strains, fractures) to limit postinjury swelling and bleeding.

1b. *Explain the systemic effects of cold.* With extensive cold applications and vasoconstriction, a client's blood pressure can increase because blood is shunted from the cutaneous circulation to the internal blood vessels. Shivering, a generalized effect of prolonged cold, is a normal response as the body attempts to warm itself.

1c. *List some indications for applying ice to the injured ankle.* Indicators include muscle spasms, inflammation, pain, and traumatic injury.

1d. *Summarize the guidelines a nurse should follow for all local cold applications.*

- Determine the client's ability to tolerate the therapy.
- Identify conditions that might contraindicate treatment (e.g., bleeding, circulatory impairment).
- Explain the application to the client.
- Assess the skin area to which the cold will be applied.
- Ask the client to report any discomfort.
- Return to the client 15 minutes after starting the cold application and observe the local skin area for any untoward signs (e.g., redness). Stop the application if any problems occur.
- Remove the equipment at the designated time, and dispose of it appropriately.
- Examine the area to which the heat or cold was applied, and record the client's response.

Review Question Answers

1. ***Answer:*** 1 (Objective: 6) ***Rationale:*** A purulent exudate is thicker than serous exudate because of the presence of pus, which consists of leukocytes, liquefied dead tissue debris, and dead and living bacteria. A serosanguineous (consisting of clear and blood-tinged drainage) exudate is commonly seen in surgical incisions. A serous exudate consists chiefly of serum (the clear portion of the blood) derived from blood and the serous membranes of the body, such as the peritoneum. It looks watery and has few cells. A sanguineous (hemorrhagic) exudate consists of large amounts of red blood cells, indicating damage to capillaries that is severe enough to allow the escape of red blood cells from plasma. This type of exudate is frequently seen in open wounds. ***Nursing Process:*** Assessment ***Client Need:*** Physiological Integrity

2. ***Answer:*** 3 (Objective: 16) ***Rationale:*** In applying electric pads, the nurse needs to teach the client the following guidelines:

   - Do not insert sharp objects (e.g., pins) into the pad. The pin could damage a wire and cause an electric shock.
   - Ensure that the body area is dry unless there is a waterproof cover on the pad. Electricity in the presence of water can cause a shock.
   - Use pads with a preset heating switch so a client cannot increase the heat.
   - Do not place the pad under the client. Heat will not dissipate, and the client may be burned. ***Nursing Process:*** Implementation ***Client Need:*** Safe, Effective Care Environment.

3. ***Answer:*** 4 (Objective: 16) ***Rationale:*** The following temperatures of the water in the bag are considered safe in most situations and provide the desired effect: normal adult and child over 2 years, 46°C to 52°C (115°F to 125°F); debilitated or unconscious adult, or child under 2 years, 40.5°C to 46°C (105°F to 115°F). The client fills the bag two thirds full with water. After filling the bag with water the client dries the bag and holds it upside down to test it for leakage. The client expels the remaining air out of the bag before securing the top. ***Nursing Process:*** Implementation ***Client Need:*** Safe, Effective Care Environment

4. ***Answer:*** 4 (Objective: 13) ***Rationale:*** The bandage should be firm, but not too tight. Ask the client if the bandage feels comfortable. A tight bandage can interfere with blood circulation, whereas a loose bandage does not provide adequate protection. Bandages can be used to support a wound (e.g., a fractured bone). Bandages can also be used to immobilize a wound (e.g., a strained shoulder). Bandages can be used to apply pressure (e.g., elastic bandages on the lower extremities to improve venous blood flow). ***Nursing Process:*** Evaluation ***Client Need:*** Physiological Integrity

5. ***Answer:*** 3 (Objective: 13) ***Rationale:*** Dressings are applied for the following purposes: to protect the wound from mechanical

injury, to prevent hemorrhage (when applied as a pressure dressing or with elastic bandages), to provide thermal insulation, and to protect the wound from microbial contamination. ***Nursing Process:*** Planning ***Client Need:*** Physiological Integrity

6. ***Answer:*** 3 (Objective: 13) ***Rationale:*** Transparent dressings are often applied to wounds including ulcerated or burned skin areas. These dressings offer several advantages: they are elastic; they can be placed over a joint without disrupting the client's mobility; they act as temporary skin; and they are nonporous, nonabsorbent, self-adhesive dressings that do not require changing as other dressings do. They are often left in place until healing has occurred or as long as they remain intact, and adhere only to the skin area around the wound and not to the wound itself because they keep the wound moist. ***Nursing Process:*** Implementation ***Client Need:*** Physiological Integrity

7. ***Answer:*** 3 (Objective: 14) ***Rationale:*** Black wounds are covered with thick necrotic tissue, or eschar. Black wounds require debridement (removal of the necrotic material). Removal of nonviable tissue from a wound must occur before the wound can be staged or heal. Wounds that are red are usually in the late regeneration phase of tissue repair (i.e., developing granulation tissue). They need to be protected to avoid disturbance to regenerating tissue. Yellow wounds are characterized primarily by liquid to semiliquid "slough" that is often accompanied by purulent drainage or previous infection. The nurse cleanses yellow wounds to remove nonviable tissue. Blue is not part of the RYB color code of wounds. ***Nursing Process:*** Assessment ***Client Need:*** Physiological Integrity

8. ***Answer:*** 2 (Objective: 10) ***Rationale:*** Any at-risk client confined to bed—even when a special support mattress is used—should be repositioned at least every 2 hours, depending on the client's need, to allow another body surface to bear the weight. Six body positions can usually be used: prone, supine, right and left lateral (side-lying), and right and left Sims positions. When a lateral position is used, the nurse should avoid positioning the client directly on the trochanter and instead position the client on a 30° angle. A written schedule should be established for turning and repositioning. A knee–chest position would not be appropriate. ***Nursing Process:*** Implementation ***Client Need:*** Physiological Integrity

9. ***Answer:*** 1 (Objective: 8) ***Rationale:*** Albumin is an important indicator of nutritional status. A value below 3.5 g/dL indicates poor nutrition and may increase the risk of poor healing and infection. ***Nursing Process:*** Assessment ***Client Need:*** Physiological Integrity

10. ***Answer:*** 2 (Objective: 8) ***Rationale:*** Check the medical orders, not the progress notes, to determine if the specimen is to be collected for an aerobic (growing only in the presence of oxygen) or anaerobic (growing only in the absence of oxygen) culture. Aerobic organisms are generally found on the surface of the wound, whereas anaerobic organisms would be found in deep wounds, tunnels, and cavities. Administer an analgesic 30 minutes before the procedure if the client is complaining of pain at the wound site. ***Nursing Process:*** Assessment ***Client Need:*** Physiological Integrity

CHAPTER 37

Key Term Review

1. t 2. f 3. w 4. k 5. n 6. b

7. p 8. a 9. q 10. y 11. d 12. h

13. r 14. m 15. u 16. c 17. i 18. s

19. e 20. l 21. b 22. o 23. x 24. j

25. g

Key Topic Review Answers

1. b. The preoperative phase begins when the decision to have surgery is made and ends when the client is transferred to the operating table.

2. a

3. b. Adequate nutrition is required for normal tissue repair.

4. a

5. a

6. circulatory

7. suture

8. sedation

9. clot

10. closed

11. ____c____ Begins with the admission of the client to the postanesthesia area and ends when healing is complete

____i____ A technique in which the anesthetic agent is injected into and around a nerve or small nerve group that supplies sensation to a small area of the body

____g____ Used most often for procedures involving the arm, wrist, and hand

____h_____ An injection of an anesthetic agent into the epidural space, the area inside the spinal column but outside the dura mater

____f_____The passage of blood through the vessels

____a_____ Begins when the decision to have surgery is made and ends when the client is transferred to the operating table

____e____ (Infiltration) is injected into a specific area and is used for minor surgical procedures such as suturing a small wound or performing a biopsy

____j____ Applied directly to the skin and mucous membranes, open skin surfaces, wounds, and burns

____d____ The temporary interruption of the transmission of nerve impulses to and from a specific area or region of the body

____b____ Begins when the client is transferred to the operating table and ends when the client is admitted to the postanesthesia care unit (PACU), also called the postanesthetic room or recovery room

12. d

13. c

14. b

15. a

16. c

Case Study Answers

1a. *Define major surgery and minor surgery.* Major surgery involves a high degree of risk for a variety of reasons: It may be complicated or prolonged, large losses of blood may occur, vital organs may be involved, or postoperative complications may be likely. Minor surgery normally involves little risk, produces few complications, and is often performed in an outpatient setting.

1b. *Give two examples of major surgery and two examples of minor surgery.* Major surgery examples are organ transplant and open heart surgery. Minor surgery examples are breast biopsy and knee surgery.

1c. *Why would you need to remove the hair on the client's abdomen before surgery?* Hair would be removed from the surgical site only if it interferes with the surgical procedure. Remove hair from the surgical site only when necessary or according to the primary care practitioner's orders or institutional policies and procedures. Personnel skilled in hair removal should remove hair using techniques that preserve skin integrity. Electric clippers or a depilatory cream should be used to reduce the risk of traumatizing the skin during hair removal. If a depilatory is used, hypersensitivity testing is performed prior to applying it to the surgical site. Skin trauma and abrasions increase the risk of microorganisms colonizing the surgical site. If hair is to be removed, it is done as close to the time of surgery as possible and not in the vicinity of the sterile field to avoid dispersal of loose hair and potential contamination of the sterile field.

Review Question Answers

1. ***Answer:*** 2 (Objective: 2) ***Rationale:*** The intraoperative phase begins when the client is transferred to the operating table and ends when the client is admitted to the postanesthesia care unit (PACU), also called the postanesthetic room or recovery room. The preoperative phase begins when the decision to have surgery is made and ends when the client is transferred to the operating table. The postoperative phase begins with the admission of the client to the postanesthesia area and ends when healing is complete. Surgery is a unique experience of a planned physical alteration encompassing three phases: preoperative, intraoperative, and postoperative. These three phases are together referred to as the perioperative period. ***Nursing Process:*** Planning ***Client Need:*** Safe, Effective Care Environment

2. ***Answer:*** 4 (Objective: 10) ***Rationale:*** Antibiotics would not be as much of a risk as the other medications listed. The regular use of certain medications can increase surgical risk. Consider these examples:

   - Anticoagulants increase blood coagulation time.
   - Tranquilizers may interact with anesthetics, increasing the risk of respiratory depression.
   - Diuretics may affect fluid and electrolyte balance.
   - Corticosteroids may interfere with wound healing and increase the risk of infection.

   Clients may be unaware of the potential adverse interactions of medications and may fail to report the use of medications for conditions unrelated to the indication for surgery. The astute nurse interviewer should question the client and family about the use of commonly prescribed medications, over-the-counter preparations, and any herbal remedies for specific conditions mentioned during the nursing history. ***Nursing Process:*** Assessment ***Client Need:*** Safe, Effective Care Environment

3. ***Answer:*** 1 (Objective: 7) ***Rationale:*** Clean the surgical site and surrounding areas. This can be accomplished before the surgical prep by having the client shower and shampoo or wash the surgical site before arriving in the surgical setting, or by washing the surgical site in the surgical setting immediately before applying an antimicrobial agent. Prepare the surgical site and surrounding area with an antimicrobial agent when indicated. A nontoxic antimicrobial agent

with a broad range of germicidal action is used to inhibit the growth of microorganisms during and following the surgical procedure. The agent selected depends on the client's history of hypersensitivity reactions, the location of the surgical site, and the skin condition. The area prepared needs to be large enough to accommodate an extension of the incision and any potential drain sites or additional incisions if needed. Remove hair from the surgical site only when necessary or according to the primary care practitioner's orders or institutional policies and procedures. Document surgical skin preparation in the client's record. Documentation should include the skin condition, including any growths, abrasions, or rashes; hair removal and the techniques used, if performed; the skin preparation, including cleansing and antimicrobial agent applied; who performed the preoperative skin preparation; and any adverse or hypersensitivity responses noted. ***Nursing Process:*** Assessment ***Client Need:*** Safe, Effective Care Environment

4. ***Answer:*** 4 (Objective: 11) ***Rationale:*** The nurse wears sterile gloves, not exam gloves. Before removing skin sutures, the nurse needs to verify the orders for suture removal (in many instances, only alternate interrupted sutures are removed one day, and the remaining sutures are removed a day or two later) and whether a dressing is to be applied following the suture removal. The nurse will grasp the suture at the knot with a pair of forceps. Sutures are cut as close to the skin as possible on one side of the visible part because the suture material that is visible to the eye is in contact with resident bacteria of the skin and must not be pulled beneath the skin during removal. Suture material that is beneath the skin is considered free from bacteria. ***Nursing Process:*** Implementation ***Client Need:*** Physiological Integrity

5. ***Answer:*** 3 (Objective: 9) ***Rationale:*** Instruct the client to report promptly to the primary care practitioner any increasing redness, swelling, pain, or discharge from the incision or drain sites. Instruct the client to use pain medications as ordered, not allowing pain to become severe before taking the prescribed dose. Teach the client to avoid using alcohol or other central nervous system depressants while taking narcotic analgesics. Emphasize the importance of adequate rest for healing and immune function. ***Nursing Process:*** Planning ***Client Need:*** Health Promotion and Maintenance

6. ***Answer:*** 2 (Objective: 10) ***Rationale:*** The proper technique is to place the bulk of the dressing over the drain area and below the drain, depending on the client's usual position. Sterile gloves must be worn during the procedure. The dressing should be secured with tape or ties. The sterile dressings are applied one at a time over the drain and the incision. ***Nursing Process:*** Evaluation ***Client Need:*** Physiological Integrity

7. ***Answer:*** 1 (Objective: 9) ***Rationale:*** The client should hold his or her breath for 2 to 3 seconds. The client should be in a sitting position. The client should exhale slowly through the mouth. The client should inhale slowly and evenly through the nose until the greatest chest expansion is achieved. ***Nursing Process:*** Evaluation ***Client Need:*** Physiological Integrity

8. ***Answer:*** 1 (Objective: 12) ***Rationale:*** Draw up the ordered volume of irrigating solution in the syringe; 30 mL of solution per instillation is usual, but up to 60 mL may be given per instillation if ordered. Attach the syringe to the nasogastric tube and slowly inject the solution. Gently aspirate the solution. Forceful withdrawal could damage the gastric mucosa. ***Nursing Process:*** Implementation ***Client Need:*** Physiological Integrity

9. ***Answer:*** 1 (Objective: 6) ***Rationale:*** The student nurse should assist the client to a lying position in bed. Reach inside the stocking from the top and, grasping the heel, turn the upper portion of the stocking inside out so the foot portion is inside the stocking leg. Have the client point his or her toes, then position the stocking on the client's foot. Ease the stocking over the toes, taking care to place the toe and heel portions of the stocking appropriately. ***Nursing Process:*** Evaluation ***Client Need:*** Physiological Integrity

10. ***Answer:*** 4 (Objective: 6) ***Rationale:*** Atelectasis is a condition in which alveoli collapse and are not ventilated. Thrombophlebitis is inflammation of the veins, usually of the legs and associated with a blood clot. Pulmonary embolism is a blood clot that has moved to the lungs and blocks a pulmonary artery, thus obstructing blood flow to a portion of the lung. Pneumonia is inflammation of the alveoli. ***Nursing Process:*** Planning ***Client Need:*** Physiological Integrity

CHAPTER 38

Key Term Review

1. n 2. i 3. o 4. a 5. m 6. d

7. e 8. s 9. q 10. j 11. b 12. r

13. h 14. k 15. p 16. g 17. c 18. f

19. l

Key Topic Review Answers

1. a

2. b. Stereognosis refers to the ability to perceive and understand an object through touch by its size, shape, and texture.

3. a

4. a

5. b. Sensory deprivation is generally thought of as a decrease in or lack of meaningful stimuli.

6. perception

7. stress

8. culture

9. attention

10. overload

11. c

12. b

13. a

14. c

15. d

Case Study Answers

1a. *What actions should you take to help with the client's visual impairment?*

- Orient the client to the arrangement of room furnishings and maintain an uncluttered environment.
- Keep pathways clear and do not rearrange furniture without orienting the client. Ensure that housekeeping personnel are informed about this.
- Organize self-care articles within the client's reach and orient the client to her location.
- Keep the call light within easy reach and place the bed in the low position.
- Assist with ambulation by standing at the client's side, walking about 1 foot ahead, and allowing her to grasp your arm. Confirm whether the client prefers grasping your arm with the dominant or nondominant hand.

1b. *What actions should you take to help with the client's hearing impairments?* Clients with hearing impairments who are unable to hear the alarms of IV pumps and cardiac monitors need to be assessed frequently. They can be taught to use their visual sense to identify kinks in the IV tubing or a loose ECG lead, and so on. For home safety, clients with impaired hearing need to obtain devices that either amplify sounds or respond with flashing lights to sounds such as a doorbell or smoke detector, a baby crying, or a burglar alarm. The sounds of doorbells and alarm clocks may be amplified or changed to a lower frequency or buzzer-like sound. These devices can be obtained from hearing aid dealers, telephone companies, and appliance stores. An important consequence of a decline in hearing as an individual ages is difficulty understanding speech. Factors that influence this difficulty are the environment, rate of speech, and presence of an accent. Environments that are noisy and reverberant (echoing, hollow sounds) cause difficulty for old adult listeners. Older adult clients with a hearing loss have difficulty understanding fast speech. Research indicates that the older adult's ability to process fast verbal information is slower and that rapid speech allows for less time for the older adult to recognize the acoustic or auditory cues of the speech. An individual who speaks with an accent can also affect speech understanding by the older adult. Nonnative English speakers may vary their pronunciation of syllables and/or words, making it challenging for the older adult.

1c. *How can environmental stimuli be adjusted for this client?* The client functions best when the environment is somewhat similar to that of the individual's ordinary daily life. Sometimes nurses need to take steps to adjust the client's environment to prevent either sensory overload or sensory deprivation.

Review Question Answers

1. ***Answer:*** 2 (Objective: 8) ***Rationale:*** The following guidelines should be adhered to by nurses:

   - Always announce your presence when entering the client's room and identify yourself by name.
   - Speak in a warm and pleasant tone of voice. Some people tend to speak louder than necessary when talking to a blind person.
   - Always explain what you are about to do before touching the person.
   - Explain the sounds in the environment.
   - Stay in the client's field of vision if the client has a partial vision loss.
   - Indicate when the conversation has ended and when you are leaving the room.

   The nurse should not speak in an overly loud voice in an attempt for the client to hear the nurse.

   Nursing Process: Evaluation ***Client Need:*** Physiological Integrity

2. ***Answer:*** 2 (Objective: 5) ***Rationale:*** Delirium alertness fluctuates. The client may be alert and oriented during the day but become confused and disoriented at night. The level of alertness of a client with dementia is generally normal. Delusions and hallucinations are not described in terms of fluctuating alertness. ***Nursing Process:*** Planning ***Client Need:*** Physiological Integrity

3. ***Answer:*** 1 (Objective: 7) ***Rationale:*** The nurse should teach the client the following: wear protective eye goggles when using power tools, riding motorcycles, spraying chemicals, and so on. Wear ear protectors when working in an environment with high noise levels or brief loud impulse noises (e.g., blasting). Wear dark glasses with UV protection to avoid damage from ultraviolet rays and never look directly into the sun. Have regular health examinations. ***Nursing Process:*** Planning ***Client Need:*** Health Promotion and Maintenance

4. ***Answer:*** 4 (Objectives: 7, 8) ***Rationale:*** Eliminate unnecessary noise. Reinforce reality by interpreting unfamiliar sounds, sights, and smells; correct any misconceptions of events or situations. Address the person by name and introduce yourself frequently: "Good morning, Mr. Richards. I am Betty Brown. I will be your nurse today." Identify time and place as indicated: "Today is December 5, and it is 8:00 in the morning." Ask the client, "Can you tell me where you are right now?" and orient the client to place (e.g., nursing home) if indicated. ***Nursing Process:*** Implementation ***Client Need:*** Psychosocial Integrity

5. ***Answer:*** 2 (Objective: 7) ***Rationale:*** The spouse should get the following: a phone dialer with large numbers, reading material with large noncursive print, an amplified telephone, and a magnifying glass. ***Nursing Process:*** Evaluation ***Client Need:*** Physiological Integrity

6. ***Answer:*** 2, 4 (Objective: 3) ***Rationale:*** The nurse should inform the client beforehand of the care to be provided, not during the care. The nurse should also provide oral care, perform range-of-motion exercises, and provide aromatic stimuli. Too much environmental stimuli can be very distressing to a client. The client is unconscious and should not be assisted to the commode. ***Nursing Process:*** Planning ***Client Need:*** Physiological Integrity

7. ***Answer:*** 2 (Objective: 1) ***Rationale:*** Stereognosis is the ability to perceive and understand an object through touch by its size, shape, and texture. Sensory reception is the process of receiving stimuli or data. Sensory perception involves the conscious organization and translation of data or stimuli into meaningful information. Sensoristasis is the term used to describe when an individual is in optimal arousal. ***Nursing Process:*** Assessment ***Client Need:*** Physiological Integrity

8. ***Answer:*** 1 (Objectives: 7, 8) ***Rationale:*** Encourage the client to use eyeglasses and hearing aids during waking hours. Address the client by name and touch the client while speaking if this is not culturally offensive. Provide a telephone, radio and/or TV, clock, and calendar. Encourage the use of self-stimulation techniques such as singing, humming, whistling, or reciting. ***Nursing Process:*** Planning ***Client Need:*** Safe, Effective Care Environment

9. ***Answer:*** 3 (Objective: 4) ***Rationale:*** Gustatory—"Have you experienced any changes in taste?" Visual—"When did you last visit an eye doctor?" Auditory—"Have you experienced any dizziness or vertigo?" Olfactory—"Can you distinguish foods by their odors and tell when something is burning?" ***Nursing Process:*** Assessment ***Client Need:*** Physiological Integrity

10. ***Answer:*** 2 (Objective: 1) ***Rationale:*** Specific sensory tests include:
    - Visual acuity—use a Snellen chart or other reading material, such as a newspaper, and visual fields.
    - Hearing acuity—observe the client's conversation with others and perform the whisper test and the Weber and Rinne tuning fork tests.
    - Olfactory sense— identification of specific aromas.
    - Gustatory sense—identification of three tastes such as lemon, salt, and sugar.
    - Tactile sense—test light touch, sharp and dull sensation, two-point discrimination, hot and cold sensation, vibration sense, position sense, and stereognosis.

    Nursing Process: Assessment ***Client Need:*** Physiological Integrity

CHAPTER 39

Key Term Review

1. k 2. g 3. m 4. h 5. n 6. a

7. f 8. b 9. l 10. j 11. c 12. p

13. e 14. i 15. d 16. o

Key Topic Review Answers

1. a
2. b. A client's attitude to a newly acquired disability is often the determining factor in successful rehabilitation.
3. a
4. a
5. a
6. positive
7. self
8. Specific
9. strength
10. ideal
11. a
12. a
13. d
14. a
15. d
16. d

Case Study Answers

1a. *What nursing techniques may help clients analyze the problem and enhance self-concept?*

- Encourage clients to appraise the situation and express their feelings.
- Encourage clients to ask questions.
- Provide accurate information.
- Become aware of distortions, inappropriate or unrealistic standards, and faulty labels in clients' speech.
- Explore clients' positive qualities and strengths.
- Encourage clients to express positive self-evaluation more than negative self-evaluation.
- Avoid criticism.
- Teach clients to substitute negative self-talk ("I can't walk to the store anymore") with positive self-talk ("I can walk half a block each morning"). Negative self-talk reinforces a negative self-concept.

1b. *List five stressors that affect self-concept. (Student will choose five.)*

- Change in physical appearance (e.g., facial wrinkles)
- Declining physical, mental, or sensory abilities
- Inability to achieve goals
- Relationship concerns
- Sexuality concerns
- Unrealistic ideal self

1c. *During your assessment, what questions should you ask the client?*

- How would you describe your personal characteristics? *or* How do you see yourself as a person?
- How do others describe you as a person?
- What do you like about yourself?
- What do you do well?
- What are your personal strengths, talents, and abilities?
- What would you change about yourself if you could?
- Does it bother you a great deal if you think someone doesn't like you?

Review Question Answers

1. ***Answer:*** 1 (Objective: 1) ***Rationale:*** Nurses can employ the following specific strategies to reinforce strengths:

- Stress positive thinking rather than self-negation.
- Notice and verbally reinforce client strengths.
- Provide honest, positive feedback.
- Encourage the setting of attainable goals.

Nursing Process: Planning ***Client Need:*** Psychosocial Integrity

2. ***Answer:*** 1 (Objective: 2) ***Rationale:*** Guidelines for conducting a psychosocial assessment include the following:

- Create a quiet, private environment.
- Minimize interruptions if possible.
- Maintain appropriate eye contact.
- Sit at eye level with the client.

Nursing Process: Assessment ***Client Need:*** Psychosocial Integrity

3. ***Answer:*** 1 (Objective: 4) ***Rationale:*** Guidelines for conducting a psychosocial assessment include the following:

- Indicate acceptance of the client by not criticizing, frowning, or demonstrating shock.
- Ask open-ended questions to encourage the client to talk rather than close-ended questions that tend to block free sharing.
- Minimize the writing of detailed notes during the interview because this can create client concern that confidential material is being "recorded" as well as interfere with your ability to focus on what the client is saying.
- Avoid asking more personal questions than are actually needed.

Nursing Process: Assessment ***Client Need:*** Psychosocial Integrity

4. ***Answer:*** 4 (Objective: 5) ***Rationale:*** The question "What are your responsibilities in the family?" is used to assess role performance and family relationships.

The following are questions to determine a client's self-esteem:

- Are you satisfied with your life?
- How do you feel about yourself?
- Are you accomplishing what you want?

Nursing Process: Assessment ***Client Need:*** Psychosocial Integrity

5. ***Answer:*** 1 (Objective: 5) ***Rationale:*** To enhance her son's self-esteem she would take the following actions:

- Give him opportunities to "practice" who he is.
- Allow him to explore and experiment with the world around him.
- Allow him to express himself as a unique individual.

- Encouraging him to stay connected with all memories would not be the best answer. This would be more appropriate for an elderly patient.

Nursing Process: Evaluation *Client Need:* Psychosocial Integrity

6. ***Answer:*** 2 (Objective: 5) ***Rationale:*** The question "What are your relationships like with your other relatives?" is used to assess family relationships. The following questions are appropriate to ask a client when assessing body image:

- Is there any part of your body you would like to change?
- Are you comfortable discussing your surgery?
- How do you feel about your appearance?

Nursing Process: Assessment *Client Need:* Psychosocial Integrity

7. ***Answer:*** 3 (Objective: 3) ***Rationale:*** The ideal self is the individual's perception of how one should behave based on certain personal standards, aspirations, goals, and values. Global self refers to the collective beliefs and images one holds about oneself. Body image is how a person perceives the size, appearance, and functioning of the body and its parts. Self-concept is one's mental image of oneself. *Nursing Process:* Assessment *Client Need:* Psychosocial Integrity

8. ***Answer:*** 4 (Objective: 2) ***Rationale:*** Erikson's stages of psychosocial development are as follows:

- Middle adulthood stage: generativity vs. stagnation
- Adolescence: identity vs. role confusion
- Early adulthood: intimacy vs. isolation
- Older adults: integrity vs. despair

Nursing Process: Assessment *Client Need:* Psychosocial Integrity

9. ***Answer:*** 2 (Objective: 4) ***Rationale:*** People undergoing role strain are frustrated because they feel or are made to feel inadequate or unsuited to a role. Role strain is often associated with sex-role stereotypes. Role conflicts arise from opposing or incompatible expectations. Role ambiguity occurs when expectations are unclear, and people do not know what to do or how to do it and are unable to predict the reactions of others to their behavior. Role development involves socialization into a particular role. *Nursing Process:* Assessment *Client Need:* Psychosocial Integrity

10. ***Answer:*** 1 (Objective: 4) ***Rationale:*** Change or loss of job or other significant role, loss of financial security, abusive relationship, and unrealistic expectations are considered stressors affecting self-concept. *Nursing Process:* Assessment *Client Need:* Psychosocial Integrity

CHAPTER 40

Key Term Review

1.	v	2.	d	3.	l	4.	p	5.	i	6.	s
7.	c	8.	b	9.	g	10.	n	11.	e	12.	t
13.	q	14.	k	15.	r	16.	x	17.	u	18.	a
19.	f	20.	w	21.	m	22.	o	23.	y	24.	h
25.	j										

Key Topic Review Answers

1. b. The development of sexuality begins with conception and continues throughout the life span.
2. a
3. b. Once gender identity is established, it cannot be easily changed.
4. a
5. a
6. responsibilities
7. condom
8. brain
9. arousal
10. Androgyny
11. __g__ Painful menstruation

    __a__ How one values oneself as a sexual being

    __j__ One's self-image as a female or male

    __b__ The outward expression of a person's sense of maleness or femaleness as well as the expression of what is perceived as gender-appropriate behavior

    __i__ Flexibility in gender roles, the belief that most characteristics and behaviors are human qualities that should not be limited to one specific gender or the other

    __h__ One's attraction to people of the same sex, other sex, or both sexes

____c____ The ongoing love affair that each of us has with ourselves throughout our lifetime

____e____ The involuntary climax of sexual tension, accompanied by physiological and psychological release

____f____ The period of return to the unaroused state; may last 10 to 15 minutes after orgasm, or longer if there is no orgasm

____d____ A severe distaste for sexual activity or the thought of sexual activity, which then leads to a phobic avoidance of sex

12. b

13. b

14. c

Case Study Answers

1a. *Explain how to provide client teaching for testicular self-examination.*

- Choose one day of each month (e.g., the first or last day of each month) to examine yourself.
- Examine yourself when you are taking a warm shower or bath.
- Support the testicle underneath with one hand. Place the fingers of the other hand under the testicle and the thumb on top (this may be easier to do if the leg on that side is raised).
- Roll each testicle between the thumb and fingers of your hand, feeling for lumps, thickening, or a hardening in consistency.
- The testes should feel smooth. Palpate the epididymis, a cordlike structure on the top and back of the testicle. The epididymis feels soft and not as smooth as a testicle.
- Locate the spermatic cord, or vas deferens, which extends upward from the scrotum toward the base of the penis. It should feel firm and smooth.
- Using a mirror, inspect your testicles for swelling, any enlargement, or lumps in the skin of the testicle.
- Promptly report any lumps or other changes to your health care provider.

1b. *Explain how to prevent the transmission of STIs and HIV.*

- Limit the number of sexual partners.
- Use condoms in nonmonogamous and homosexual relationships or other relationships that have the potential for STI transmission.
- Follow safe sex practices during oral sex, including the use of a latex dental dam during cunnilingus to prevent STI transmission.
- Talk openly with sexual partners about how to have "safer sex" and be honest about any history of an STI.
- Abstain from high-risk sexual activity with a partner known to have or suspected of having an STI.
- Report to a health care facility for examination whenever in doubt about possible exposure or when signs of an STI are evident.
- When an STI is diagnosed, notify all partners and encourage them to seek treatment.
- Avoid transfusions of banked blood or blood products. Use autologous transfusions (donation of own blood before surgery) for elective surgery whenever possible.

1c. *Summarize the nursing strategies to deal with the client's inappropriate sexual behavior.*

- Communicate that the behavior is not acceptable by saying, for example, "I really do not like the things you are saying," or "I see you are not dressed. I will be back in 10 minutes and will help you with breakfast when you get your clothes on."
- Tell the client how the behavior makes you feel: "When you act like that toward me, I am very uncomfortable. It embarrasses me and makes it hard for me to give you the kind of nursing care you need."
- Identify the behavior you expect: "Please call me by my name, not 'Honey'" or "I expect you to keep yourself covered when I am in the room. If you are feeling hot or something is uncomfortable, let me know, and I will try to make you more comfortable."
- Set firm limits: Take the client's hand and move it away, use direct eye contact, and say, "Don't do that!"
- Try to refocus clients from the inappropriate behavior to their real concerns and fears; offer to discuss sexuality concerns: "All morning you have been making very personal sexual comments about yourself. Sometimes people talk like that when they are concerned about the sexual part of their life and how their illness will affect them. Are there things that you have questions about or would like to talk about?"
- Report the incident to your nursing instructor, charge nurse, or clinical nurse specialist. Discuss the incident, your feelings, and possible interventions.
- Assign a nurse who will confront the behavior and relate to the client in a consistent manner.
- Clarify the consequences of continued inappropriate behavior (avoidance, withdrawal of services, no chance to help resolve underlying concerns of client).

Review Question Answers

1. ***Answer:*** 4 (Objective: 8) ***Rationale:*** When an STI is diagnosed, notify all partners and encourage them to seek treatment. Use of condoms should occur in nonmonogamous and homosexual relationships, or other relationships that have the potential for STI transmission. Follow safe sex practices during oral sex, including the use of a latex dental dam during cunnilingus to prevent STI transmission. Report to a health care facility for examination whenever in doubt about possible exposure or when signs of an STI are evident. ***Nursing Process:*** Planning ***Client Need:*** Health Promotion and Maintenance

2. ***Answer:*** 2 (Objective: 9) ***Rationale:*** Press the breast tissue against the chest wall firmly enough to know how your breast feels. A ridge of firm tissue in the lower curve of each breast is normal. Use the finger pads (tips) of the three middle fingers (held together) on your left hand to feel for lumps. Use small circular motions systematically all the way around the breast as many times as necessary until the entire breast is covered. Look for any change in size or shape; lumps or thickenings; any rashes or other skin irritations; dimpled or puckered skin; any discharge or change in the nipples. ***Nursing Process:*** Evaluation ***Client Need:*** Health Promotion and Maintenance

3. ***Answer:*** 4 (Objective: 8) ***Rationale:*** The correct statement should have been: "I will report the incident to my nursing instructor, charge nurse, or clinical nurse specialist." The following statements would be correct: "I will communicate that the behavior is not acceptable." "I will identify the behavior I expect." "I will set firm limits with the client." ***Nursing Process:*** Evaluation ***Client Need:*** Psychosocial Integrity

4. ***Answer:*** 1 (Objective: 9) ***Rationale:*** ***Vaginal diaphragms, cervical caps, and condoms are mechanical barriers of contraception, not chemical ones.*** Chemical barriers include insertion of spermicidal foams, creams, jellies, or suppositories into the vagina before intercourse. Surgical sterilization—tubal ligation and vasectomy, is an effective contraception method. Intrauterine devices (IUDs) may be used for contraception. ***Nursing Process:*** Planning ***Client Need:*** Physiological Integrity

5. ***Answer:*** 2 (Objective: 9) ***Rationale:*** The following statement by the nurse would be correct: "Diuretics decrease vaginal lubrication." The following statements would be correct: "Antipsychotics decrease sexual desire." "Narcotics inhibit sexual desire and response." "Barbiturates in large amounts decrease sexual desire." ***Nursing Process:*** Planning ***Client Need:*** Physiological Integrity

6. ***Answer:*** 4 (Objective: 9) ***Rationale:*** "Alcohol is a sexual stimulant" is an incorrect statement. Alcohol is a relaxant and central nervous system depressant. The following statements would be correct: "Sexual ability is not lost due to age." "There is no evidence that sexual activity weakens a person." "Chronic alcoholism is associated with erectile dysfunction." ***Nursing Process:*** Evaluation ***Client Need:*** Physiological Integrity

7. ***Answer:*** 2 (Objective: 1) ***Rationale:*** The orgasmic phase is the involuntary climax of sexual tension, accompanied by physiological and psychological release. The response cycle starts in the brain, with conscious sexual desires called the desire phase. The resolution phase, the period of return to the unaroused state, may last 10 to 15 minutes after orgasm, or longer if there is no orgasm. Myotonia, an increase of tension in muscles, may increase until released by orgasm, or it may also simply fade away. ***Nursing Process:*** Assessment ***Client Need:*** Physiological Integrity

8. ***Answer:*** 1 (Objective: 1) ***Rationale:*** Body image, a central part of the sense of self, is constantly changing. Gender identity is one's self-image as a female or male. Gender-role behavior is the outward expression of a person's sense of maleness or femaleness as well as the expression of what is perceived as gender-appropriate behavior. Androgyny, or flexibility in gender roles, is the belief that most characteristics and behaviors are human qualities that should not be limited to one specific gender or the other. ***Nursing Process:*** Assessment ***Client Need:*** Physiological Integrity

9. ***Answer:*** 2 (Objective: 9) ***Rationale:*** "Preorgasmic women have experienced an orgasm" is an incorrect statement. The following statements would not need any further education: "*Preorgasmic* women have never experienced an orgasm." "*Rapid ejaculation* is one of the most common sexual dysfunctions among men." "*Vulvodynia* is constant, unremitting burning that is localized to the vulva with an acute onset." "*Vestibulitis* causes severe pain only on touch or attempted vaginal entry." ***Nursing Process:*** Evaluation ***Client Need:*** Health Promotion and Maintenance

10. ***Answer:*** 1 (Objective: 3) ***Rationale:*** One technique nurses can use to help clients with altered sexual function is the PLISSIT model, developed by Annon (1974) for this purpose. The model involves four progressive levels represented by the acronym PLISSIT:

P	Permission giving
LI	Limited information
SS	Specific suggestions
IT	Intensive therapy

The following are incorrect choices: PLIISIT, PLLISSIT, PLISIT. ***Nursing Process:*** Assessment ***Client Need:*** Physiological Integrity

CHAPTER 41

Key Term Review

1.	f	2.	j	3.	m	4.	b	5.	l	6.	h
7.	a	8.	i	9.	c	10.	n	11.	d	12.	k
13.	e	14.	g								

Key Topic Review Answers

1. b. Spirituality generally involves a belief in a relationship with some higher power, creative force, divine being, or infinite source of energy.

2. a

3. a

4. a

5. a

6. kosher

7. Presencing

8. planning

9. Sacred

10. forgiveness

11. ____f___ To believe in or be committed to something or someone

____g____ A concept that incorporates spirituality

___d___ The belief in more than one God

___h___ The belief in the existence of one God

___c___ One without belief in a God

____i__ A person who doubts the existence of God or a supreme being or believes the existence of God has not been proved

___b___ An organized system of beliefs and practices

___a___ A challenge to the spiritual well-being or to the belief system that provides strength, hope, and meaning to life

____j__ Is manifested by a feeling of being "generally alive, purposeful, and fulfilled"

___e_____ Refers to that part of being human that seeks meaningfulness through intra-, inter-, and transpersonal connection

12. d

13. a

14. c

15. b

16. d

Case Study Answers

1a. *The client asks you to pray with him. Describe some of the guidelines you should follow.*

- Prayers with clients should only be done when there is mutual agreement between the clients and those praying with them.
- Nurses who are unaccustomed to praying aloud or in public may find it helpful to have a formal prayer or a scriptural passage readily available.
- Because prayer can evoke deep feelings, the nurse may need to spend time with the client following a prayer to enable the client to express these feelings.
- The nurse's goal when praying with the client is to facilitate the client's prayer and not to self-disclose his or her own religious beliefs.

1b. *Summarize the practice guidelines you should follow to support the client's religious practices.*

- Create a trusting relationship with the client so that any religious concerns or practices can be openly discussed and addressed.
- If unsure of client religious needs, ask how nurses can assist in having these needs met. Avoid relying on personal assumptions when caring for clients.
- Do not discuss personal spiritual beliefs with a client unless the client requests it.
- Inform clients and family caregivers about spiritual support available at your institution (e.g., chapel or meditation room, chaplain services).
- Remember the difference between facilitating/supporting a client's religious practice and participating in it yourself.
- All spiritual interventions must be done within agency guidelines.

1c. *Give some examples of spiritual needs that would be related to others.*

- Need to forgive or be forgiven by others.
- Need to cope with loss of loved ones

Review Question Answers

1. ***Answer:*** 4 (Objective: 5) ***Rationale:*** It is important for nurses to understand health-related information about specific religions. Seventh-Day Adventists—Avoid unnecessary treatments on Saturday (Sabbath). Sabbath begins Friday sundown, ends Saturday sundown. Adventists prefer restful, spirit-nurturing, family activities on Sabbaths. Buddhists—Facilitate meditation (may desire

incense, visual focal point, use breathing or chanting, etc.). Jehovah's Witnesses—Abstain from most blood products; need to discuss alternative treatments such as blood conservation strategies, autologous techniques, hematopoietic agents, nonblood volume expanders, and so on; contact local Jehovah's Witness hospital liaison committee. Latter-Day Saints (LDS or Mormons)—Avoid alcohol, caffeine, smoking. Prefer to wear temple undergarments. Arrange for priestly blessing if requested. ***Nursing Process:*** Assessment ***Client Need:*** Psychosocial Integrity

2. ***Answer:*** 1 (Objective: 2) ***Rationale:*** Religion is an organized system of beliefs and practices. It offers a way of spiritual expression that provides guidance for believers in responding to life's questions and challenges. Spiritual distress refers to a challenge to the spiritual well-being or to the belief system that provides strength, hope, and meaning to life. Spiritual health, or spiritual well-being, is manifested by a feeling of being "generally alive, purposeful, and fulfilled." Spirituality refers to that part of being human that seeks meaningfulness through intra-, inter-, and transpersonal connection. ***Nursing Process:*** Assessment ***Client Need:*** Psychosocial Integrity

3. ***Answer:*** 2 (Objective: 1) ***Rationale:*** An atheist is an individual without belief in a God. An agnostic is an individual who doubts the existence of God or a supreme being or believes the existence of God has not been proved. Monotheism is the belief in the existence of one God, while polytheism is the belief in more than one god. ***Nursing Process:*** Assessment ***Client Need:*** Psychosocial Integrity

4. ***Answer:*** 2 (Objective: 5) ***Rationale:*** Orthodox Jews do not eat shellfish or pork. Buddhists and Hindus are generally vegetarian, not wanting to take life to support life. Members of the Church of Jesus Christ of Latter-Day Saints (LDS or Mormons) do not drink caffeinated or alcoholic beverages. ***Nursing Process:*** Assessment ***Client Need:*** Psychosocial Integrity

5. ***Answer:*** 2 (Objective: 1) ***Rationale:*** "Being there in a way that is meaningful to yourself" is incorrect. The following statements are correct: "Being there in a way that is meaningful to another person." "Giving of self in the present moment." "Listening, with full awareness of the privilege of doing so." "Being available with all of the self." ***Nursing Process:*** Implementation ***Client Need:*** Psychosocial Integrity

6. ***Answer:*** 3 (Objective: 1) ***Rationale:*** "Always discuss personal spiritual beliefs with a client" is incorrect. The following statements would demonstrate practice guidelines that support religious practices: "Do not discuss personal spiritual beliefs with a client unless the client requests it." "Create a trusting relationship with the client so that any religious concerns or practices can be openly discussed and addressed." "If unsure of client religious needs, ask how nurses can assist in having these needs met." "Acquaint yourself with the religions, spiritual practices, and cultures of the area in which you are working." ***Nursing Process:*** Evaluation ***Client Need:*** Psychosocial Integrity

7. ***Answer:*** 4 (Objective: 1) ***Rationale:*** Personalizing the prayer is an appropriate practice guideline for praying with clients. The following statements are also appropriate practice guidelines for praying with clients: "Clients' preferences for prayer reflect their personalities." "Before praying, assess what they would like for you to pray." "Prayer may be the springboard to further discussion or catharsis." ***Nursing Process:*** Implementation ***Client Need:*** Psychosocial Integrity

8. ***Answer:*** 3 (Objective: 5) ***Rationale:*** Muslims follow the practice of prayer fives times a day, and the Muslim client may need assistance to maintain this commitment. ***Nursing Process:*** Assessment ***Client Need:*** Psychosocial Integrity

9. ***Answer:*** 4 (Objective: 1) ***Rationale:*** Planning in relation to spiritual needs should be designed to do one or more of the following:

   - Promote a sense of hope.
   - Help the client fulfill religious obligations.
   - Help the client draw on and use inner resources more effectively to meet the present situation.
   - Help the client find meaning in existence and the present situation.

   Nursing Process: Planning ***Client Need:*** Psychosocial Integrity

10. ***Answer:*** 4 (Objective: 3) ***Rationale:*** The need to cope with loss of loved ones is a need related to others. Needs related to the self include:

    - Need for meaning and purpose
    - Need to express creativity
    - Need for hope

    Nursing Process: Planning ***Client Need:*** Psychosocial Integrity

CHAPTER 42

Key Term Review

1.	g	2.	o	3.	u	4.	p	5.	b	6.	j
7.	c	8.	q	9.	d	10.	m	11.	a	12.	t
13.	v	14.	l	15.	r	16.	i	17.	n	18.	s
19.	f	20.	h	21.	e	22.	k				

Key Topic Review Answers

1. a

2. a

3. a

4. b. Self-control (discipline) is assuming a manner and facial expression that convey a sense of being in control or in charge.

5. b. Structuring is the arrangement or manipulation of a situation so that threatening events do not occur.

6. Suppression

7. Fantasy

8. Coping

9. intervention

10. strategy

11. ____e____ Unconscious psychological adaptive mechanisms or, according to Sigmund Freud (1946), mental mechanisms that develop as the personality attempts to defend itself, establish compromises among conflicting impulses, and calm inner tensions

___f___ An extreme feeling of sadness, despair, dejection, lack of worth, or emptiness; affects millions of Americans a year

____c____ An emotional state consisting of a subjective feeling of animosity or strong displeasure

____j____ An emotion or feeling of apprehension aroused by impending or seeming danger, pain, or other perceived threat

___h_____ A state of mental uneasiness, apprehension, dread, or foreboding or a feeling of helplessness related to an impending or anticipated unidentified threat to self or significant relationships

___b_____ When the body's adaptation takes place

___i_____ When the changes produced in the body during the shock phase are reversed

___a_____ The stressor may be perceived consciously or unconsciously by the person

____g____ One organ or a part of the body reacts alone

____d____ Any event or stimulus that causes an individual to experience stress

12. c

13. a

14. d

15. a

16. c

Case Study Answers

1a. *What level of anxiety is the client most likely experiencing?* The client is most likely experiencing severe anxiety—see Table 42–2 in the text.

1b. *Describe various methods you could teach the client to minimize stress and anxiety.*

- Listen attentively; try to understand the client's perspective on the situation.
- Provide an atmosphere of warmth and trust; convey a sense of caring and empathy.
- Determine if it is appropriate to encourage the client's participation in the plan of care; give the client choices about some aspects of care but do not overwhelm the client with choices.
- Stay with the client as needed to promote safety and feelings of security and to reduce fear.
- Control the environment to minimize additional stressors, such as by reducing noise, limiting the number of individuals in the room, and providing care by the same nurse as much as possible.
- Implement suicide precautions if indicated.
- Communicate in short, clear sentences.
- Help the client to
  a. Determine situations that precipitate anxiety and identify signs of anxiety.
  b. Verbalize feelings, perceptions, and fears as appropriate. Some cultures discourage the expression of feelings.
  c. Identify personal strengths.
  d. Recognize usual coping patterns and differentiate positive from negative coping mechanisms.
  e. Identify new strategies for managing stress (e.g., exercise, massage, progressive relaxation).
  f. Identify available support systems.
- Teach the client about:
  a. The importance of adequate exercise, a balanced diet, and rest and sleep to energize the body and enhance coping abilities.

b. Support groups available such as Alcoholics Anonymous, Weight Watchers or Overeaters Anonymous, and parenting and child abuse support groups.

c. Educational programs available such as time management, assertiveness training, and meditation groups.

1c. *Explain the difference between anxiety and fear.* The source of anxiety may not be identifiable; the source of fear is identifiable. Anxiety is related to the future, that is, to an anticipated event. Fear is related to the present. Anxiety is vague, whereas fear is definite. Anxiety is the result of psychological or emotional conflict; fear is the result of a discrete physical or psychological entity.

Review Question Answers

1. ***Answer:*** 2 (Objective: 3) ***Rationale:*** The client is experiencing moderate anxiety as evidenced by voice tremors and pitch changes, facial twitches, shakiness, and slightly elevated respiratory and heart rates, and she told you "I feel like I have butterflies in my stomach." Mild anxiety would be characterized by mild restlessness, sleeplessness, increased verbalization, feelings of increased arousal and alertness, and no changes in respiratory and heart rates. Severe anxiety is characterized by communication difficulties; increased motor activity; inability to relax, focus, and concentrate; ease of distractibility; tachycardia; and hyperventilation. Panic anxiety is characterized by increased motor activity, agitation, unpredictable responses, distorted or exaggerated perception, dyspnea, palpitations, choking, chest pain, and a feeling of impending doom. ***Nursing Process:*** Assessment ***Client Need:*** Psychosocial Integrity

2. ***Answer:*** 1 (Objective: 3) ***Rationale:*** The source of anxiety may not be identifiable; the source of fear is identifiable. Anxiety is related to the future, that is, to an anticipated event. Fear is related to the present. Anxiety is vague, whereas fear is definite. Anxiety is the result of psychological or emotional conflict; fear is the result of a discrete physical or psychological entity. ***Nursing Process:*** Evaluation ***Client Need:*** Psychosocial Integrity

3. ***Answer:*** 1 (Objective: 7) ***Rationale:*** Try to understand the meaning of the client's anger. After the interaction is completed, take time to process your feelings and your responses to the client with your colleagues. Let clients talk about their anger. Listen to the client, and act as calmly as possible. ***Nursing Process:*** Implementation ***Client Need:*** Psychosocial Integrity

4. ***Answer:*** 3 (Objective: 9) ***Rationale:*** Nurses can prevent burnout by using the techniques to manage stress discussed for clients. Nurses must first recognize their stress and become attuned to such responses as feelings of being overwhelmed, fatigue, angry outbursts, physical illness, and increases in coffee drinking, smoking, or substance abuse. Once attuned to stress and personal reactions, it is necessary to identify which situations produce the most pronounced reactions so that steps may be taken to reduce the stress. Suggestions include:

   - Develop collegial support groups to deal with feelings and anxieties generated in the work setting.
   - Get involved in constructive change efforts if organizational policies and procedures cause stress.
   - Learn to say no.
   - Establish a regular exercise program to direct energy outward.

   Nursing Process: Implementation ***Client Need:*** Psychosocial Integrity

5. ***Answer:*** 2 (Objective: 8) ***Rationale:***

   - The adolescent is characterized by changing physique, relationships involving sexual attraction, exploring independence, choosing a career.
   - The young adult is characterized by getting married, leaving home, managing a home, getting started in an occupation, continuing one's education, having children.
   - The middle adult is characterized by physical changes of aging, maintaining social status and standard of living, helping teenage children to become independent, aging parents.
   - The older adult is characterized by decreasing physical abilities and health, changes in residence, retirement and reduced income, death of spouse and friends.

   Nursing Process: Assessment ***Client Need:*** Psychosocial Integrity

6. ***Answer:*** 1 (Objective: 5) ***Rationale:*** Displacement is the transferring or discharging of emotional reactions from one object or person to another object or person. An example would be when a husband and wife have an argument, the husband becomes so angry he hits a door instead of his wife. Denial is an attempt to screen or ignore unacceptable realities by refusing to acknowledge them. An example would be a woman who, though told her father has metastatic cancer, continues to plan a family reunion 18 months in advance. Projection is a process in which blame is attached to others or the environment for unacceptable desires, thoughts, shortcomings, and mistakes. An example would be a mother who is told that her child must repeat a grade in school, and the mother blames this on the teacher's poor instruction. Substitution is the replacement of a highly valued, unacceptable, or unavailable object by a less valuable, acceptable, or available object. An example would be a woman who wants to marry a man exactly like her deceased father, and settles for someone whose appearance resembles her father's. . ***Nursing Process:*** Assessment ***Client Need:*** Psychosocial Integrity

7. ***Answer:*** 2 (Objective: 5) ***Rationale:*** Regression is resorting to an earlier, more comfortable level of functioning that is characteristically less demanding and responsible. An example

would be an adult who throws a temper tantrum when he does not get his own way. Repression is an unconscious mechanism by which threatening thoughts, feelings, and desires are kept from becoming conscious; the repressed material is denied entry into consciousness. An example would be a teenager who, having seen his best friend killed in a car crash, becomes amnesic about the circumstances surrounding the accident. Reaction formation is a mechanism that causes people to act exactly opposite to the way they feel. An example would be an executive who resents his bosses for calling in a consulting firm to make recommendations for change in his department, but verbalizes complete support of the idea and is exceedingly polite and cooperative. Rationalization is justification of certain behaviors by faulty logic and ascribing motives that are socially acceptable but did not in fact inspire the behavior. An example would be a mother who spanks her toddler too hard and says it was all right because he couldn't feel it through the diaper anyway. ***Nursing Process:*** Assessment ***Client Need:*** Psychosocial Integrity

8. ***Answer:*** 4 (Objective: 9) ***Rationale:*** To minimize stress and anxiety the nurse should communicate in short, clear sentences; provide an atmosphere of warmth and trust; convey a sense of caring and empathy; listen attentively; try to understand the client's perspective on the situation; and control the environment to minimize additional stressors, such as by reducing noise, limiting the number of individuals in the room, and providing care by the same nurse as much as possible. ***Nursing Process:*** Planning ***Client Need:*** Psychosocial Integrity

9. ***Answer:*** 3 (Objective: 7) ***Rationale:*** Common characteristics of crises include:

   - All crises are experienced as sudden. The person is usually not aware of a warning signal, even if others could "see it coming." The individual or family may feel that they had little or no preparation for the event or trauma.
   - The crisis is often experienced as ultimately life threatening, whether this perception is realistic or not.
   - Communication with significant others is often decreased or cut off.
   - There may be perceived or real displacement from familiar surroundings or loved ones.
   - All crises have an aspect of loss, whether actual or perceived. The losses can include an object, a person, a hope, a dream, or any significant factor for that individual.

   Nursing Process: Planning ***Client Need:*** Psychosocial Integrity

10. ***Answer:*** 1 (Objective: 3) ***Rationale:*** The clinical manifestations of stress include:

    - Pupils dilate to increase visual perception when serious threats to the body arise.
    - Sweat production (diaphoresis) increases to control elevated body heat due to increased metabolism.
    - Heart rate and cardiac output increase to transport nutrients and by-products of metabolism more efficiently.
    - Skin is pallid because of constriction of peripheral blood vessels, an effect of norepinephrine.

    Nursing Process: Evaluation ***Client Need:*** Psychosocial Integrity

CHAPTER 43

Key Term Review

1.	r	2.	d	3.	w	4.	u	5.	n	6.	l
7.	a	8.	i	9.	v	10.	s	11.	j	12.	p
13.	t	14.	f	15.	o	16.	x	17.	g	18.	m
19.	h	20.	c	21.	k	22.	q	23.	e	24.	b

Key Topic Review Answers

1. a
2. b. Anticipatory loss is experienced before the loss actually occurs.
3. a
4. a
5. a
6. mortis
7. Algor
8. mortician/undertaker
9. shroud
10. Hopelessness
11. c
12. c
13. d
14. c

15. b

11. c

12. c

13. d

14. c

15. b

Case Study Answers

1. *Which type of loss is the client experiencing?* The client is experiencing an actual loss because it can be recognized by others.

2. *Explain grief, bereavement, and mourning.* Grief is the total response to the emotional experience related to loss. Grief is manifested in thoughts, feelings, and behaviors associated with overwhelming distress or sorrow. Bereavement is the subjective response experienced by the surviving loved ones after the death of a person with whom they have shared a significant relationship. Mourning is the behavioral process through which grief is eventually resolved or altered; it is often influenced by culture, spiritual beliefs, and custom. Grief and mourning are experienced not only by the individual who faces the death of a loved one, but also by the individual who suffers other kinds of losses. Grieving is essential for good mental and physical health. It permits the individual to cope with the loss gradually and to accept it as part of reality. Grief is a social process; it is best shared and carried out with the assistance of others.

3. *List four appropriate questions to ask during the assessment.*

   - Are you having trouble sleeping? Eating? Concentrating? Breathing?
   - Do you have any pain or other new physical problems?
   - What are you doing to help you deal with this loss?
   - Are you taking any drugs or medications to help you cope with this loss?

Review Question Answers

1. ***Answer:*** 2 (Objective: 1) ***Rationale:*** Bereavement is the subjective response experienced by the surviving loved ones after the death of a person with whom they have shared a significant relationship. Grief is the total response to the emotional experience related to loss. Grief is manifested in thoughts, feelings, and behaviors associated with overwhelming distress or sorrow. Mourning is the behavioral process through which grief is eventually resolved or altered; it is often influenced by culture, spiritual beliefs, and custom. Loss is an actual or potential situation in which something that is valued is changed or no longer available. ***Nursing Process:*** Assessment ***Client Need:*** Psychosocial Integrity

2. ***Answer:*** 1 (Objective: 9) ***Rationale:*** Rigor mortis is the stiffening of the body that occurs about 2 to 4 hours after death. It results from a lack of adenosine triphosphate (ATP), which causes the muscles to contract, which in turn immobilizes the joints. Rigor mortis starts in the involuntary muscles (heart, bladder, and so on), then progresses to the head, neck, and trunk, and finally reaches the extremities. All other times are incorrect. ***Nursing Process:*** Assessment ***Client Need:*** Physiological Integrity

3. ***Answer:*** 1 (Objective: 2) ***Rationale:*** Denial occurs when an individual refuses to believe that loss is happening, or is unready to deal with practical problems, such as a prosthesis after loss of leg. A client in denial may assume artificial cheerfulness to prolong denial. Anger is when a client or family is hostile toward a staff member about matters that normally would not bother them. Bargaining occurs when one seeks to bargain to avoid loss. The bargaining client may express feelings of guilt or fear of punishment for past sins, real or imagined. Depression occurs when one grieves over what has happened and what cannot be. The depressed client may talk freely (e.g., reviewing past losses such as money or job) or may withdraw. ***Nursing Process:*** Assessment ***Client Need:*** Psychosocial Integrity

4. ***Answer:*** 1 (Objective: 2) ***Rationale:*** During the shock and disbelief stage, the client refuses to accept loss, has stunned feelings, and accepts the situation intellectually but denies it emotionally. During the developing awareness stage, reality of loss begins to penetrate consciousness, and anger may be directed at the agency, nurses, or others. During the restitution stage, the client conducts rituals of mourning (e.g., funeral). During the stage of resolving the loss, the client attempts to deal with the painful void, is still unable to accept a new love object to replace the lost person or object, may accept a more dependent relationship with a support person, and thinks over and talks about memories of the lost person or object. ***Nursing Process:*** Assessment ***Client Need:*** Psychosocial Integrity

5. ***Answer:*** 2 (Objective: 2) ***Rationale:*** Conservation/withdrawal—during this phase, survivors feel a need to be alone to conserve and replenish both physical and emotional energy. The social support available to the bereaved has decreased, and they may experience despair and helplessness. The healing phase is the turning point. During this phase, the bereaved move from distress about living without their loved one to learning to live more independently. Awareness of loss—during this phase the friends and family resume normal activities. The bereaved experience the full significance of their loss. Shock—during this phase the survivors are left with feelings of confusion, unreality, and disbelief that the loss has occurred. They are often unable to process the normal

thought sequences. This phase may last from a few minutes to many days. ***Nursing Process:*** Assessment ***Client Need:*** Psychosocial Integrity

6. ***Answer:*** 1 (Objective: 7) ***Rationale:*** For an unconscious client experiencing airway clearance problems, the nursing student would put the client in a lateral position. For a conscious client with an airway clearance problem, the nursing student would place him in Fowler's position. If the client is diaphoretic, the nursing student would give the client frequent baths, change the linen, and regularly change the client's position. The nursing student would provide skin care to the client in response to incontinence of urine or feces. ***Nursing Process:*** Implementation ***Client Need:*** Physiological Integrity

7. ***Answer:*** 4 (Objective: 6) ***Rationale:*** The dying person's bill of rights includes:

   - I have the right not to die alone.
   - I have the right to express my feelings and emotions about my approaching death in my own way.
   - I have the right to expect continuing medical and nursing attention even though cure goals must be changed to comfort goals.
   - I have the right to be free from pain.

   Nursing Process: Planning ***Client Need:*** Psychosocial Integrity

8. ***Answer:*** 4 (Objective: 6) ***Rationale:*** Clinical manifestations of impending clinical death include:

   - Slower and weaker pulse
   - Difficulty swallowing and gradual loss of the gag reflex
   - Mottling and cyanosis of the extremities
   - Rapid, shallow, irregular, or abnormally slow respirations

   Nursing Process: Implementation ***Client Need:*** Physiological Integrity

9. ***Answer:*** 1 (Objective: 4) ***Rationale:***

   - Infancy to 5 years—Does not understand concept of death. Infant's sense of separation forms basis for later understanding of loss and death. Believes death is reversible, a temporary departure, or sleep. Emphasizes immobility and inactivity as attributes of death.
   - 5 to 9 years—Understands that death is final. Believes own death can be avoided. Associates death with aggression or violence. Believes wishes or unrelated actions can be responsible for death.
   - 9 to 12 years—Understands death as the inevitable end of life. Begins to understand own mortality, expressed as interest in afterlife or as fear of death.
   - 12 to 18 years—Fears a lingering death.

   Nursing Process: Assessment ***Client Need:*** Psychosocial Integrity

10. ***Answer:*** 3 (Objective: 9) ***Rationale:*** Nursing personnel may be responsible for care of a body after death. Normally the body is placed in a supine position with the arms either at the sides, palms down, or across the abdomen. Dentures are usually inserted to help give the face a natural appearance. The mouth is then closed. One pillow is placed under the head and shoulders to prevent blood from discoloring the face by settling in it. The eyelids are closed and held in place for a few seconds so they remain closed. All jewelry is removed, except a wedding band in some instances, which is taped to the finger. ***Nursing Process:*** Implementation ***Client Need:*** Physiological Integrity

CHAPTER 44

Key Term Review

1. d 2. l 3. g 4. f 5. i 6. c

7. a 8. e 9. h 10. j 11. u 12. n

13. o 14. m 15. p 16. b 17. v 18. s

19. q 20. r 21. w 22. k 23. x

Key Topic Review Answers

1. a 2. a 3. a 4. a 5. a

1. a

2. a

3. a

4. a

5. a

6. Hypertrophy

7. Osteoporosis

8. atrophy

9. contracture

10. ankylosed

11. ____e____ The ability to move freely, easily, rhythmically, and purposefully in the environment; is an essential part of living

____a____ Bodily movement produced by skeletal muscle contraction that increases energy expenditure

____b____ A type of physical activity defined as a planned, structured, and repetitive bodily movement performed to improve or maintain one or more components of physical fitness

___c_____ Exercise in which the muscle shortens to produce muscle contraction and active movement

____j____ Exercise in which there is muscle contraction without moving the joint (muscle length does not change)

_____g___ Involve muscle contraction or tension against resistance; thus, they can be either isotonic or isometric

____d____ Activity during which the amount of oxygen taken in by the body is greater than that used to perform the activity

____f____ Involves activity in which the muscles cannot draw out enough oxygen from the bloodstream, and anaerobic pathways are used to provide additional energy for a short time

____i____ Air circulating into and out of the lungs

____h____ A condition in which the bones become brittle and fragile due to calcium depletion

12. d

13. a

14. a

15. a

Case Study Answers

1. *Provide the client and the client's family education about the following topics:*

Maintaining Musculoskeletal Function

- Teach the systematic performance of passive or assistive ROM exercises to maintain joint mobility.
- Demonstrate, as appropriate, the proper way to perform isotonic, isometric, or isokinetic exercises to maintain muscle mass and tone (collaborate with the physical therapist about these). Incorporate ADLs into exercise program if appropriate.
- Provide a written schedule for the type, frequency, and duration of exercises; encourage the use of a progress graph or chart to facilitate adherence with the therapy.
- Offer an ambulation schedule.
- Instruct in the availability of assistive ambulatory devices and correct use of them.
- Discuss pain control measures required before exercise.

Preventing Injury

- Provide assistive devices for moving and transferring, whenever possible, and teach safe transfer and ambulation techniques.
- Discuss safety measures to avoid falls (e.g., locking wheelchairs, wearing appropriate footwear, using rubber tips on crutches, keeping the environment safe, and using mechanical aids such as a raised toilet seat, grab bars, urinal, and bedpan or commode to facilitate toileting).
- Teach the use of proper body mechanics, especially for those times when assistive equipment is not used.
- Teach ways to prevent postural hypotension.

Managing Energy to Prevent Fatigue

- Discuss activity and rest patterns and develop a plan as indicated; intersperse rest periods with activity periods.
- Discuss ways to minimize fatigue such as performing activities more slowly and for shorter periods, resting more often, and using more assistance as required.
- Provide information about available resources to help with ADLs and home maintenance management.
- Teach ways to increase energy (e.g., increasing intake of high-energy foods, ensuring adequate rest and sleep, controlling pain, sharing feelings with a trusted listener).
- Teach techniques to monitor activity tolerance as appropriate.

Preventing Back Injuries

- Understand that the use of body mechanics will not necessarily prevent injury if manually handling a load greater than 51 pounds without the use of assistive devices.
- Avoid lifting anything greater than 51 pounds—use assistive equipment, get help from coworkers, and participate in the purchasing/ordering process of appropriate assistive equipment for your work setting.
- Become consciously aware of your posture and body mechanics.
- When standing for a period of time, periodically move legs and hips, and flex one hip and knee and rest your foot on an object if possible.
- When sitting, keep your knees slightly higher than your hips.
- Use a firm mattress and soft pillow that provide good body support at natural body curvatures.
- Exercise regularly to maintain overall physical condition and regulate weight; include exercises that strengthen the pelvic, abdominal, and spinal muscles.

- Avoid movements that cause pain or require spinal flexion with straight legs (e.g., toe-touching and sit-ups) or spinal rotation (twisting).
- When moving an object, spread your feet apart to provide a wide base of support.
- When lifting an object, distribute the weight between the large muscles of the legs and arms, limiting the load to 15 to 25 pounds held at elbow height.
- Wear comfortable low-heeled shoes that provide good foot support and reduce the risk of slipping, stumbling, or turning your ankle.

Review Question Answers

1. ***Answer:*** 4 (Objective: 3) ***Rationale:*** The following statements would be correct when providing client teaching about preventing back injuries:

   - Exercise regularly to maintain overall physical condition and regulate weight; include exercises that strengthen the pelvic, abdominal, and spinal muscles.
   - When standing for a period of time, periodically move legs and hips, flex one hip and knee and rest your foot on an object if possible.
   - When sitting, keep your knees slightly higher than your hips.
   - Use a firm mattress and soft pillow that provide good body support at natural body curvatures.

   Nursing Process: Planning ***Client Need:*** Physiological Integrity

2. ***Answer:*** 2 (Objective: 7) ***Rationale:*** Practice guidelines for wheelchair safety include:

   - Raise the footplates before transferring the client into the wheelchair.
   - Always lock the brakes on both wheels of the wheelchair when the client transfers in or out of it.
   - Lower the footplates after the transfer, and place the client's feet on them.
   - Ensure the client is positioned well back in the seat of the wheelchair.

   Nursing Process: Evaluation ***Client Need:*** Safe, Effective Care Environment

3. ***Answer:*** 3 (Objective: 7) ***Rationale:*** The following are correct statements that indicate understanding of stretcher safety:

   - Maneuver the stretcher when entering the elevator so that the client's head goes in first.
   - Never leave a client unattended on a stretcher unless the wheels are locked and the side rails are raised on both sides and/or the safety straps are securely fastened across the client.
   - Always push a stretcher from the end where the client's head is positioned. This position protects the client's head in the event of a collision.
   - Fasten safety straps across the client on a stretcher, and raise the side rails.

   Nursing Process: Evaluation ***Client Need:*** Safe, Effective Care Environment

4. ***Answer:*** 1 (Objective: 2) ***Rationale:*** Active ROM exercises guidelines include:

   - Perform each ROM exercise as taught to the point of slight resistance, but not beyond, and never to the point of discomfort.
   - Perform the movements systematically, using the same sequence during each session.
   - Perform each exercise three times.
   - Perform each series of exercises twice daily.

   Nursing Process: Implementation ***Client Need:*** Safe, Effective Care Environment

5. ***Answer:*** 3 (Objective: 5) ***Rationale:*** During client teaching about controlling postural hypotension, the client should verbalize the following:

   - Use a rocking chair to improve circulation in the lower extremities.
   - Never bend down all the way to the floor or stand up too quickly after stooping.
   - Wear elastic stockings at night to inhibit venous pooling in the legs.
   - Get out of a hot bath very slowly, because high temperatures can lead to venous pooling.

   Nursing Process: Planning ***Client Need:*** Safe, Effective Care Environment

6. ***Answer:*** 4 (Objective: 2) ***Rationale:*** Isotonic (dynamic) exercises are those in which the muscle shortens to produce muscle contraction and active movement. Isometric (static or setting) exercises are those in which there is muscle contraction without moving the joint (muscle length does not change). Isokinetic (resistive) exercises involve muscle contraction or tension against resistance; thus, they can be either isotonic or isometric. Aerobic exercise is activity during which the amount of oxygen taken in by the body is greater than that used to perform the activity. ***Nursing Process:*** Implementation ***Client Need:*** Physiological Integrity

7. *Answer:* 1 (Objective: 7) ***Rationale:*** Positioning a client in good body alignment and changing the position regularly (every 2 hours) and systematically are essential aspects of nursing practice. Any position, correct or incorrect, can be detrimental if maintained for a prolonged period. For all clients, it is important to assess the skin and provide skin care before and after a position change. Frequent change of position helps to prevent muscle discomfort, undue pressure resulting in pressure ulcers, damage to superficial nerves and blood vessels, and contractures. ***Nursing Process:*** Evaluation ***Client Need:*** Physiological Integrity

8. *Answer:* 1 (Objective: 4) ***Rationale:*** Fowler's position, or a semisitting position, is a bed position in which the head and trunk are raised 45° to 60°. In the dorsal recumbent (back-lying) position, the client's head and shoulders are slightly elevated on a small pillow. In the prone position, the client lies on the abdomen with the head turned to one side. In the lateral (side-lying) position, the person lies on one side of the body. Flexing the top hip and knee and placing this leg in front of the body creates a wider, triangular base of support and achieves greater stability. ***Nursing Process:*** Implementation ***Client Need:*** Safe, Effective Care Environment

9. *Answer:* 2 (Objective: 7) ***Rationale:*** Always support or hold the client rather than the equipment and ensure the client's safety and dignity. Obtain essential equipment before starting (e.g., transfer belt, wheelchair), and check its function. Remove obstacles from the area used for the transfer. Explain the transfer to the nursing personnel who are helping; specify who will give directions (one person needs to be in charge). Nursing Process: Implementation ***Client Need:*** Safe, Effective Care Environment

10. *Answer:* 2 (Objective: 7) ***Rationale:*** When nurses measure clients for axillary crutches, it is most important to obtain the correct length for the crutches and the correct placement of the hand piece. The nurse must measure for the crutches and determine the correct placement of the hand bar. The nurse measures the angle of elbow flexion. It should be about 30°. The client lies in a supine position and the nurse measures from the anterior fold of the axilla to the heel of the foot and adds 2.5 cm (1 in.). The client stands erect and positions the crutch. The nurse makes sure the shoulder rest of the crutch is at least three fingerwidths, that is, 2.5 to 5 cm (1 to 2 in.), below the axilla. The client stands upright and supports the body weight by the hand grips of the crutches. ***Nursing Process:*** Implementation ***Client Need:*** Safe, Effective Care Environment

CHAPTER 45

Key Term Review

1. h 2. k 3. n 4. p 5. d 6. j

7. e 8. a 9. l 10. o 11. f 12. g

13. b 14. i 15. c 16. m

Key Topic Review Answers

1. a

2. b. Stage 3 is the deepest stage of sleep.

3. a

4. a

5. b. Sleep hygiene is a term referring to interventions used to promote sleep.

6. Sleep

7. rhythms

8. 90

9. Insomnia

10. Narcolepsy

11. ____j____ The study of sleep

____i____ The basic organization of normal sleep

____a____ A pattern of symptoms (e.g., agitation, anxious, aggressive, and sometimes delusional) that occur in the late afternoon

____d____ A subjective characteristic, often determined by whether or not a person wakes up feeling energetic or not

____g____ The total time the individual sleeps

___b___ The most common sleep complaint in America

____c__ Learning to develop positive thoughts and beliefs about sleep

____h____ Creating a sleep environment that promotes sleep

___f_____ Conditions where the affected individual obtains sufficient sleep at night but still cannot stay awake during the day

___e_____ A disorder of excessive daytime sleepiness caused by the lack of the chemical hypocretin in the area of the central nervous system that regulates sleep

12. d

13. a

14. a

15. b

16. c

Case Study Answers

1a. *Explain the two types of sleep.* The two types of sleep are NREM (non–rapid-eye-movement) sleep and REM (rapid-eye-movement) sleep. During sleep, NREM and REM sleep alternate in cycles. NREM sleep occurs when activity in the RAS is inhibited. About 75% to 80% of sleep during a night is NREM sleep. NREM sleep is divided into four stages, each associated with distinct brain activity and physiology. Stage 1 is the stage of very light sleep and lasts only a few minutes. During this stage, the individual feels drowsy and relaxed, the eyes roll from side to side, and the heart and respiratory rates drop slightly. The individual can be readily awakened and may deny that he or she was sleeping. Stage 2 is the stage of light sleep during which body processes continue to slow down. The eyes are generally still, the heart and respiratory rates decrease slightly, and body temperature falls. Stage 2 lasts only about 10 to 15 minutes but constitutes 44% to 55% of total sleep. An individual in stage 2 requires more intense stimuli than in stage 1 to awaken. Stages 3 and 4 are the deepest stages of sleep, differing only in the percentage of delta waves recorded during a 30-second period. During deep sleep or delta sleep, the individual's heart and respiratory rates drop 20% to 30% below those exhibited during waking hours. The sleeper is difficult to arouse. The individual is not disturbed by sensory stimuli, the skeletal muscles are very relaxed, reflexes are diminished, and snoring is most likely to occur. Even swallowing and saliva production are reduced during delta sleep. These stages are essential for restoring energy and releasing important growth hormones. REM sleep usually recurs about every 90 minutes and lasts 5 to 30 minutes. Most dreams take place during REM sleep, but usually will not be remembered unless the individual arouses briefly at the end of the REM period. During REM sleep, the brain is highly active, and brain metabolism may increase as much as 20%. For example, during REM sleep, levels of acetylcholine and dopamine increase, with the highest levels of acetylcholine release occurring during REM sleep. Since both of these neurotransmitters are associated with cortical activation, it makes sense that these neurotransmitter levels would be high during dreaming sleep. This type of sleep is also called paradoxical sleep because EEG activity resembles that of wakefulness. Distinctive eye movements occur, voluntary muscle tone is dramatically decreased, and deep tendon reflexes are absent. In this phase, the individual may be difficult to arouse or may wake spontaneously, gastric secretions increase, and heart and respiratory rates often are irregular. It is thought that the regions of the brain that are used in learning, thinking, and organizing information are stimulated during REM sleep.

1b. *Describe factors that affect sleep.* Both the quality and the quantity of sleep are affected by a number of factors. Sleep quality is a subjective characteristic and is often determined by whether or not an individual wakes up feeling energetic or not. Quantity of sleep is the total time the individual sleeps. Illness, environment, lifestyle, emotional stress, stimulants and alcohol, diet, smoking, motivation, and medications are some of the factors that affect sleep.

1c. *Explain the information that should be included in a sleep diary.* A sleep diary may include all or selected aspects of the following information that pertain to the client's specific problem:

- Time of (a) going to bed, (b) trying to fall asleep, (c) falling asleep (approximate time), (d) any instances of waking up and duration of these periods, (e) waking up in the morning, and (f) time and duration of any naps
- Activities performed 2 to 3 hours before going to bed (type, duration, and time)
- Consumption of caffeinated beverages and alcohol and amounts of those beverages
- Any prescribed and over-the-counter medications, and herbal remedies, taken during the day
- Bedtime rituals before bed
- Any difficulties remaining awake during the day and times when difficulties occurred
- Any worries that the client believes may affect sleep
- Factors that the client believes have a positive or negative effect on sleep

Review Question Answers

1. ***Answer:*** 2 (Objective: 7) ***Rationale:*** Clients may be asked to keep a sleep diary or log for 1 to 2 weeks in order to get a more complete picture of their sleep complaints. A sleep diary may include all or selected aspects of the following information that pertain to the client's specific problem: consumption of caffeinated beverages and alcohol and amounts of those beverages; activities performed 2 to 3 hours before going to bed (type, duration, and time); bedtime rituals before bed; any prescribed and over-the-counter medications, and herbal remedies taken during the day. ***Nursing Process:*** Planning ***Client Need:*** Physiological Integrity

2. ***Answer:*** 4 (Objective: 7) ***Rationale:*** "When I'm in pain, I will take the prescribed analgesics 30 minutes before I go to sleep" would have been a correct statement. The following statements by the client would be correct: "I should wear loose-fitting nightwear." "I will void before bedtime." "I will perform hygienic routines prior to bedtime." ***Nursing Process:*** Evaluation ***Client Need:*** Physiological Integrity

3. ***Answer:*** 3 (Objective: 8) ***Rationale:*** Sleep medications affect REM sleep more than NREM sleep. The following statements are correct: Antianxiety medications decrease levels of arousal by facilitating the action of neurons in the CNS that suppress responsiveness to stimulation. Sleep medications vary in their onset and duration of action and will impair waking function as long as they are chemically active. Initial doses of medications should be low and increases added gradually, depending on the

client's response. ***Nursing Process:*** Evaluation ***Client Need:*** Physiological Integrity

4. ***Answer:*** 1 (Objective: 5) ***Rationale:*** Hypersomnia refers to a condition in which the affected individual obtains sufficient sleep at night but still cannot stay awake during the day. Narcolepsy is a disorder of excessive daytime sleepiness caused by the lack of the chemical hypocretin in the area of the central nervous system that regulates sleep. Sleep apnea is characterized by frequent short breathing pauses during sleep. A parasomnia is behavior that may interfere with sleep and/or occurs during sleep. ***Nursing Process:*** Assessment ***Client Need:*** Physiological Integrity

5. ***Answer:*** 2 (Objective: 2) ***Rationale:*** NREM sleep is divided into four stages, each associated with distinct brain activity and physiology. Stage 2 lasts only about 10 to 15 minutes but constitutes 44% to 55% of total sleep. An individual in stage 2 requires more intense stimuli than in stage I to awaken. Stage 1 is the stage of very light sleep and lasts only a few minutes. Stage 2 is the stage of light sleep during which body processes continue to slow down. The eyes are generally still, the heart and respiratory rates decrease slightly, and body temperature falls. Stages 3 and 4 are the deepest stages of sleep, differing only in the percentage of delta waves recorded during a 30-second period. During deep sleep or delta sleep, the individual's heart and respiratory rates drop 20% to 30% below those exhibited during waking hours. The individual is difficult to arouse. ***Nursing Process:*** Assessment ***Client Need:*** Physiological Integrity

6. ***Answer:*** 3 (Objective: 2) ***Rationale:*** Physiological changes during NREM sleep include:

   - Peripheral blood vessels dilate.
   - Arterial blood pressure falls.
   - Pulse rate decreases.
   - Cardiac output decreases.

   Nursing Process: Evaluation ***Client Need:*** Physiological Integrity

7. ***Answer:*** 4 (Objective: 8) ***Rationale:*** To reduce environmental distractions in hospitals the following should be practiced: Perform only essential noisy activities during sleeping hours; lower the ring tone of nearby telephones; discontinue use of the paging system after a certain hour (e.g., 2100 hours) or reduce its volume; keep required staff conversations at low levels; conduct nursing reports or other discussions in a separate area away from client rooms. ***Nursing Process:*** Assessment ***Client Need:*** Physiological Integrity

8. ***Answer:*** 1 (Objective: 8) ***Rationale:*** The following are suggestions to promote sleep: Establish a regular bedtime and wake-up time for all days of the week to enhance biological rhythm; avoid performing office work or discussing family problems before bedtime; get adequate exercise during the day to reduce stress, but avoid excessive physical exertion at least 3 hours before bedtime; establish a regular bedtime routine before sleep such as reading, listening to relaxing music, and taking a warm bath or shower. ***Nursing Process:*** Planning ***Client Need:*** Physiological Integrity

9. ***Answer:*** 1 (Objective: 8) ***Rationale:*** Interventions to promote sleep can include the following: Create a sleep-conducive environment that is dark, quiet, comfortable, and cool. Give analgesics before bedtime to relieve aches and pains. If a bedtime snack is necessary, give only low-carbohydrate snack or a milk drink. Avoid giving the client heavy meals 2 to 3 hours before bedtime. ***Nursing Process:*** Planning ***Client Need:*** Physiological Integrity

10. ***Answer:*** 4 (Objective: 1) ***Rationale:*** Night terrors are partial awakenings from non-REM stage 3 or 4 sleep. They are usually seen in children 3 to 6 years of age. The child may sleepwalk, or may sit up in bed screaming and thrashing about. Children experiencing night terrors usually cannot be wakened, but should be protected from injury, helped back to bed, and soothed back to sleep. Baby-sitters should be alerted to the possibility of a night terror occurring. Children do not remember the incident the next day, and there is no indication of a neurologic or emotional problem. Excessive fatigue and a full bladder may contribute to the problem. Having the child take an afternoon nap and empty the bladder before going to sleep at night may be helpful. ***Nursing Process:*** Evaluation ***Client Need:*** Physiological Integrity

CHAPTER 46

Key Term Review

1.	g	2.	r	3.	n	4.	u	5.	d	6.	s
7.	w	8.	a	9.	l	10.	f	11.	j	12.	c
13.	i	14.	b	15.	e	16.	t	17.	x	18.	k
19.	q	20.	o	21.	h	22.	m	23.	p	24.	v
25.	y										

Key Topic Review Answers

1. b. Sympathetically maintained pain occurs occasionally when abnormal connections between pain fibers and the sympathetic nervous system perpetuate problems with both the pain and sympathetically controlled functions (e.g., edema, temperature, and blood flow regulation).

2. b. Pain threshold is the least amount of stimulus that is needed for an individual to label a sensation as pain.

3. a

4. a

5. b. Pain tolerance is the maximum amount of painful stimuli that a person is willing to withstand without seeking avoidance of the pain or relief.

6. analgesic

7. ceiling

8. Equianalgesia

9. Placebo

10. Transdermal

11. __f_____ Appear to arise in different areas

__h_____ Pain arising from organs or hollow viscera

__j_____ When pain lasts only through the expected recovery period

__a_____ Prolonged, usually recurring or persisting over 6 months or longer, and interferes with functioning

__b_____ Pain in the 1–3 range of a 0-10 scale

__c_____ Experienced when an intact, properly functioning nervous system sends signals that tissues are damaged, requiring attention and proper care

___g____ Originates in the skin, muscles, bone, or connective tissue

___e____ Experienced by people who have damaged or malfunctioning nerves

__d___ Follow damage and/or sensitization of peripheral nerves

__i_____ Pain in the 4–6 range of a 0-10 scale

12. d

13. c

14. b

15. d

Case Study Answers

1a. *As the fifth vital sign, pain should be screened for every time vital signs are evaluated. Define pain.* Pain is an unpleasant and highly personal experience that may be imperceptible to others, while consuming all parts of the person's life. The widely agreed-on definition of pain is "Pain is an unpleasant sensory and emotional experience associated with actual or potential tissue damage, or described in terms of such damage." Three parts of this definition have important implications for nurses. First, pain is a physical *and* emotional experience, not all in the body or all in the mind. Second, it is in response to actual *or* potential tissue damage, so there may not be abnormal lab or radiographic reports, despite real pain. Finally, pain is described in terms of such damage. This final component is aligned with McCaffery's often-quoted definition of pain: "Pain is whatever the experiencing person says it is, existing whenever he says it does." Given that some clients are reluctant to disclose the presence of pain unless prompted, nurses will not know of the client's pain until they assess for it. Additionally, it is clear that even nonverbal clients (e.g., preverbal children, intubated clients, the cognitively impaired) experience pain that demands nursing assessment and treatment even if clients are unable to "describe in terms" the nature of their discomfort.

1b. *Identify the two major components of a pain assessment.* Pain assessments consist of two major components: (1) a pain history to obtain facts from the client and (2) direct observation of behaviors, physical signs of tissue damage, and secondary physiological responses of the client.

1c. *Explain the pain intensity scale.* The use of pain intensity scales is an easy and reliable method of determining the client's pain intensity. Such scales provide consistency for nurses to communicate with the client and other health care providers. To avoid confusion, pain scales should use a 0 to 10 range with 0 indicating "no pain" and the highest number indicating the "worst pain possible" for that individual.

Review Question Answers

1. ***Answer:*** 3 (Objective: 1) ***Rationale:*** Severe pain is viewed as an emergency situation deserving attention and prompt professional treatment. Pain is more than a symptom of a problem; it is a high-priority problem in itself. Pain presents both physiological and psychological dangers to health and recovery. ***Nursing Process:*** Assessment ***Client Need:*** Physiological Integrity

2. ***Answer:*** 2 (Objective: 1) ***Rationale:*** When pain lasts only through the expected recovery period, it is described as acute pain, whether it has a sudden or slow onset and regardless of the intensity. Chronic pain, on the other hand, is prolonged, usually recurring or persisting over 6 months or longer, and interferes with functioning. Pain may be referred (appear to arise in different areas) to other parts of the body. Visceral pain (pain arising from organs or hollow

viscera) often presents this way, being perceived in an area remote from the organ causing the pain. ***Nursing Process:*** Assessment ***Client Need:*** Physiological Integrity

3. ***Answer:*** 2 (Objective: 1) ***Rationale:*** Pain tolerance is the maximum amount of painful stimuli that an individual is willing to withstand without seeking avoidance of the pain or relief. Pain threshold is the least amount of stimuli that is needed for a person to feel a sensation he or she labels as pain. Dysesthesia is an unpleasant abnormal sensation. Allodynia is the condition in which nonpainful stimuli (e.g., contact with linen, water, or wind) produce pain. ***Nursing Process:*** Assessment ***Client Need:*** Physiological Integrity

4. ***Answer:*** 1 (Objective: 1) ***Rationale:*** Linking the rating to health and functioning scores, pain in the 1 to 3 range is deemed mild pain, a rating of 4 to 6 is moderate pain, and pain reaching 7 to 10 is ranked severe pain and is associated with the worst outcomes. ***Nursing Process:*** Assessment ***Client Need:*** Physiological Integrity

5. ***Answer:*** 3 (Objective: 1) ***Rationale:***

Acute Pain

Mild to severe

Sympathetic nervous system responses:

- Increased pulse rate
- Increased respiratory rate
- Elevated blood pressure
- Diaphoresis
- Dilated pupils

Related to tissue injury; resolves with healing

Client appears restless and anxious

Client reports pain

Client exhibits behavior indicative of pain: crying, rubbing area, holding area

Chronic Pain

Mild to severe

Parasympathetic nervous system responses:

- Vital signs normal
- Dry, warm skin
- Pupils normal or dilated

Continues beyond healing

Client appears depressed and withdrawn

Client often does not mention pain unless asked

Pain behavior often absent

Nursing Process: Assessment ***Client Need:*** Physiological Integrity

6. ***Answer:*** 4 (Objective: 5) ***Rationale:*** That the amount of tissue damage is directly related to the amount of pain is a misconception about pain. The following are correct statements about pain: The individual who experiences the pain is the only authority about its existence and nature. Pain is a subjective experience, and the intensity and duration of pain vary considerably among individuals. Even with severe pain, periods of physiological and behavioral adaptation can occur. ***Nursing Process:*** Assessment ***Client Need:*** Physiological Integrity

7. ***Answer:*** 4 (Objective: 10) ***Rationale:*** Giving a dose of nonopioid at the same time as a dose of opioid poses no more danger than giving the doses at different times. In fact, many opioids are compounded with a nonopioid (e.g., Percocet [oxycodone and acetaminophen]). It is safe to administer a nonopioid and opioid at the same time. The following statements are true about nonopioids: Nonopioids alone are rarely sufficient to relieve severe pain, but they are an important part in the total analgesic plan. Side effects from long-term use of NSAIDs are considerably more severe and life threatening than the side effects from daily doses of oral morphine or other opioids. ***Nursing Process:*** Assessment ***Client Need:*** Physiological Integrity

8. ***Answer:*** 4 (Objective: 7) ***Rationale: The*** COLDERR mnemonic for pain assessment is defined as follows:

Character:	Describe the sensation (e.g., sharp, aching, burning)
Onset:	When it started, how it has changed
Location:	Where it hurts (all locations)
Duration:	Constant versus intermittent in nature
Exacerbation:	Factors that make it worse
Relief:	Factors that make it better (medications and other factors)
Radiation:	Pattern of shooting/ spreading/location of pain away from its origin

Nursing Process: Planning ***Client Need:*** Physiological Integrity

9. ***Answer:*** 3 (Objective: 3) ***Rationale:*** The Puerto Rican culture tends to be loud and outspoken in their expressions of pain. Do not judge or disapprove. This is a socially learned way to cope with the pain. The Asian American culture values silence. Some clients may be quiet when in pain. Becoming verbally loud may be viewed as causing dishonor to themselves and their family. The African American culture believes pain and suffering is a part of life and is to be endured. The Mexican American culture believes that enduring pain is a sign of strength. Native Americans are quiet, less expressive verbally and nonverbally, and may tolerate a high level of pain. ***Nursing Process:*** Assessment ***Client Need:*** Psychosocial Integrity

10. ***Answer:*** 4 (Objective: 8) ***Rationale:*** Maintain an unbiased attitude (open mind) about what may relieve the pain. New ways to relieve pain are continually being developed. It is not always

possible to explain the effectiveness of particular pain relief measures; however, the use of approaches the patient believes will work should be considered. Provide measures to relieve pain before it becomes severe. Consider the client's ability and willingness to participate actively in pain relief measures. Clients who are excessively fatigued, sedated, or have altered levels of consciousness are less able to participate actively. Establish a trusting relationship. Convey your concern, and acknowledge that you believe that the client is experiencing pain. A trusting relationship promotes expression of the client's thoughts and feelings and enhances effectiveness of planned pain therapies. ***Nursing Process:*** Assessment ***Client Need:*** Physiological Integrity

CHAPTER 47

Key Term Review

1. a 2. e 3. r 4. m 5. b 6. c

7. t 8. j 9. d 10. f 11. l 12. p

13. x 14. y 15. v 16. h 17. g 18. k

19. l 20. n 21. s 22. u 23. w 24. q

25. o

Key Topic Review Answers

1. a

2. a

3. a

4. b. Sugars, the simplest of all carbohydrates, are water soluble and are produced naturally by both plants and animals.

5. b. Of the three monosaccharides (glucose, fructose, and galactose), glucose is by far the most abundant simple sugar.

6. Nutrition

7. Nutrients

8. Starches

9. Fiber

10. Enzymes

11. __c_____ Organic molecules made up primarily of carbon, hydrogen, oxygen, and nitrogen, which combine to form proteins

___j___ Those that cannot be manufactured in the body and must be supplied as part of the protein ingested in the diet

___f___ Those that the body can manufacture

___a___ Contain all of the essential amino acids plus many nonessential ones

__b_____ Lack one or more essential amino acids (most commonly lysine, methionine, or tryptophan) and are usually derived from vegetables

___i___ Organic substances that are greasy and insoluble in water but soluble in alcohol or ether

___g___ Lipids that are solid at room temperature

___d___ Lipids that are liquid at room temperature

___h___ Made up of carbon chains and hydrogen; are the basic structural units of most lipids

___e___ Fatty acids with one double bond

12. d

13. a

14. d

15. a

16. a

Case Study Answers

1a. *Explain the combinations of plant proteins that provide complete proteins*. The combinations of plant proteins that provide complete proteins are grains plus legumes; legumes plus nuts or seeds; and grains, legumes, nuts or seeds plus milk or milk products.

1b. *Identify ways this client can improve his or her appetite.*

- Provide familiar food that the individual likes. Often the relatives of clients are pleased to bring food from home but may need some guidance about special diet requirements.
- Select small portions so as not to discourage the client.
- Avoid unpleasant or uncomfortable treatments immediately before or after a meal.

- Provide a tidy, clean environment that is free of unpleasant sights and odors. A soiled dressing, a used bedpan, an uncovered irrigation set, or even used dishes can negatively affect the appetite.
- Encourage or provide oral hygiene before mealtime. This improves the client's ability to taste.
- Relieve illness symptoms that depress appetite before mealtime; for example, give an analgesic for pain or an antipyretic for a fever or allow rest for fatigue.
- Reduce psychological stress. A lack of understanding of therapy, the anticipation of an operation, and fear of the unknown can cause anorexia. Often, the nurse can help by discussing feelings with the client, giving information and assistance, and allaying fears.

1c. *Discuss possible variations in nutritional practices and preferences among this client's culture.*

- Gifts of food are common and should never be rejected.
- Diets are often high in fat, cholesterol, and sodium.
- Being overweight is viewed as positive.

Review Question Answers

1. ***Answer:*** 4 (Objective: 1) ***Rationale:*** Micronutrients—vitamins and minerals—are those required in small amounts (e.g., milligrams or micrograms) to metabolize the energy-providing nutrients. Carbohydrates, fats, and protein are referred to as macronutrients, because they are needed in large amounts (e.g., hundreds of grams) to provide energy. ***Nursing Process:*** Assessment ***Client Need:*** Physiological Integrity

2. ***Answer:*** 4 (Objective: 1) ***Rationale:*** Fiber is present in the outer layer of grains and bran, and in the skin, seeds, and pulp of many vegetables and fruits. Starches are the insoluble, nonsweet forms of carbohydrate. Most sugars are produced naturally by plants, especially fruits, sugar cane, and sugar beets. Fiber, a complex carbohydrate derived from plants, supplies roughage, or bulk, to the diet. ***Nursing Process:*** Assessment ***Client Need:*** Physiological Integrity

3. ***Answer:*** 2 (Objective: 2) ***Rationale:*** Nonessential amino acids include alanine, aspartic acid, cystine, glutamic acid, glycine, hydroxyproline, proline, serine, and tyrosine. The nine essential amino acids are histidine, isoleucine, leucine, lysine, methionine, phenylalanine, tryptophan, threonine, and valine. Essential amino acids are those that cannot be manufactured in the body and must be supplied as part of the protein ingested in the diet. Nonessential amino acids are those that the body can manufacture. Most animal proteins, including meats, poultry, fish, dairy products, and eggs, are complete proteins. ***Nursing Process:*** Assessment ***Client Need:*** Physiological Integrity

4. ***Answer:*** 2 (Objective: 2) ***Rationale:*** In common use, the terms *fats* and *lipids* are used interchangeably. Lipids are organic substances that are greasy and insoluble in water but soluble in alcohol or ether. Fats are lipids that are solid at room temperature. Oils are lipids that are liquid at room temperature. ***Nursing Process:*** Assessment ***Client Need:*** Physiological Integrity

5. ***Answer:*** 1 (Objective: 4) ***Rationale:***

   To calculate the BMI use the following formula:

   $$\text{BMI} = \frac{\text{Weight in kilograms}}{(\text{Height in meters})^2}$$

   or

   $$\frac{70 \text{ kilograms}}{1.5 \times 1.5 \text{ (meters)}^2} = 31.11$$

   Nursing Process: Assessment ***Client Need:*** Physiological Integrity

6. ***Answer:*** 2 (Objective: 5) ***Rationale:*** The following suggestions may help parents meet the child's nutritional needs and promote effective parent–child interactions: (a) Make mealtime a pleasant time by avoiding tensions at the table and discussions of bad behavior; (b) offer a variety of simple, attractive foods in small portions, and avoid meals that combine foods into one dish, such as a stew; (c) do not use food as a reward or punish a child who does not eat; (d) schedule meals, sleep, and snack times that will allow for optimum appetite and behavior; and (e) avoid the routine use of sweet desserts. ***Nursing Process:*** Implementation ***Client Need:*** Physiological Integrity

7. ***Answer:*** 2 (Objective: 8) ***Rationale:*** A food diary is a detailed record of measured amounts (portion sizes) of all food and fluids a client consumes during a specified period, usually 3 to 7 days. For a 24-hour food recall, the nurse asks the client to recall all the food and beverages the client consumes during a typical 24-hour period when at home. A diet history is a comprehensive, time-consuming assessment of a client's food intake that involves an extensive interview by a nutritionist or dietitian. A food frequency record is a checklist that indicates how often general food groups or specific foods are eaten. ***Nursing Process:*** Implementation ***Client Need:*** Physiological Integrity

8. ***Answer:*** 4 (Objective: 11) ***Rationale: The*** statement, "Note that the word "clear" in clear diet means "colorless" is not correct. A clear liquid diet is limited to water, tea, coffee, clear broths, ginger ale, or other carbonated beverages, strained and clear juices, and plain gelatin. A full liquid diet contains only liquids or foods that turn to liquid at body temperature, such as ice cream. The soft diet is easily chewed and digested. ***Nursing Process:*** Evaluation ***Client Need:*** Physiological Integrity

9. *Answer:* 3 (Objective: 12) ***Rationale:*** Enteral feedings can be given intermittently or continuously. Intermittent feedings are the administration of 300 to 500 mL of enteral formula several times per day. The stomach is the preferred site for these feedings, which are usually administered over at least 30 minutes. The other amounts given are incorrect. ***Nursing Process:*** Implementation ***Client Need:*** Physiological Integrity

10. *Answer:* 4 (Objective: 13) ***Rationale:*** Provide a tidy, clean environment that is free of unpleasant sights and odors. Avoid unpleasant or uncomfortable treatments immediately before or after a meal. Provide familiar food that the client likes. Encourage or provide oral hygiene before mealtime. ***Nursing Process:*** Planning ***Client Need:*** Physiological Integrity

CHAPTER 48

Key Term Review

1. c 2. t 3. f 4. m 5. k 6. l

7. y 8. q 9. a 10. v 11. h 12. n

13. x 14. o 15. j 16. e 17. d 18. r

19. b 20. s 21. g 22. w 23. p 24. i

25. u

Key Topic Review Answers

1. a

2. b. Urinary tract infections (UTIs) are the second most common infection in children, after respiratory infections.

3. a

4. a

5. a

6. Diuretics

7. flaccid

8. Irrigation

9. nephrostomy

10. vesicostomy

11. __c____ Bed-wetting

___b___ The production of abnormally large amounts of urine by the kidneys, often several liters more than the client's usual daily output

___i___ Low urine output

___a___ Refers to a lack of urine production

___j___ Voiding two or more times at night

___g___ Voiding that is either painful or difficult

__d__ Urine remaining in the bladder following the voiding

__f____ A test that uses 24-hour urine and serum creatinine levels to determine the glomerular filtration rate, a sensitive indicator of renal function

__e____ Requires that the client postpone voiding, resist or inhibit the sensation of urgency, and void according to a timetable rather than according to the urge to void

___h___ Referred to as timed voiding or scheduled toileting, attempts to keep clients dry by having them void at regular intervals

12. a

13. d

14. a

15. b

16. d

Case Study Answers

1a. *List the steps a nurse must follow to measure fluid output.*

- Wear clean gloves to prevent contact with microorganisms or blood in the urine.
- Ask the client to void in a clean urinal, bedpan, commode, or toilet collection device ("hat").
- Instruct the client to keep the urine separate from feces and to avoid putting toilet paper in the urine collection container.
- Pour the voided urine into a calibrated container.
- Holding the container at eye level, read the amount in the container. Containers usually have a measuring scale on the inside.
- Record the amount on the fluid intake and output sheet, which may be at the bedside or in the bathroom.

- Rinse the urine collection and measuring containers with cool water and store appropriately.
- Remove gloves and perform hand hygiene.
- Calculate and document the total output on the client's chart at the end of each shift and at the end of 24 hours.

1b. *Identify various goals for clients with urinary elimination problems.* The goals established will vary according to the diagnosis and defining characteristics. Examples of overall goals for clients with urinary elimination problems may include the following:

- Maintain or restore a normal voiding pattern.
- Regain normal urine output.
- Prevent associated risks such as infection, skin breakdown, fluid and electrolyte imbalance, and lowered self-esteem.
- Perform toilet activities independently with or without assistive devices.
- Contain urine with the appropriate device, catheter, ostomy appliance, or absorbent product.

1c. *Explain how this client can maintain normal urinary elimination.* Most interventions to maintain normal urinary elimination are independent nursing functions. These include promoting adequate fluid intake, maintaining normal voiding habits, and assisting with toileting.

Review Question Answers

1. ***Answer:*** 1 (Objective: 2) ***Rationale:*** Oliguria is low urine output, usually less than 500 mL a day or 30 mL an hour for an adult. Polyuria (or diuresis) refers to the production of abnormally large amounts of urine by the kidneys, often several liters more than the client's usual daily output. Polydipsia is excessive fluid intake. Anuria refers to a lack of urine production. ***Nursing Process:*** Assessment ***Client Need:*** Physiological Integrity

2. ***Answer:*** 2 (Objective: 2) ***Rationale:*** Urinary frequency is voiding at frequent intervals, that is, more than four to six times per day. Nocturia is voiding two or more times at night. Urgency is the sudden strong desire to void. Dysuria means voiding that is either painful or difficult. ***Nursing Process:*** Assessment ***Client Need:*** Physiological Integrity

3. ***Answer:*** 4 (Objective: 7) ***Rationale:*** Ways to prevent a recurrence of a UTI include the following: Avoid tight-fitting pants or other clothing that creates irritation to the urethra and prevents ventilation of the perineal area. Drink eight 8-ounce glasses of water per day to flush bacteria out of the urinary system. Wear cotton rather than nylon underclothes. Girls and women should always wipe the perineal area from front to back following urination or defecation in order to prevent introduction of gastrointestinal bacteria into the urethra. ***Nursing Process:*** Planning ***Client Need:*** Physiological Integrity

4. ***Answer:*** 4 (Objective: 8) ***Rationale:*** Intermittent self-catheterization protects the upper urinary tract from reflux, reduces the incidence of urinary tract infection, enables the client to retain independence and gain control of the bladder, and allows normal sexual relations without incontinence. ***Nursing Process:*** Evaluation ***Client Need:*** Physiological Integrity

5. ***Answer:*** 3 (Objective: 4) ***Rationale:*** The normal color or clarity of urine is straw, amber, or transparent. Abnormal color or clarity of urine is dark amber, dark orange, red, dark brown, cloudy, mucous plugs, viscid, thick. ***Nursing Process:*** Assessment ***Client Need:*** Physiological Integrity

6. ***Answer:*** 3 (Objective: 6) ***Rationale:*** Normal results for a urine specific gravity should be in the range of 1.010 to 1.025. All other results not in this range are considered abnormal. ***Nursing Process:*** Assessment ***Client Need:*** Physiological Integrity

7. ***Answer:*** 3 (Objective: 8) ***Rationale:*** Lubricate the catheter 6 to 7 inches for males. If this is not done, the entire part of the catheter that is inserted into the male penis will not be lubricated. This will make the procedure very uncomfortable for the client as well as cause harm to the client. The following statements are correct steps: Pick up a cleansing ball with the forceps in your dominant hand and wipe from the center of the meatus in a circular motion around the glans. Grasp the catheter firmly 2 to 3 in. from the tip. Ask the client to take a slow deep breath and insert the catheter as the client exhales. ***Nursing Process:*** Implementation ***Client Need:*** Physiological Integrity

8. ***Answer:*** 3 (Objective: 6) ***Rationale:*** Facilitating and promoting urinary elimination includes the following: Emphasize the importance of drinking eight to ten 8-ounce glasses of water daily. Advise the client and family to install grab bars and elevated toilet seats as needed. Teach the client to empty the bladder completely at each voiding. Suggest clothing that is easily removed for toileting, such as elastic-waist pants or pants with Velcro closures. ***Nursing Process:*** Evaluation ***Client Need:*** Physiological Integrity

9. ***Answer:*** 3 (Objective: 7) ***Rationale:*** Develop a schedule that will help remind you to do these exercises, for example, before getting out of bed in the morning. Initially perform each contraction 10 times, three times daily. Gradually increase the count to a full 10 seconds for both contraction and relaxation. To control episodes of stress incontinence, perform a pelvic muscle contraction when initiating any activity that increases intra-abdominal pressure, such as coughing, laughing, sneezing, or lifting. Contract your pelvic muscles whereby you pull your rectum, urethra, and vagina up inside, and hold for a count of 3 to 5 seconds. Then relax the same muscles for a count of 3 to 5 seconds. ***Nursing Process:*** Planning ***Client Need:*** Health Promotion and Maintenance

10. *Answer:* 2 (Objective: 8) ***Rationale:*** For preventing catheter-associated urinary infections the following guidelines should be practiced: Do not disconnect the catheter and drainage tubing unless absolutely necessary. Maintain a sterile closed-drainage system. Provide routine perineal hygiene, including cleansing with soap and water after defecation. Prevent contamination of the catheter with feces. ***Nursing Process:*** Evaluation ***Client Need:*** Preventing Catheter-Associated Urinary Infections

CHAPTER 49

Key Term Review

1.	p	2.	f	3.	s	4.	n	5.	w	6.	c
7.	j	8.	d	9.	u	10.	x	11.	b	12.	q
13.	g	14.	l	15.	k	16.	m	17.	y	18.	h
19.	a	20.	o	21.	i	22.	v	23.	e	24.	r
25.	t										

Key Topic Review Answers

1. a

2. b. The large intestine extends from the ileocecal (ileocolic) valve, which lies between the small and large intestines, to the anus.

3. b. Normal feces are made of about 75% water and 25% solid materials.

4. a

5. a

6. Flatulence

7. ostomy

8. bedpan

9. enema

10. Cathartics

11. __h__ The act of eating food

__j__ Waste products leaving the stomach through the small intestine and then passing through the ileocecal valve

__a__ A condition that can occur when the veins become distended, as can occur with repeated pressure

__f__ The expulsion of feces from the anus and rectum

__i__ Increased peristalsis of the colon after food has entered the stomach

__b__ Medications that stimulate bowel activity and so assist fecal elimination

__d__ Fewer than three bowel movements per week

__g__ A mass or collection of hardened feces in the folds of the rectum

__e__ The passage of liquid feces and an increased frequency of defecation

__c__ The loss of voluntary ability to control fecal and gaseous discharges through the anal sphincter

12. c

13. b

14. d

15. d

Case Study Answers

1a. *Identify ways for the client to manage diarrhea.*

- Drink at least eight glasses of water per day to prevent dehydration. Consider drinking a few glasses of electrolyte replacement fluids each day.
- Eat foods with sodium and potassium. Most foods contain sodium. Potassium is found in meats and many vegetables and fruits, especially purple grape juice, tomatoes, potatoes, bananas, cooked peaches, and apricots.
- Increase foods containing soluble fiber, such as rice, oatmeal, and skinless fruits and potatoes.
- Avoid alcohol and beverages with caffeine, which aggravate the problem.
- Limit foods containing insoluble fiber, such as high-fiber whole-wheat and whole-grain breads and cereals, and raw fruits and vegetables.
- Limit fatty foods.
- Thoroughly clean and dry the perianal area after passing stool to prevent skin irritation and breakdown. Use soft toilet tissue to clean and dry the area. Apply a dimethicone-based cream or alcohol-free barrier film as needed.

- If possible, discontinue medications that cause diarrhea.
- When diarrhea has stopped, reestablish normal bowel flora by eating fermented dairy products, such as yogurt or buttermilk.
- Seek a primary care provider consultation right away if weakness, dizziness, or loose stools persist for more than 48 hours.

1b. *Provide the client with information about healthy defecation.*

- Establish a regular exercise regimen.
- Include high-fiber foods, such as vegetables, fruits, and whole grains, in the diet.
- Maintain fluid intake of 2,000 to 3,000 mL a day.
- Do not ignore the urge to defecate.
- Allow time to defecate, preferably at the same time each day.
- Avoid over-the-counter medications to treat constipation and diarrhea.

1c. *Identify three major causes of diarrhea.* Some causes of diarrhea include psychological stress (e.g., anxiety); medications; antibiotics; cathartics; allergy to food, fluid, or drugs; intolerance of food or fluid.

Review Question Answers

1. ***Answer:*** 1 (Objective: 1) ***Rationale:*** A gastrostomy is an opening through the abdominal wall into the stomach. A jejunostomy opens through the abdominal wall into the jejunum. A colostomy opens into the colon (large bowel). An ileostomy opens into the ileum (small bowel). ***Nursing Process:*** Assessment ***Client Need:*** Physiological Integrity

2. ***Answer:*** 2 (Objective: 8) ***Rationale:*** A carminative enema is given primarily to expel flatus. A retention enema introduces oil or medication into the rectum and sigmoid colon. A return-flow enema is used occasionally to expel flatus. Cleansing enemas may also be described as high or low. ***Nursing Process:*** Assessment ***Client Need:*** Physiological Integrity

3. ***Answer:*** 2 (Objective: 6) ***Rationale:*** Ask the client to assume a left side-lying position, with the knees flexed and the back toward the nurse. Place a bed pad under the client's buttocks and a bedpan nearby to receive stool. Drape the client for comfort and to avoid unnecessary exposure of the body. Gently insert the index finger into the rectum and move the finger along the length of the rectum. ***Nursing Process:*** Implementation ***Client Need:*** Physiological Integrity

4. ***Answer:*** 2 (Objectives: 2, 7) ***Rationale:*** Client teaching for healthy defecation: maintain fluid intake of 2,000 to 3,000 mL a day; include high-fiber foods, such as vegetables, fruits, and whole grains, in the diet; allow time to defecate, preferably at the same time each day; avoid over-the-counter medications to treat constipation and diarrhea. ***Nursing Process:*** Evaluation ***Client Need:*** Physiological Integrity

5. ***Answer:*** 3 (Objectives: 2, 7) ***Rationale:*** Limit foods containing insoluble fiber, such as high-fiber whole-wheat and whole-grain breads and cereals, and raw fruits and vegetables. Drink at least eight glasses of water per day to prevent dehydration. Eat foods with sodium and potassium. Limit fatty foods. ***Nursing Process:*** Planning ***Client Need:*** Physiological Integrity

6. ***Answer:*** 2 (Objective: 9) ***Rationale:*** Ostomy appliances can be applied for up to 7 days. The pouch is emptied when it is one-third to one-half full. Most pouches contain odor barrier material. If the pouch overfills, it can cause separation of the skin barrier from the skin, and stool can come in contact with the skin. ***Nursing Process:*** Evaluation ***Client Need:*** Physiological Integrity

7. ***Answer:*** 4 (Objective: 9) ***Rationale:*** The divided colostomy is often used in situations where spillage of feces into the distal end of the bowel needs to be avoided. The single stoma is created when one end of bowel is brought out through an opening onto the anterior abdominal wall. In the loop colostomy, a loop of bowel is brought out onto the abdominal wall and supported by a plastic bridge, or a piece of rubber tubing. The divided colostomy consists of two edges of bowel brought out onto the abdomen but separated from each other. ***Nursing Process:*** Evaluation ***Client Need:*** Physiological Integrity

8. ***Answer:*** 3 (Objective: 2) ***Rationale:*** Although the squatting position best facilitates defecation, the best position for most clients seems to be leaning forward while on a toilet seat. A client should be encouraged to defecate when the urge is recognized. Regular exercise helps clients develop a regular defecation pattern. For clients who have difficulty sitting down and getting up from the toilet, an elevated toilet seat can be attached to a regular toilet. ***Nursing Process:*** Implementation ***Client Need:*** Physiological Integrity

9. ***Answer:*** 2 (Objective: 3) ***Rationale:***

Orange or green-colored stools are indications of an intestinal infection. Additional abnormal colors to stools include:

Adult: brown, clay or white, absence of bile pigment (bile obstruction); diagnostic study using barium

Infant: yellow, black or tarry, drug (e.g., iron); bleeding from upper gastrointestinal tract (e.g., stomach, small intestine); diet high in red meat and dark green vegetables (e.g., spinach)

Red, bleeding from lower gastrointestinal tract (e.g., rectum); some foods (e.g., beets)

White, malabsorption of fats; diet high in milk and milk products and low in meat

Nursing Process: Assessment ***Client Need:*** Physiological Integrity

10. *Answer:* 3 (Objective: 8) ***Rationale:*** Oil solutions lubricate the feces and the colonic mucosa. Isotonic solutions distend the colon, stimulate peristalsis, and soften feces. Hypertonic solutions draw water into the colon. Hypotonic solutions distend the colon, stimulate peristalsis, and soften feces. Soapsuds solutions irritate the mucosa and distend the colon. Nursing Process: Evaluation *Client Need:* Physiological Integrity

CHAPTER 50

Key Term Review

1. l 2. a 3. c 4. e 5. f 6. r

7. j 8. o 9. g 10. i 11. u 12. y

13. v 14. m 15. w 16. q 17. k 18. x

19. t 20. h 21. d 22. b 23. s 24. p

25. n

Key Topic Review Answers

1. a

2. a

3. b. Hyperinflation involves giving the client breaths that are 1 to 1.5 times the tidal volume set on the ventilator through the ventilator circuit or via a manual resuscitation bag.

4. b. When air collects in the pleural space, it is known as a pneumothorax.

5. b. Hyperoxygenation can be done with a manual resuscitation bag or through the ventilator and is performed by increasing the oxygen flow (usually to 100%) before suctioning and between suction attempts.

6. Oxygen

7. Intrapulmonary

8. Atelectasis

9. Diffusion

10. Apnea

11. __a__ A lipoprotein produced by specialized alveolar cells; acts like a detergent, reducing the surface tension of alveolar fluid

__e__ Oxygen-carrying red pigment

__j__ Red blood cells (RBCs)

__h__ A condition of insufficient oxygen anywhere in the body, from the inspired gas to the tissues

__c__ Bluish discoloration of the skin, nail beds, and mucous membranes, due to reduced hemoglobin-oxygen saturation

__f__ An abnormally slow respiratory rate

__i__ The inability to breathe except in an upright or standing position

__b__ Coughed-up material

__d__ Spit out

__g__ Devices that add water vapor to inspired air

12. d

13. b

14. a

15. c

16. d

Case Study Answers

1a. *Which factors does adequate ventilation depend on?*

Adequate ventilation depends on several factors:

- Clear airways
- An intact central nervous system and respiratory center
- An intact thoracic cavity capable of expanding and contracting
- Adequate pulmonary compliance and recoil.

1b. *Which factors affect the rate of oxygen transport from the lungs to the tissues?*

The following factors can affect the rate of oxygen transport from the lungs to the tissues:

- Cardiac output
- Number of erythrocytes and blood hematocrit
- Exercise.

1c. *Which factors that influence oxygenation affect the cardiovascular system as well as the respiratory system?* These factors include age, environment, lifestyle, health status, medications, and stress.

1d. *What are oxygen therapy safety precautions?*

- For home oxygen use or when the facility permits smoking, teach family members and roommates to smoke only outside or in provided smoking rooms away from the client and oxygen equipment.
- Place cautionary signs reading "No Smoking: Oxygen in Use" on the client's door, at the foot or head of the bed, and on the oxygen equipment.
- Instruct the client and visitors about the hazard of smoking with oxygen in use.
- Make sure that electric devices (such as razors, hearing aids, radios, televisions, and heating pads) are in good working order to prevent the occurrence of short-circuit sparks.
- Avoid materials that generate static electricity, such as woolen blankets and synthetic fabrics. Cotton blankets should be used, and clients and caregivers should be advised to wear cotton fabrics.
- Avoid the use of volatile, flammable materials, such as oils, greases, alcohol, ether, and acetone (e.g., nail polish remover) near clients receiving oxygen.
- Be sure that electric monitoring equipment, suction machines, and portable diagnostic machines are all electrically grounded.
- Make known the location of fire extinguishers, and make sure personnel are trained in their use.

Review Question Answers

1. ***Answer:*** 3 (Objective: 1) ***Rationale:*** Adequate ventilation depends on several factors:

   - An intact central nervous system and respiratory center
   - Clear airways
   - Adequate pulmonary compliance and recoil
   - An intact thoracic cavity capable of expanding and contracting

   Nursing Process: Assessment ***Client Need:*** Physiological Integrity

2. ***Answer:*** 1 (Objective: 5) ***Rationale:*** Normal respiration (eupnea) is quiet, rhythmic, and effortless. Tachypnea (rapid rate) is seen with fevers, metabolic acidosis, pain, and with hypercapnia or hypoxemia. Bradypnea is an abnormally slow respiratory rate, which may be seen in clients who have taken drugs such as morphine, who have metabolic alkalosis, or who have increased intracranial pressure (e.g., from brain injuries). Apnea is the cessation of breathing. ***Nursing Process:*** Assessment ***Client Need:*** Physiological Integrity

3. ***Answer:*** 3 (Objective: 5) ***Rationale:*** Cheyne-Stokes respirations are the marked rhythmic waxing and waning of respirations from very deep to very shallow breathing and temporary apnea; common causes include congestive heart failure, increased intracranial pressure, and overdose of certain drugs. Biot's (cluster) respirations are shallow breaths interrupted by apnea; may be seen in clients with central nervous system disorders. Orthopnea is the inability to breathe except in an upright or standing position. Difficult or uncomfortable breathing is called dyspnea. ***Nursing Process:*** Assessment ***Client Need:*** Physiological Integrity

4. ***Answer:*** 4 (Objective: 7) ***Rationale:*** The nonrebreather mask delivers the highest oxygen concentration possible—95% to 100%—by means other than intubation or mechanical ventilation, at liter flows of 10 to 15 L per minute. The other answers are incorrect. ***Nursing Process:*** Assessment ***Client Need:*** Physiological Integrity

5. ***Answer:*** 2 (Objective: 7) ***Rationale:*** The Venturi mask delivers oxygen concentrations varying from 24% to 40% or 50% at liter flows of 4 to 10 L per minute. The nonrebreather mask delivers the highest oxygen concentration possible—95% to 100%—by means other than intubation or mechanical ventilation, at liter flows of 10 to 15 L per minute. One-way valves on the mask and between the reservoir bag and the mask prevent the room air and the client's exhaled air from entering the bag so only the oxygen in the bag is inspired. The simple face mask delivers oxygen concentrations from 40% to 60% at liter flows of 5 to 8 L per minute, respectively. The partial rebreather mask delivers oxygen concentrations of 60% to 90% at liter flows of 6 to 10 L per minute, respectively. The oxygen reservoir bag that is attached allows the client to rebreathe about the first third of the exhaled air in conjunction with oxygen. ***Nursing Process:*** Assessment ***Client Need:*** Physiological Integrity

6. ***Answer:*** 4 (Objective: 7) ***Rationale:*** Because an endotracheal tube passes through the epiglottis and glottis, the client is unable to speak while it is in place; however, the client is still able to swallow. Endotracheal tubes are most commonly inserted for clients who have had general anesthetics or for those in emergency situations where mechanical ventilation is required. An endotracheal tube is inserted by the primary care provider, nurse, or respiratory therapist with specialized education. An endotracheal tube is inserted through the mouth or the nose and into the trachea with the guide of a laryngoscope. The tube terminates just superior to the bifurcation of the trachea into the bronchi. The tube may have an air-filled cuff to prevent air leakage around it. ***Nursing Process:*** Assessment ***Client Need:*** Physiological Integrity

7. ***Answer:*** 2 (Objective: 6) ***Rationale:***

   Residual volume (RV): the amount of air remaining in the lungs after maximal exhalation

   Total lung capacity (TLC): the total volume of the lungs at maximum inflation; calculated by adding the V_T, IRV, ERV, and RV

Vital capacity (VC): total amount of air that can be exhaled after a maximal inspiration; calculated by adding the V_T, IRV, and ERV

Expiratory reserve volume (ERV): maximum amount of air that can be exhaled following a normal exhalation

Nursing Process: Assessment ***Client Need:*** Physiological Integrity

8. ***Answer:*** 2 (Objective: 1) ***Rationale:*** The cough reflex consists of the following:

   - Nerve impulses are sent through the vagus nerve to the medulla.
   - A large inspiration of approximately 2.5 L occurs.
   - The epiglottis and glottis (vocal cords) close.
   - A strong contraction of abdominal and internal intercostal muscles dramatically raises the pressure in the lungs.
   - The epiglottis and glottis open suddenly.
   - Air rushes outward with great velocity.
   - Mucus and any foreign particles are dislodged from the lower respiratory tract and are propelled up and out.

   Nursing Process: Assessment ***Client Need:*** Physiological Integrity

9. ***Answer:*** 4 (Objective: 7) ***Rationale:*** Oxygen therapy safety precautions include:

   - Avoid the use of volatile, flammable materials, such as oils, greases, alcohol, ether, and acetone (e.g., nail polish remover) near clients receiving oxygen.
   - For home oxygen use or when the facility permits smoking, teach family members and roommates to smoke only outside or in provided smoking rooms away from the client and oxygen equipment.
   - Place cautionary signs reading "No Smoking: Oxygen in Use" on the client's door, at the foot or head of the bed, and on the oxygen equipment.
   - Instruct the client and visitors about the hazard of smoking with oxygen in use.
   - Make sure that electric devices (such as razors, hearing aids, radios, televisions, and heating pads) are in good working order to prevent the occurrence of short-circuit sparks.
   - Avoid materials that generate static electricity, such as woolen blankets and synthetic fabrics. Cotton blankets should be used, and clients and caregivers should be advised to wear cotton fabrics.
   - Be sure that electric monitoring equipment, suction machines, and portable diagnostic machines are all electrically grounded.
   - Make known the location of fire extinguishers, and make sure personnel are trained in their use.

   Nursing Process: Assessment ***Client Need:*** Physiological Integrity

10. ***Answer:*** 4 (Objective: 7) ***Rationale:*** Put on sterile gloves. Keep your dominant hand sterile during the procedure. Clean the lumen and entire inner cannula thoroughly using a brush or pipe cleaners moistened with sterile normal saline. Rinse the inner cannula thoroughly in the sterile normal saline. After rinsing, gently tap the cannula against the inside edge of the sterile saline container. ***Nursing Process:*** Implementation ***Client Need:*** Physiological Integrity

CHAPTER 51

Key Term Review

1. w 2. n 3. h 4. f 5. c 6. p

7. t 8. y 9. q 10. k 11. j 12. e

13. u 14. a 15. v 16. r 17. s 18. g

19. x 20. b 21. l 22. d 23. o 24. i

25. m

Key Topic Review Answers

1. a
2. b. Heart rates are highest and most variable in newborns.
3. a
4. b. The AHA recommends at least 150 minutes per week of moderate exercise or 75 minutes per week of vigorous exercise for adults.
5. a
6. Ischemia
7. heart
8. stroke volume (SV)
9. Preload
10. Afterload

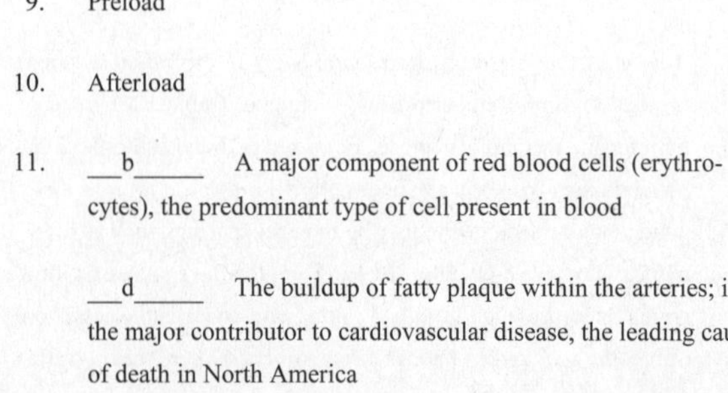

11. __b_____ A major component of red blood cells (erythrocytes), the predominant type of cell present in blood

    __d_____ The buildup of fatty plaque within the arteries; is the major contributor to cardiovascular disease, the leading cause of death in North America

___c_____ Serves as the transport medium within the cardiovascular system, bringing oxygen and nutrients from the environment (via the lungs and gastrointestinal system) to the cells

___j_____ A ________ arrest (pulmonary arrest) is the cessation of breathing.

___g_____ The study of the forces or pressures involved in blood circulation

____i____ A lack of blood supply due to obstructed circulation

____h____ The molecule that oxygen attaches to; it gives an indication of the oxygen-carrying capacity of the blood

____f____ The heart and the blood vessels make up the ________ system that, together with blood, is the major system for transporting oxygen and nutrients to the tissues, and waste products away from the tissues for elimination.

____e____ A type of blood vessel that carries blood to the tissues through a system of arteries, arterioles, and capillaries and returns it to the heart through the venules, veins, and the venae cavae

____a____ The force exerted on arterial walls by the blood flowing within the vessel

12. d

13. a

14. a

15. d

16. d

Case Study Answers

1a. *Why is the health care provider concerned about my lipid levels being elevated?* A strong link exists between elevated serum lipid levels and the development of coronary heart disease. Lipoproteins circulate in the blood and are made up of cholesterol, triglycerides, and phospholipids. A high dietary intake of saturated fats is the most critical factor for the development of elevated serum lipids. The average American diet often contains more than 40% of its calories in fats. The American Heart Association recommends that less than 30% of total calories come from fats.

1b. *What is hypertension?* Hypertension (or increased blood pressure) increases the risk of coronary heart disease in several ways. First, it increases the workload of the heart, increasing oxygen demand and coronary blood flow. The increased workload also causes hypertrophy of the ventricles. Over time this can contribute to heart failure. Second, hypertension causes endothelial damage to the blood vessels, which stimulates the development of atherosclerosis.

1c. *What are the risk factors for coronary heart disease?* Nonmodifiable risk factors are heredity, age, and gender (women's risk increases after menopause); modifiable risk factors are elevated serum lipid level, hypertension, cigarette smoking, diabetes, obesity, and sedentary lifestyle; other risk factors are previous health status, stress and coping, dietary factors, alcohol intake, and elevated homocysteine level.

Review Question Answers

1. ***Answer:*** 1 (Objective: 2) ***Rationale:*** Modifiable risk factors for coronary heart disease include elevated serum lipid level; hypertension; cigarette smoking; diabetes; obesity; sedentary lifestyle. Nonmodifiable risk factors include heredity; age; gender (women's risk increases post-menopause). Other risk factors include previous health status; stress and coping; dietary factors; alcohol intake; elevated homocysteine level. ***Nursing Process:*** Assessment ***Client Need:*** Physiological Integrity

2. ***Answer:*** 3 (Objective: 4) ***Rationale:*** Homocysteine does not increase the cholesterol level of an individual. Homocysteine is an amino acid that has been shown to be increased in many people with atherosclerosis, increasing the risk for developing cardiovascular disease. It is thought that individuals can reduce their homocysteine level by taking a multivitamin that provides folate, vitamin B_6, vitamin B_{12}, and riboflavin. ***Nursing Process:*** Assessment ***Client Need:*** Physiological Integrity

3. ***Answer:*** 4 (Objective: 2) ***Rationale:*** Normal changes of aging may contribute to problems of circulation in elders, even when there is no actual pathology:

   - There is a decrease in baroreceptor response to blood pressure changes, making the heart and blood vessels less responsive to exercise and stress. This often results in dizziness, falls, orthostatic hypotension, and mental changes.
   - A decrease of muscle tone in the heart results in a decrease in cardiac output.
   - Blood vessels become less elastic and have an increase in calcification. This results in a restricted blood flow and a decrease of oxygen and nutrients to tissues (heart, peripheral, and cerebral).
   - Impaired valve function in the heart is often the result of increased stiffness and calcification and results in a decrease in cardiac output.

   Nursing Process: Assessment ***Client Need:*** Physiological Integrity

4. ***Answer:*** 2 (Objective: 7) ***Rationale:*** Promoting a healthy heart includes exercising regularly, participating in at least 20 minutes (40 minutes is preferred) of vigorous exercise four to five times a week; not smoking; eating a diet low in total fat, saturated fats, and cholesterol; reducing stress; and managing anger. ***Nursing Process:*** Planning ***Client Need:*** Physiological Integrity

5. *Answer:* 4 (Objective: 1) ***Rationale:*** Deoxygenated blood from the veins enters the right side of the heart through the superior and inferior venae cavae. Four hollow chambers within the heart, two upper atria and two lower ventricles, are separated longitudinally by the interventricular septum, forming two parallel pumps. The heart is a hollow, cone-shaped organ about the size of a fist. The heart is located in the mediastinum, between the lungs and underlying the sternum. ***Nursing Process:*** Evaluation ***Client Need:*** Physiological Integrity

6. *Answer:* 2 (Objective: 1) ***Rationale:*** With each heartbeat, the myocardium goes through a cycle of contraction (systole) and relaxation (diastole). Systole is when the heart ejects (propels) the blood into the pulmonary and systemic circulations. Diastole is when the ventricles fill with blood. The diastolic phase of the cardiac cycle is twice as long as the systolic phase. This is important because diastole (or ventricular filling) is largely a passive process. The longer diastolic phase allows this filling to occur. At the end of the diastolic phase the atria contract, adding an additional volume to the ventricles. This volume is sometimes called atrial kick. ***Nursing Process:*** Assessment ***Client Need:*** Physiological Integrity

7. *Answer:* 1 (Objective: 1) ***Rationale:*** The primary pacemaker of the heart is the sinoatrial (SA or sinus) node, located where the superior venae cavae enters the right atrium. The SA node normally initiates electrical impulses that are conducted throughout the heart and result in ventricular contraction. In adults, it usually discharges impulses at a regular rate of 60 to 100 times per minute, the "normal" heart rate. The impulse then spreads throughout the atria via the interatrial pathways. These conduction pathways converge and narrow through the atrioventricular (AV) node, slightly delaying transmission of the impulse to the ventricles. This delay allows the atria to contract slightly before ventricular contraction occurs. From the AV node, the impulse then progresses down through the intraventricular septum to the ventricular conduction pathways: the bundle of His, the right and left bundle branches, and the Purkinje fibers. ***Nursing Process:*** Assessment ***Client Need:*** Physiological Integrity

8. *Answer:* 4 (Objective: 1) ***Rationale:*** Resistance is opposition to flow; peripheral vascular resistance impedes or opposes blood flow to the tissues. PVR is determined by:

   - Blood vessel length
   - Blood vessel diameter
   - The viscosity, or thickness, of the blood

   Nursing Process: Assessment ***Client Need:*** Physiological Integrity

9. *Answer:* 1 (Objective: 9) ***Rationale:*** Signs of heart failure may include:

   - Pulmonary congestion; adventitious lung sounds
   - Shortness of breath
   - Increased heart rate
   - Increased respiratory rate
   - Peripheral vasoconstriction; cold, pale extremities
   - Distended neck veins

   Nursing Process: Assessment ***Client Need:*** Physiological Integrity

CHAPTER 52

Key Term Review

1.	c	2.	f	3.	q	4.	e	5.	g	6.	m
7.	l	8.	h	9.	u	10.	j	11.	n	12.	d
13.	o	14.	r	15.	s	16.	t	17.	v	18.	p
19.	b	20.	x	21.	k	22.	i	23.	w	24.	y
25.	a										

Key Topic Review Answers

1. b. Approximately 60% of the average healthy adult's weight is water, the primary body fluid.
2. a
3. a
4. b. Osmotic pressure is the power of a solution to pull water across a semipermeable membrane.
5. a
6. calcium
7. hypervolemia
8. blood
9. drip
10. Butterfly
11. ___c___ The chemical combining power of the ion, or the capacity of cations to combine with anions to form molecules

    ___j___ The continual intermingling of molecules in liquids, gases, or solids brought about by the random movement of the molecules

    ___a___ Found outside the cells and accounts for about one third of total body fluid

____i____ Have a low hydrogen ion concentration and can accept hydrogen ions in solution

____h____ Also known as hyperosmolar imbalance, this occurs when water is lost from the body, leaving the client with excess sodium

____f____ Prevent excessive changes in pH by removing or releasing hydrogen ions

____g____ A sodium deficit, or serum sodium level of less than 135 mEq/L,

___e___ A substance that releases hydrogen ions (H^+) in solution

___d_____ A process whereby fluid and solutes move together across a membrane from one compartment to another

___b___ Ions that carry a positive charge

12. a

13. b

14. c

15. d

16. b

Case Study Answers

1a. *Why is water vital to health and normal cellular function?* Water is vital to health and normal cellular function because it serves as a medium for metabolic reactions within cells; a transporter for nutrients, waste products, and other substances; a lubricant; an insulator and shock absorber; and one means of regulating and maintaining body temperature.

1b. *Explain the thirst mechanism.* The thirst mechanism is the primary regulator of fluid intake. The thirst center is located in the hypothalamus of the brain. A number of stimuli trigger this center, including the osmotic pressure of body fluids, vascular volume, and angiotensin (a hormone released in response to decreased blood flow to the kidneys). For example, a long-distance runner loses significant amounts of water through perspiration and rapid breathing during a race, increasing the concentration of solutes and the osmotic pressure of body fluids. This increased osmotic pressure stimulates the thirst center, causing the runner to experience the sensation of thirst and the desire to drink to replace lost fluids. Thirst is normally relieved immediately after drinking a small amount of fluid, even before it is absorbed from the gastrointestinal tract. However, this relief is only temporary, and the thirst returns in about 15 minutes. The thirst is again temporarily relieved after the ingested fluid distends the upper gastrointestinal tract. These mechanisms protect the individual from drinking too much, because it takes from 30 minutes to 1 hour for the fluid to be absorbed and distributed throughout the body.

1c. *List the four routes of fluid output.* The four routes of fluid output are (1) urine, (2) insensible loss through the skin as perspiration and through the lungs as water vapor in the expired air, (3) noticeable loss through the skin, and (4) loss through the intestines in feces.

Review Question Answers

1. ***Answer:*** 3 (Objective: 1) ***Rationale:*** Women have a lower percentage of body water than men. Approximately 60% of the average healthy adult's weight is water, the primary body fluid. In good health, this volume remains relatively constant and the individual's weight varies by less than 0.2 kg (0.5 lb) in 24 hours, regardless of the amount of fluid ingested. Infants have the highest proportion of water, accounting for 70% to 80% of their body weight. Water makes up a greater percentage of a lean individual's body weight than an obese individual's. ***Nursing Process:*** Assessment ***Client Need:*** Physiological Integrity

2. ***Answer:*** 1 (Objective: 1) ***Rationale:*** Diffusion is the continual intermingling of molecules in liquids, gases, or solids brought about by the random movement of the molecules. Osmosis is an important mechanism for maintaining homeostasis and fluid balance. Osmosis occurs when the concentration of solutes on one side of a selectively permeable membrane, such as the capillary membrane, is higher than on the other side. Osmolality is determined by the total solute concentration within a fluid compartment and is measured as parts of solute per kilogram of water. ***Nursing Process:*** Assessment ***Client Need:*** Physiological Integrity

3. ***Answer:*** 3 (Objective: 3) ***Rationale:*** Hyponatremia is a sodium deficit, or serum sodium level of less than 135 mEq/L, and is, in acute care settings, a common electrolyte imbalance. Hypernatremia is excess sodium in ECF, or a serum sodium of greater than 145 mEq/L. Hypokalemia is a potassium deficit or a serum potassium level of less than 3.5 mEq/L. Hyperkalemia is a potassium excess or a serum potassium level greater than 5.0 mEq/L. ***Nursing Process:*** Assessment ***Client Need:*** Physiological Integrity

4. ***Answer:*** 3 (Objective: 5) ***Rationale:*** When an individual hyperventilates, the pH rises to greater than 7.45. In addition, more carbon dioxide than normal is exhaled (not oxygen) and carbonic acid levels fall. ***Nursing Process:*** Assessment ***Client Need:*** Physiological Integrity

5. ***Answer:*** 1 (Objective: 5) ***Rationale:*** The normal values of arterial blood gases are:

PaO_2	80–100 mm Hg
pH	7.35–7.45
$PaCO_2$	35–45 mm Hg
HCO_3^-	22–26 mEq/L
Base excess	–2 to +2 mEq/L
O_2 saturation	95%–98%

Nursing Process: Assessment ***Client Need:*** Physiological Integrity

6. *Answer:* 2 (Objective: 7) ***Rationale:*** The following steps are appropriate for the nurse who is starting an intravenous infusion: Partially fill the drip chamber with solution. Adjust the IV pole so that the container is suspended about 1 m (3 ft) above the client's head. Use the client's nondominant arm, unless contraindicated. Clean the skin at the site of entry with a topical antiseptic swab. ***Nursing Process:*** Implementation ***Client Need:*** Physiological Integrity

7. *Answer:* 2, 3, 4 (Objective: 6) ***Rationale:*** The following pertain to wellness care and promoting fluid and electrolyte balance: Consume six to eight glasses of water daily; limit alcohol intake because it has a diuretic effect; avoid excess amounts of foods or fluids high in salt, sugar, and caffeine; increase fluid intake before, during, and after strenuous exercise, particularly when the environmental temperature is high; and replace lost electrolytes from excessive perspiration as needed with commercial electrolyte solutions. ***Nursing Process:*** Planning ***Client Need:*** Physiological Integrity

8. *Answer:* 3 (Objective: 8) ***Rationale:*** Avoid using veins that are highly visible, because they tend to roll away from the needle. Also avoid using veins damaged by previous use, phlebitis, infiltration, or sclerosis; those in areas of flexion (e.g., the antecubital fossa); and those continually distended with blood, or knotted or tortuous or in a surgically compromised or injured extremity (e.g., following a mastectomy), because of possible impaired circulation and discomfort for the client. ***Nursing Process:*** Assessment ***Client Need:*** Physiological Integrity

9. *Answer:* 4 (Objective: 8) ***Rationale:*** Human blood is commonly classified into four main groups: A, B, AB, and O. A blood transfusion is the introduction of whole blood or blood components into the venous circulation. To avoid transfusing incompatible red blood cells, both blood donor and recipient are typed and their blood is crossmatched. Stop the transfusion immediately if signs of a reaction develop. ***Nursing Process:*** Assessment ***Client Need:*** Physiological Integrity

10. *Answer:* 4 (Objective: 8) ***Rationale:*** Special precautions are necessary when administering blood. A Y-type blood transfusion set with an in-line or add-on filter is used when administering blood. Blood is usually administered through a #18- to #20-gauge intravenous needle or catheter; using a smaller needle may slow the infusion and damage blood cells (although a smaller gauge needle may be necessary for small children or clients with small, fragile veins). Saline is used to prime the set and flush the needle before administering blood. Once blood or a blood product is removed from the refrigerator, there is a limited amount of time to administer it (e.g., packed RBCs should not hang for more than 4 hours after being removed from the refrigerator). ***Nursing Process:*** Implementation ***Client Need:*** Physiological Integrity